T0074565

DEATH AND DYING

SOURCEBOOK

FIFTH EDITION

Health Reference Series

DEATH AND DYING
SOURCEBOOK

FIFTH EDITION

Basic Consumer Information about End-of-Life Care and Related Perspectives,
Including End-of-Life Symptoms and Treatments, Effective Pain Management,
Quality-of-Life Considerations, Patients' Rights and Privacy Matters, Advance
Directives, Physician-Assisted Suicide, Caregiving, Organ Donation, Funeral
Arrangements, and Grief Support

Along with Statistical Data, Information about the Leading Causes of Death,
a Glossary, and Directories of Support Groups and Additional Resources

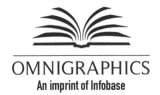

OMNIGRAPHICS
An imprint of Infobase

OMNIGRAPHICS
An imprint of Infobase
132 W. 31st St.
New York, NY 10001
www.infobase.com
James Chambers, *Editorial Director*

* * *

Copyright © 2024 Infobase
ISBN 978-0-7808-2090-6
E-ISBN 978-0-7808-2091-3

Library of Congress Cataloging-in-Publication Data

Names: Chambers, James (Editor), editor.

Title: Death and dying sourcebook: provides basic consumer information about end-of-life care and related perspectives, including end-of-life symptoms and treatments, pain management, quality-of-life concerns, patients' rights and privacy issues, advance directives, physician-assisted suicide, caregiving, organ donation, funeral arrangements, and others, along with information about the leading causes of death, a glossary, and directories of resources for more information / edited by James Chambers.

Description: Fifth edition. | New York, NY: Omnigraphics, an imprint of Infobase, [2024] | Series: Health reference series | Includes index. | Summary: "Provides basic consumer information about end-of-life care and related perspectives, including end-of-life symptoms and treatments, pain management, quality-of-life concerns, patients' rights and privacy issues, caregiving, organ donation, funeral arrangement, and legal and economic issues associated with end-of-life. Includes index, glossary of related terms, and other resources"-- Provided by publisher.

Identifiers: LCCN 2023038912 (print) | LCCN 2023038913 (ebook) | ISBN 9780780820906 (library binding) | ISBN 9780780820913 (ebook)

Subjects: LCSH: Death. | Terminal care.

Classification: LCC R726.8.D3785 2024 (print) | LCC R726.8 (ebook) | DDC 616.02/9--dc23/eng/20230829

LC record available at https://lccn.loc.gov/2023038912
LC ebook record available at https://lccn.loc.gov/2023038913

Table of Contents

Part 5. End-of-Life Caregiving

Part 6. Death and Children: A Guide for Parents and Caregivers

Part 7. Legal and Economic Considerations at the End of Life

Part 8. Funerals and Grief

Part 9. Mortality Statistics

Preface

ABOUT THIS BOOK

While death is often a sensitive subject, it's a universal part of life. Some individuals experience sudden passing, while others face extended battles with chronic disabilities or illnesses. Considering the dying process in advance enables people to engage in conversations about their preferences for end-of-life medical care. These discussions can be challenging, but thoughtful planning empowers individuals to maintain control over their health care even when they are unable to make decisions. Furthermore, being aware of the preferences of loved ones can assist friends and families in navigating the profound shock and grief that follows a loss.

Death and Dying Sourcebook, Fifth Edition provides information about end-of-life perspectives and the medical management of symptoms that can occur as death approaches. It discusses palliative care, end-of-life care complexities, and the intricacies of the organ donation process. The book also addresses caregiver concerns and provides information about children and death. Facts about legal and economic matters related to the end of life, funeral preparations and other end-of-life arrangements, and grief are also included, along with statistical data, a glossary, and directories of support groups and additional resources.

HOW TO USE THIS BOOK

This book is divided into parts and chapters. Parts focus on broad areas of interest. Chapters are devoted to single topics within a part.

Part 1: Preparing for End-of-Life Care begins with defining and discussing end-of-life care and emphasizing its necessity of end-of-life planning. Grief reactions and spiritual considerations that influence decisions related to end-of-life care are discussed and ways to manage chronic conditions in older adults are also described.

Part 2: Managing End-of-Life Symptoms and Providing Comfort offers an overview of both palliative care and end-of-life care. It provides detailed discussions on pain management and assessment, along with information on effectively managing and treating fatigue in the context of end-of-life care.

Part 3: Medical Decisions and End-of-Life Care presents personalization of end-of-life care preferences. It also offers specialized guidance for individuals with dementia and young cancer patients. It provides information for commonly encountered end-of-life issues related to advanced cancer and human immunodeficiency virus/acquired immune deficiency syndrome (HIV/AIDS).

Part 4: End-of-Life Care Facilities offers guidance for assessing and choosing end-of-life care facilities tailored to the requirements of patients and caregivers. It discusses various options, including home care, long-term care, palliative care, hospice care, as well as telemedicine and virtual support.

Part 5: End-of-Life Caregiving provides practical information for caregivers on effectively managing communication among patients, families, and health-care and support service providers. It covers various topics, including providing assistance during the end of life, navigating the steps to take when death occurs, and self-care tips for caregivers.

Part 6: Death and Children: A Guide for Parents and Caregivers provides insights and tips to parents, helping them navigate the challenges of stillbirth, miscarriage, infant death, and sudden infant death syndrome. It also provides guidance on caring for terminally ill children and grieving the loss of a child. Parents will find valuable information on how to support children in coping with death, navigating funerals, and managing grief. Additionally, it covers pediatric critical care research.

Part 7: Legal and Economic Considerations at the End of Life provides guidance on navigating the legal and financial aspects of end-of-life planning. It covers topics such as advance directives, financial assistance, taxes, and Social Security issues. It also talks about patients' legal rights, the Family and Medical Leave Act (FMLA), and the responsibilities of an executor.

Part 8: Funerals and Grief provides practical information and guidance on funeral and cremation services, planning meaningful funerals or memorial services. It also includes chapters on grief, addressing bereavement, providing support to grieving individuals, and offering tips for navigating the grieving process.

Part 9: Mortality Statistics includes global and national mortality trends and presents statistics on the leading causes of death in the United States, as well as life expectancy at birth. It also addresses disparities in deaths from suicide and alcohol-related causes.

Part 10: Additional Help and Information includes a glossary of end-of-life terms, a directory of support groups for those dealing with end-of-life issues, and a directory of organizations offering additional information on topics related to death and dying.

BIBLIOGRAPHIC NOTE

This volume contains documents and excerpts from publications issued by the following U.S. government agencies: Administration for Community Living (ACL); Agency for Healthcare Research and Quality (AHRQ); Benefits.gov; Centers for Disease Control and Prevention (CDC); Centers for Medicare & Medicaid Services (CMS); Eldercare Locator; *Eunice Kennedy Shriver* National Institute of Child Health and Human Development (NICHD); Federal Communications Commission (FCC); Federal Trade Commission (FTC); Health Resources and Services Administration (HRSA); Internal Revenue Service (IRS); MedlinePlus; National Cancer Institute (NCI); National Institute of Nursing Research (NINR); National Institute on Aging (NIA); National Institute on Alcohol Abuse and Alcoholism (NIAAA); *NIH News in Health*; Office on Women's Health (OWH); Organdonor.gov; U.S. Bureau of Labor Statistics (BLS); U.S. Department of Health and Human Services (HHS); U.S. Department of Labor (DOL); U.S. Department of Veterans Affairs (VA); U.S. Environmental Protection Agency (EPA); U.S. Food and Drug Administration (FDA); U.S. Social Security Administration (SSA); and United States Census Bureau.

It also contains original material produced by Infobase and reviewed by medical consultants.

ABOUT THE *HEALTH REFERENCE SERIES*

The *Health Reference Series* is designed to provide basic medical information for patients, families, caregivers, and the general public. Each volume provides comprehensive coverage on a particular topic. This is especially important for people who may be dealing with a newly diagnosed disease or a chronic disorder in themselves or in a family member. People looking for preventive guidance, information about disease warning signs, medical statistics, and risk factors for health problems will also find answers to their questions in the *Health Reference Series*. The *Series*, however, is not intended to serve as a tool for diagnosing illness, in prescribing treatments, or as a substitute for the physician–patient relationship. All people concerned about medical symptoms or the possibility of disease are encouraged to seek professional care from an appropriate health-care provider.

A NOTE ABOUT SPELLING AND STYLE

Health Reference Series editors use *Stedman's Medical Dictionary* as an authority for questions related to the spelling of medical terms and *The Chicago Manual of Style* for questions related to grammatical structures, punctuation, and other editorial concerns. Consistent adherence is not always possible, however, because the individual volumes within the *Series* include many documents from a wide variety of different producers, and the editor's primary goal is to present material from each source as accurately as is possible. This sometimes means that information in different chapters or sections may follow other guidelines and alternate spelling authorities. For example, occasionally a copyright holder may require that eponymous terms be shown in possessive forms (Crohn's disease vs. Crohn disease) or that British spelling norms be retained (leukaemia vs. leukemia).

MEDICAL REVIEW

Infobase contracts with a team of qualified, senior medical professionals who serve as medical consultants for the *Health Reference Series*. As necessary, medical consultants review reprinted and originally written material for currency and accuracy. Medical consultation services are provided to the *Health Reference Series* editors by:

Dr. Vijayalakshmi, MBBS, DGO, MD
Dr. Senthil Selvan, MBBS, DCH, MD
Dr. K. Sivanandham, MBBS, DCH, MS (Research), PhD

HEALTH REFERENCE SERIES UPDATE POLICY

The inaugural book in the *Health Reference Series* was the first edition of *Cancer Sourcebook* published in 1989. Since then, the *Series* has been enthusiastically received by librarians and in the medical community. In order to maintain the standard of providing high-quality health information for the layperson, the editorial staff felt it was necessary to implement a policy of updating volumes when warranted.

Medical researchers have been making tremendous strides, and it is the purpose of the *Health Reference Series* to stay current with the most recent advances. Each decision to update a volume is made on an individual basis. Some of the considerations include how much new information is available and the feedback we receive from people who use the books. If there is a topic you would like to see added to the update list, or an area of medical concern you feel has not been adequately addressed, please write to: custserv@infobaselearning.com.

Part 1 | **Preparing for End-of-Life Care**

Chapter 1 | **Understanding End-of-Life Care**

Not all end-of-life experiences are alike. Death can come suddenly, or a person may linger in a near-death state for days. For some older adults at the end of life, the body weakens while the mind stays clear. Others remain physically strong while cognitive function declines. It is common to wonder what happens when someone is dying. You may want to know how to provide comfort, what to say, or what to do.

WHAT IS END-OF-LIFE CARE?

End-of-life care is the term used to describe the support and medical care given during the time surrounding death. This type of care does not happen only in the moments before breathing ceases and the heart stops beating. Older people often live with one or more chronic illnesses and need significant care for days, weeks, and even months before death.

The end of life may look different depending on the person's preferences, needs, or choices. Some people may want to be at home when they die, while others may prefer to seek treatment in a hospital or facility until the very end. Many want to be surrounded by family and friends, but it is common for some to slip away while their loved ones are not in the room. When possible, there are steps you can take to increase the likelihood of a peaceful death for your loved one: Follow their end-of-life wishes and treat them with respect while they are dying.

Generally speaking, people who are dying need care in four areas: physical comfort, mental and emotional needs, spiritual

3

needs, and practical tasks. Of course, the family of the dying person needs support as well, with practical tasks and emotional distress.

END OF LIFE: PROVIDING PHYSICAL COMFORT

Discomfort during the dying process can come from a variety of sources. Depending on the cause of the discomfort, there are things you or a health-care provider can do to help make the dying person more comfortable. For example, the person may be uncomfortable because of the following reasons.

Pain

Not everyone who is dying experiences pain. For those who do, experts believe that care should focus on relieving pain without worrying about possible long-term problems of drug dependence or abuse.

Struggling with severe pain can be draining and make the dying person understandably angry or short-tempered. This can make it even harder for families and other loved ones to communicate with the person in a meaningful way.

Caregivers and other family members can play significant roles in managing a dying person's pain. But knowing how much pain someone is in can be difficult. Watch for clues, such as trouble sleeping, showing increased agitation, or crying. Do not be afraid of giving as much pain medicine as is prescribed by the doctor.

Pain is easier to prevent than to relieve, and severe pain is hard to manage. Try to make sure that the level of pain does not get ahead of pain-relieving medicines. Tell the health-care professionals if the pain is not controlled because medicines can be increased or changed. Palliative medical specialists are experienced in pain management for seriously ill patients; consider consulting with one if they are not already involved.

Breathing Problems

Shortness of breath or the feeling that breathing is difficult is a common experience at the end of life. The doctor might call this "dyspnea." To help ease breathing for your loved one, try raising the head of the bed, opening a window, using a humidifier, or using a fan to circulate air in the room. Sometimes, morphine or other pain medications can help relieve the sense of breathlessness.

There may be times when a dying person has an abnormal breathing pattern, known as "Cheyne-Stokes breathing." The person's breathing may alternate between deep, heavy breaths and shallow or even no breaths. Some people very near death might have noisy breathing, sometimes called a "death-rattle." In most cases, this noisy breathing does not upset the dying person though it may be alarming to family and friends. You may try turning the person to rest on one side or elevating their head. Prescription medicine may also help.

Skin Irritation

Skin problems can be very uncomfortable for someone when they are dying. Keep the person's skin clean and moisturized. Gently apply alcohol-free lotion to relieve itching and dryness.

Dryness on parts of the face, such as the lips and eyes, can be a common cause of discomfort near death. The following tips may help:

- Apply a balm or petroleum jelly to the lips.
- Gently dab an eye cream or gel around the eyes.
- Try placing a damp cloth over the person's closed eyes.
- If the inside of the mouth seems dry, give ice chips (if the person is conscious) or wipe the inside of the person's mouth with a damp cloth, cotton ball, or specially treated swab that might help.

Sitting or lying in one position can put constant pressure on sensitive skin, which can lead to painful bed sores (sometimes called "pressure ulcers"). When a bed sore first forms, the skin gets discolored or darker. Watch carefully for these discolored spots, especially on the heels, hips, lower back, and back of the head.

Turning the person in bed every few hours may help prevent bed sores and stiffness. Try putting a foam pad under the person's heel or elbow to raise it off the bed and reduce pressure. Ask a member of your health-care team if a special mattress or chair cushion might also help.

Digestive Problems

Nausea, vomiting, constipation, and loss of appetite are common issues at the end of life. Swallowing may also be a problem. The causes and treatments for these symptoms vary, so talk to a doctor or nurse about what you are seeing. Medicines can control nausea or vomiting or relieve constipation, all of which are common side effects of strong pain medications.

If the person loses their appetite, try gently offering favorite foods in small amounts. Serve frequent, smaller meals rather than three larger ones. Help with feeding if the person wants to eat but is too tired or weak.

But do not force a dying person to eat. Losing one's appetite is a common and normal part of dying. Going without food and/or water is generally not painful, and eating and drinking can add to a dying person's discomfort. A conscious decision to give up food can be part of a person's acceptance that death is near.

Temperature Sensitivity

When a person is closer to death, their hands, arms, feet, or legs may be cool to the touch. Some parts of the body may become darker or blueish. People who are dying may not be able to tell you that they are too hot or too cold, so watch for clues. For example, someone who is too warm might repeatedly try to remove a blanket. You can remove the blanket and place a cool cloth on the person's head.

Hunching their shoulders, pulling the cover-ups, and shivering can be signs the person is cold. Make sure there is no draft, raise the heat, and add another blanket. Avoid electric blankets because they can get too hot.

Fatigue

It is common for people nearing the end of life to feel tired and have little or no energy. Keep things simple. For example, a bedside commode can be used instead of walking to the bathroom. Providing a stool, so the person can sit in the shower, or sponge baths in bed can also help.

END OF LIFE: MANAGING MENTAL AND EMOTIONAL NEEDS

End-of-life care can also include helping the dying person manage mental and emotional distress. Someone who is alert near the end of life might understandably feel depressed or anxious. It is important to treat emotional pain and suffering. You might want to contact a counselor, possibly one familiar with end-of-life issues, to encourage conversations about feelings. Medicine may help if the depression or anxiety is severe.

The dying person may also have some specific fears and concerns. He or she may fear the unknown or worry about those left behind. Some people are afraid of being alone at the very end. These feelings can be made worse by the reactions of family, friends, and even the medical team. For example, family and friends may not know how to help or what to say, so they stop visiting, or they may withdraw because they are already grieving. Doctors may feel helpless and avoid dying patients because they cannot help them further.

And some people may experience mental confusion and may have strange or unusual behavior, making it harder to connect with their loved ones. This can add to a dying person's sense of isolation.

The following are a few tips that may help manage mental and emotional needs:

- **Provide physical contact**. Try holding hands or a gentle massage.
- **Set a comforting mood**. Some people prefer quiet moments with less people. Use soft lighting in the room.
- **Play music at a low volume**. This can help with relaxation and lessen pain.
- **Involve the dying person**. If the person can still communicate, ask them what they need.
- **Be present**. Visit with the person. Talk or read to them, even if they cannot talk back. If they can talk, listen

attentively to what they have to say without worrying about what you will say next. Your presence can be the greatest gift you can give to a dying person.

SPIRITUAL NEEDS AT THE END OF LIFE

For people nearing the end of life, spiritual needs may be as important as their physical concerns. Spiritual needs may include finding meaning in one's life, ending disagreements with others, or making peace with life circumstances. The dying person might find comfort in resolving unsettled issues with friends or family. Visits from a social worker or a counselor may help.

Many people find solace in their faith. Others may struggle with their faith or spiritual beliefs. Praying, reading religious texts, or listening to religious music may help. The person can also talk with someone from their religious community, such as a minister, priest, rabbi, or imam.

Family and friends can talk to the dying person about the importance of their relationship. For example, adult children may share how their fathers have influenced the course of their lives. Grandchildren can let their grandfathers know how much they have meant to them. Friends can share how they value years of support and companionship. Family and friends who cannot be present in person can send a video or audio recording of what they would like to say or a letter to be read out loud.

Sharing memories of good times is another way some people find peace near death. This can be comforting for everyone. Some doctors think that dying people can still hear even if they are not conscious. Always talk to, not about, the person who is dying. When you come into the room, identify yourself to the person. You may want to ask someone to write down some of the things said at this time—both by and to the person who is dying. In time, these words might serve as a source of comfort to family and friends.

There may come a time when a dying person who has been confused suddenly seems to be thinking clearly. Take advantage of these moments but understand that they are likely temporary and not necessarily a sign of getting better. Sometimes, a dying person may appear to see or talk to someone who is not there. Resist the temptation to interrupt or correct them or say they are imagining things. Give the dying person the space to experience their own reality. Sometimes, dying people will report having dreams of meeting deceased relatives, friends, or religious figures. The dying person may have various reactions to such dreams, but often, they are quite comforting to them.

PROVIDING SUPPORT FOR PRACTICAL TASKS

Many practical jobs need to be done at the end of life—both to relieve the person who is dying and to support the caregiver. A person who is dying might be worried about who will take care of things when they are gone. A family member or friend can offer reassurance—"I'll make sure your African violets are watered," "Jessica has promised to take care of Bandit," or "Dad, we want Mom to live with us from now on"—which may help provide a measure of peace. You may also remind the dying person that their personal affairs are in good hands.

Everyday tasks can also be a source of worry for someone who is dying and can overwhelm a caregiver. A family member or friend can provide the caregiver with a much-needed break by helping with small daily chores around the house, such as picking up the mail, writing down phone messages, doing a load of laundry, feeding the family pet, or picking up medicine from the pharmacy.

Caregivers may also feel overwhelmed keeping close friends and family informed. A family member or friend can help set up an outgoing voicemail message, a blog, an email list, a private Facebook page, or even a phone tree to help reduce the number of calls the caregiver must make.

Providing comfort and care for someone at the end of life can be physically and emotionally exhausting. If you are a primary caregiver, ask for help when you need it and accept help when it is offered. Do not hesitate to suggest a specific task to someone who offers to help. Friends and family are usually eager to do something for you and the person who is dying, but they may not know what to do.

In the end, consider that there may be no "perfect" death, so just do the best you can for your loved one. The deep pain of losing someone close to you may be softened a little by knowing that when you were needed, you did what you could.

How Can Family and Friends Help Primary Caregivers?

Family and friends may wish to provide primary caregivers relief while they are focusing on the dying loved one. Keep in mind that the caregiver may not know exactly what is needed and may feel overwhelmed by responding to questions. If the caregiver is open to receiving help, the following are some questions you might ask:

- How are you doing? Do you need someone to talk with?
- Would you like to go out for an hour or two? I could stay here while you are away.
- Who has offered to help you? Do you want me to work with them to coordinate our efforts?[1]

Should There Always be Someone in the Room with a Dying Person?

Staying close to someone who is dying is often called "keeping a vigil." It can be comforting for the caregiver or other family members to always be there, but it can also be tiring and stressful. Unless your cultural or religious traditions require it, do not feel that you must stay with the person all the time. If there are other family members or friends around, try taking turns sitting in the room.

---

[1] National Institute on Aging (NIA), "Providing Care and Comfort at the End of Life," National Institutes of Health (NIH), November 17, 2022. Available online. URL: www.nia.nih.gov/health/providing-comfort-end-life. Accessed July 24, 2023.

Chapter 2 | Making Informed Health-Care Decisions at the End of Life

You may wonder how you can comfort a dying person, prevent suffering, and provide the best quality of life (QOL) possible in their remaining time. If the person can no longer communicate, you may be asked to make difficult decisions about their care and comfort. This can be overwhelming for family members, especially if they have not had a chance to discuss the person's wishes ahead of time—or if multiple family members are involved and do not agree.

ADDRESSING A PERSON'S ADVANCE CARE WISHES

If the person has written documents as part of an advance care plan, such as a do-not-resuscitate (DNR) order, tell the doctor in charge as soon as possible. If end-of-life care is given at home, you will need a special out-of-hospital order signed by a doctor to ensure that emergency medical technicians (EMTs), if called to the home, will respect the person's wishes. Hospice staff can help determine whether a medical condition is part of the normal dying process or something that needs the attention of health-care personnel.

For situations that are not addressed in a person's advance care plan or if the person does not have such a plan, you can consider different decision-making strategies to help determine the best approach for the person.

DECISION-MAKING STRATEGIES: SUBSTITUTED JUDGMENT AND BEST INTERESTS

Two approaches might be useful when you encounter decisions that have not been addressed in a person's advance care plan or in previous conversations with them. One is to put yourself in the place of the person who is dying and try to choose as they would. This is called "substituted judgment." Some experts believe that decisions should be based on substituted judgment whenever possible. Another approach, known as "best interests," is to decide what you, as their representative, think is best for the dying person. This is sometimes combined with substituted judgment.

If you are making decisions for someone at the end of life and are trying to use one of these approaches, it may be helpful to think about the following questions:

- Have they ever talked about what they would want at the end of life?
- Have they expressed an opinion about someone else's end-of-life treatment?
- What were their values, and what gave meaning to their life? Maybe it was being close to family and making memories together. Or perhaps they loved the outdoors and enjoyed nature. Are they still able to participate in these activities?

If you are making decisions without specific guidance from the dying person, you will need as much information as possible to help guide your actions. Remember that the decisions you are faced with and the questions you may ask the person's medical team can vary depending on whether the person is at home or in a care facility or hospital. You might ask the doctor the following questions:

- What might we expect to happen in the next few hours, days, or weeks if we continue our current course of treatment?
- Will treatment provide more quality time with family and friends?
- What if we do not want the treatment offered? What happens then?

- When should we begin hospice care? Can they receive this care at home or at the hospital?
- If we begin hospice, will the person be denied certain treatments?
- What medicines will be given to help manage pain and other symptoms? What are the possible side effects?
- What will happen if our family member stops eating or drinking? Will a feeding tube be considered? What are the benefits and risks?
- If we try using the ventilator to help with breathing and decide to stop, how will that be done?

It is a good idea to have someone with you when discussing these issues with medical staff. That person can take notes and help you remember details. Do not be afraid to ask the doctor or nurse to repeat or rephrase what they said if you are unclear about something they told you. Keep asking questions until you have all the information you need to make decisions. If the person is at home, make sure you know how to contact a member of the health-care team if you have a question or if the dying person needs something.

It can be difficult for doctors to accurately predict how much time someone has left to live. Depending on the diagnosis, certain conditions, such as dementia, can progress unpredictably. You should talk with the doctor about hospice care if they predict your loved one has six months or less to live.

CULTURAL CONSIDERATIONS AT THE END OF LIFE

Everyone involved in a patient's care should understand how a person's history and cultural and religious background may influence expectations, needs, and choices at the end of life. Different cultural and ethnic groups may have various expectations about what should happen and the type of care a person receives. The doctor and other members of the health-care team may have different backgrounds than you and your family. Discuss your personal and family traditions surrounding the end of life with the health-care team.

A person's cultural background may influence comfort care and pain management at the end of life, who can be present at the time of death, who makes the health-care decisions, and where they want to die.

It is crucial that the health-care team knows what is important to your family surrounding the end of life. You might say the following:

- In my religion, we… (then describe your religious traditions regarding death).
- Where we come from… (tell what customs are important to you at the time of death).
- In our family when someone is dying, we prefer… (describe what you hope to happen).

Make sure you understand how the available medical options presented by the health-care team fit into your family's desires for end-of-life care. Telling the medical staff ahead of time may help avoid confusion and misunderstandings later. Knowing that these practices will be honored could comfort the dying person and help improve the quality of care provided.

DISCUSSING A CARE PLAN

Having a care plan in place at the end of life is important in ensuring the person's wishes are respected as much as possible. A care plan summarizes a person's health conditions; medications; health-care providers; emergency contacts; end-of-life care wishes, such as advance directives; and other decisions. A care plan may also include your loved one's wishes after they die, such as funeral arrangements and what will be done with their body. It is not uncommon for the entire family to want to be involved in a person's care plan at the end of life. Maybe that is part of your family's cultural tradition. Or maybe the person dying did not pick a person to make health-care choices before becoming unable to do so, which is also not unusual.

If one family member is named as the decision-maker, it is a good idea, as much as possible, to have a family agreement about the care plan. If family members cannot agree on end-of-life care or they disagree with the doctor, your family might consider working with a mediator. A mediator is a professional trained to bring people with different opinions to a common decision. Clinicians trained in palliative care often conduct family meetings to help address disagreements around health-care decisions.

Regardless, your family should try to discuss the end-of-life care they want with the health-care team. In most cases, it is helpful for the medical staff to have one person as the main point of contact.

The following are some questions you might want to ask the medical staff when making decisions about a care plan:

- What is the best place—such as a hospital, facility, or at home—to get the type of care the dying person wants?
- What decisions should be included in our care plan? What are the benefits and risks of these decisions?
- How often should we reassess the care plan?
- What is the best way for our family to work with the care staff?
- How can I ensure I get a daily update on my family member's condition?
- Will you call me if there is a change in his or her condition?
- Where can we find help to pay for this care?

There may be other questions that arise depending on your family's situation. It is important to stay in contact with the health-care team.[1]

---

[1] National Institute on Aging (NIA), "Making Decisions for Someone at the End of Life," National Institutes of Health (NIH), November 17, 2022. Available online. URL: www.nia.nih.gov/health/making-decisions-someone-end-life. Accessed July 31, 2023.

Chapter 3 | **Understanding Grief Reactions and Duration**

To best support an individual who is grieving, it is helpful to know common ways that grief affects individuals and what an individual may go through during the grief process. This will help prevent you from pathologizing reactions that are normal and enable you to reassure individuals who are concerned about their reactions. It is crucial to keep in mind, though, that people have their own unique grief experience. In grief, each person is like everyone else in some respects while at the same time like no one else.

COMMON GRIEF REACTIONS

Grief researcher Dr. William Worden, a fellow member of the American Psychological Association (APA) has identified grief reactions that are common in acute grief and has placed them in four general categories: feelings, physical sensations, cognitions, and behaviors. All are considered normal unless they continue over a very long period of time or are especially intense. An individual might have one reaction, several, or many. Reactions might be very strong for a while and then lessen, or they might not be as strong but last for a long time.

Feelings
- sadness
- anger
- guilt and self-reproach

- anxiety
- loneliness
- fatigue
- helplessness
- shock
- yearning (pining for the person or whatever was lost, thinking if only this had not happened)
- emancipation (Not all feelings are negative. Sometimes, there is a sense of being released when a loss occurs.)
- relief (This may especially be felt after someone dies from a lengthy or painful illness or if a relationship with the deceased was a difficult one.)
- numbness, a lack of feeling (Numbness may actually protect one from a flood of feelings all occurring at the same time.)

Physical Sensations
- hollowness in the stomach
- tightness in the chest
- tightness in the throat
- oversensitivity to noise
- feeling that nothing is real, maybe even feeling that oneself is not real
- breathlessness, feeling short of breath
- muscle weakness
- lack of energy
- dry mouth

Cognitions
- disbelief, thinking the loss did not happen
- confused thinking, difficulty concentrating, and forgetfulness
- preoccupation, obsessive thoughts about the deceased or what was lost
- sensing the presence of the deceased, thinking the deceased is still there
- hallucinations, seeing and/or hearing the deceased

Behaviors

- trouble falling asleep or waking up too early
- eating too much or too little
- absent-minded behavior
- withdrawing from others; feeling less interested in the world
- dreaming of the deceased
- avoiding reminders of the deceased
- searching and calling out the name of the deceased person
- sighing
- being restlessly overactive
- crying
- visiting places or carrying objects that remind one of the deceased person
- strongly treasuring objects that belonged to the deceased

DURATION OF GRIEF

The length of time it takes to adjust to a loss is different in each circumstance for each person. Grieving often takes much longer than people think. The grieving individual will cope with many new experiences in the first year. The second year may also be difficult, as the loss becomes more real to the griever. Some have noted that grief reactions start to fade within six months although eminent specialists caution that there is no timetable to grief and that the intensity of grief does not steadily decline but rather fluctuates over time. Grief tends to come in waves, so one will not be distressed constantly. Grief reactions may pop up from time to time, even after many years. This is very common. Many things may trigger grief, such as songs, a season of the year, birthdays, holidays, anniversaries, or special events in someone's life, which they may wish the deceased could enjoy with them. Usually, these grief episodes that occur a long time subsequent to the loss are short-lived.[1]

---

[1] "Grief Reactions, Duration, and Tasks of Mourning," U.S. Department of Veterans Affairs (VA), December 4, 2020. Available online. URL: www.va.gov/WHOLEHEALTHLIBRARY/tools/grief-reactions-duration-and-tasks-of-mourning.asp. Accessed September 27, 2023.

Chapter 4 | Spirituality and Its Role in End-of-Life Care

Specific religious beliefs and practices should be distinguished from the idea of a universal capacity for spiritual and religious experiences. Although this distinction may not be salient or important on a personal basis, it is important conceptually to understand various aspects of evaluation and the role of different beliefs, practices, and experiences in coping with any critical illness.

The most useful general distinction in this context is between religion and spirituality. There is no general agreement on definitions of either term, but there is general agreement on the usefulness of this distinction.

- Religion can be viewed as a specific set of beliefs and practices associated with a recognized religion or denomination.
- Spirituality is generally recognized as encompassing experiential aspects, whether related to engaging in religious practices or acknowledging a general sense of peace and connectedness. Found in all cultures, the concept of spirituality is often considered to encompass a search for ultimate meaning through religion or other paths.

In health care, concerns about spiritual or religious well-being have sometimes been viewed as an aspect of complementary and alternative medicine (CAM), but this perception may be more characteristic of providers than of patients. In one study, virtually no patients but about 20 percent of providers said that CAM services were sought to assist with spiritual or religious issues.

Religion is highly culturally determined. Spirituality is considered a universal human capacity, usually—but not necessarily—associated with and expressed in religious practice. Most individuals consider themselves both spiritual and religious. Some may consider themselves religious but not spiritual; others, including some atheists (people who do not believe in the existence of God) or agnostics (people who believe that God cannot be shown to exist), may consider themselves spiritual but not religious.

One effort to characterize individuals by types of spiritual and religious experience identified the following three groups using cluster analytic techniques:

- **Religious individuals**. These individuals highly value religious faith, spiritual well-being, and the meaning of life.
- **Existential individuals**. These individuals highly value spiritual well-being but not religious faith.
- **Nonspiritual individuals**. These individuals have little value for religiousness, spirituality, or a sense of the meaning of life.

Individuals in the third group were far more distressed about their illness and experienced worse adjustment than the other two groups. There is not yet a consensus on the number or types of underlying dimensions of spirituality or religious engagement.

From the perspective of both the research and clinical literature on the relationships among religion, spirituality, and health, it is important to consider how investigators and authors define and use these concepts. Much of the epidemiological literature that indicates a relationship between religion and health is based on definitions of religious involvement, such as:

- membership in a religious group
- frequency of attendance at religious services

Assessing specific beliefs or religious practices such as belief in God, frequency of prayer, or reading religious material is somewhat more complex. Individuals may engage in such practices or believe in God without necessarily attending services. Terminology also carries certain connotations. The term religiosity, for example, has a history of implying fervor and perhaps undue investment in particular religious practices or beliefs. The term religiousness may be a more neutral way to refer to the "dimension of religious practice."

Spirituality and spiritual well-being are more challenging to define. Some definitions limit spirituality to mean profound mystical experiences. However, in effects on health and psychological well-being, the more helpful definitions focus on accessible feelings, such as:

- a sense of inner peace
- existential meaning
- awe when walking in nature

This discussion assumes a continuum of meaningful spiritual experiences, from the common and accessible to the extraordinary and transformative. Both type and intensity of experience may vary. Other aspects of spirituality that have been identified by those working with patients include the following:

- a sense of meaning and peace
- a sense of faith
- a sense of connectedness to others or to God

Low levels of these experiences may be associated with poorer coping.

The definition of acute spiritual distress must be considered separately. Spiritual distress may result from the belief that any critical illness reflects punishment by God or may accompany a preoccupation with the question, "Why me?" A patient may also suffer a loss of faith. Although many individuals may have such thoughts at some point after diagnosis, only a few become obsessed with these thoughts or score high on a general measure of religious and spiritual distress (such as the Negative subscale of the Religious Coping Scale). High levels of spiritual distress may contribute to poorer health and psychosocial outcomes.

MODES OF INTERVENTION

Various modes of intervention or assistance might be considered to address the spiritual concerns of patients, including the following:

- exploration by the physician or other health-care provider within the context of usual medical care
- encouragement for patients to seek assistance from their own clergy
- formal referral to a hospital chaplain
- referral to a religious or faith-based therapist
- referral to support groups known to address spiritual issues

Two survey studies found that physicians consistently underestimate the degree to which patients want spiritual concerns addressed. An Israeli study found that patients expressed the desire that 18 percent of a hypothetical 10-minute visit be spent addressing such concerns, while their providers estimated that 12 percent of the time should be spent in this way. This survey also found that while providers perceived a patient's desire to address spiritual concerns related to a broader interest in CAM modalities, patients viewed CAM-related issues and spiritual/religious concerns as quite separate.

Physicians

A task force of physicians and end-of-life specialists suggested several guidelines for physicians who wish to respond to patients' spiritual concerns:

- Respect the patient's views and follow the patient's lead.
- Make a connection by listening carefully and acknowledging the patient's concerns but avoid theological discussions or specific religious rituals.
- Maintain one's own integrity in relation to one's own religious beliefs and practices.
- Identify common goals for care and medical decisions.
- Mobilize other resources of support for the patient, such as referral to a chaplain or contact with the patient's own clergy.

Inquiring about religious or spiritual concerns may provide valuable and appreciated support to patients. Most cancer patients appear to welcome a dialogue about such concerns, regardless of diagnosis or prognosis. In a large survey, 20–35 percent of outpatients with cancer expressed the following:

- a desire for religious and spiritual resources
- help with talking about finding meaning in life
- help with finding hope
- talking about death and dying
- finding peace of mind

One trial, with a sample of 115 mixed-diagnosis patients (54% under active treatment), evaluated a five-minute semi-structured inquiry into spiritual and religious concerns. The four physicians' personal religious backgrounds included two Christians, one Hindu, and one Sikh; 81 percent of patients were Christian. Unlike the history-oriented interviews noted above, this inquiry was informed by brief patient-centered counseling approaches that view the physician as an important source of empowerment to help patients identify and address personal concerns. After three weeks, the intervention group had larger reductions in depression, had more improvement in QOL, and rated their relationship with the physician more favorably. Effects for QOL remained after statistically adjusting for changes in other variables. More improvement was also seen in patients who scored lower in spiritual well-being, as measured by the Functional Assessment of Chronic Illness Therapy-Spiritual Well-Being Scale (FACIT-Sp) at baseline. Acceptability was high with physicians rating themselves as "comfortable" in providing the intervention during 85 percent of encounters. Seventy-six percent of patients characterized the inquiry as "somewhat" to "very" useful. Physicians were twice as likely to underestimate the usefulness of the inquiry to patients rather than to overestimate it in relation to patient ratings.

A common concern is whether to offer to pray with patients. Although one study found that more than one-half of the patients surveyed expressed a desire to have physicians pray with them, a large proportion did not express this preference. A qualitative study of cancer patients found that they were concerned that physicians

25

were too busy, not interested, or even prohibited from discussing religion. At the same time, patients generally wanted their physicians to acknowledge the value of spiritual and religious issues. A suggestion was made that physicians might raise the question of prayer by asking, "Would that comfort you?"

In a study of 70 patients with advanced cancer, 206 oncology physicians, and 115 oncology nurses, all participants were interviewed about the appropriateness of patient-practitioner prayer in the advanced cancer setting. Results showed that 71 percent of patients, 83 percent of nurses, and 65 percent of physicians reported that it is occasionally appropriate for a practitioner to pray with a patient when the patient initiates the request. Similarly, 64 percent of patients, 76 percent of nurses, and 59 percent of physicians reported that they consider it appropriate for a religious/spiritual health-care practitioner to pray for a patient.

The most important guideline is to remain sensitive to the patient's preference. Asking patients about their beliefs or spiritual concerns in the context of exploring how they are coping, in general, is the most viable approach to exploring these issues.

Hospital Chaplains

Traditionally, hospital chaplains deliver religious or spiritual assistance to patients. Hospital chaplains can play a key role because they are trained to work with a wide range of issues as they arise for patients and to be sensitive to patients' diverse beliefs and concerns. Chaplains are generally available in large medical centers but may not be reliably available in smaller hospitals.

Another traditional approach in outpatient settings is having spiritual/religious resources available in waiting rooms. This activity is relatively easy to do, and many resources exist. A breadth of resources covering all faith backgrounds of patients is highly desirable.

Support Groups

Support groups may provide a setting where patients may explore spiritual concerns. The health-care provider may need to identify whether an in-person or online group addresses these issues. The published data on the specific effects of support groups on assisting with spiritual concerns are relatively sparse, partly because this aspect of adjustment has not been systematically evaluated. A randomized trial compared the effects of a mind-body-spirit group to a standard support group for women with breast cancer. Both groups showed improvement in spiritual well-being although there were appreciably more differential effects for the mind-body-spirit group in the area of spiritual integration.

A study of 97 lower-income women with breast cancer who were participating in an online support group examined the relationship between a variety of psychosocial outcomes and religious expression (as indicated by the use of religious words such as faith, God, pray, holy, or spirit). Results showed that women who communicated a deeper religiousness in their online writing to others had lower levels of negative emotions, higher levels of perceived health self-efficacy, and higher functional well-being. An exploratory study of a monthly spirituality-based support group program for African-American women with breast cancer suggested high levels of satisfaction in a sample that already had high levels of religious and spiritual engagement.

One author presents a well-developed model of adjuvant psychological therapy that uses a large group format and addresses both basic coping issues and spiritual concerns and healing, using a combination of group exploration, meditation, prayer, and other spiritually oriented exercises. In a carefully conducted, longitudinal, and qualitative study of 22 patients enrolled in this type of intervention, researchers found that patients who were more psychologically engaged with the issues presented were more likely to survive longer. Other approaches are available but have yet to be systematically evaluated, have not explicitly addressed religious and spiritual issues, or have failed to evaluate the effects of the intervention on spiritual well-being.

Other Interventions

Other therapies may also support spiritual growth and posttraumatic benefit finding. For example, in a nonrandomized comparison of mindfulness-based stress reduction (n = 60) and a healing arts program (n = 44) in cancer outpatients with a variety of diagnoses, both programs significantly improved the facilitation of positive growth in participants although improvements in spirituality, stress, depression, and anger were significantly larger for the mindfulness-based stress reduction group.[1]

[1] "Spirituality in Cancer Care (PDQ®)—Health Professional Version," National Cancer Institute (NCI), October 26, 2022. Available online. URL: www.cancer.gov/about-cancer/coping/day-to-day/faith-and-spirituality/spirituality-hp-pdq. Accessed August 1, 2023.

Chapter 5 | Managing Chronic Conditions in Older Adults

THE BURDEN OF CHRONIC DISEASE FOR OLDER ADULTS
Leading Causes of Death

During the 20th century, effective public health strategies and advances in medical treatment contributed to a dramatic increase in average life expectancy in the United States. The 30-year gain in life expectancy within the span of a century had never before been achieved. Many of the diseases that claimed our ancestors—including tuberculosis (TB), diarrhea and enteritis, and syphilis—are no longer the threats they once were. Although they may still present significant health challenges in the United States, these diseases are no longer the leading killers of American adults.

However, other diseases have continued to be the leading causes of death every year since 1900. By 1910, heart disease became the leading cause of death every year except 1918–1920 when the influenza epidemic took its disastrous toll. Since 1938, cancer has held the second position every year.

Heart disease and cancer pose their greatest risks as people age, as do other chronic diseases and conditions, such as stroke, chronic lower respiratory diseases (CLRDs), Alzheimer disease (AD), and diabetes. Influenza and pneumonia also continue to cause deaths among older adults despite the availability of effective vaccines.

Diminished Quality of Life and Loss of Independence

The burden of chronic diseases encompasses a much broader spectrum of negative health consequences than death alone. People living with one or more chronic diseases often experience diminished quality of life (QOL), generally reflected by a long period of decline and disability associated with their disease.

Chronic diseases can affect a person's ability to perform important and essential activities both inside and outside the home. Initially, they may have trouble with the instrumental activities of daily living (IADL), such as managing money, shopping, preparing meals, and taking medications as prescribed. As functional ability—physical, mental, or both—further declines, people may lose the ability to perform more basic activities, called "activities of daily living" (ADLs), such as taking care of personal hygiene, feeding themselves, getting dressed, and toileting.

The inability to perform daily activities can restrict people's engagement in life and their enjoyment of family and friends. Lack of mobility in the community or at home significantly narrows an older person's world and ability to do the things that bring enjoyment and meaning to life. Loss of the ability to care for oneself safely and appropriately means further loss of independence and can often lead to the need for care in an institutional setting.

The need for caregiving for older adults by formal, professional caregivers or by family members—and the need for long-term care services and support—will increase sharply during the next several decades, given the effects of chronic diseases on an aging population.

Major Contributor to Health-Care Costs

The nation's expenditures for health care, already the highest among developed countries, are expected to rise considerably as chronic diseases affect growing numbers of older adults. More than two-thirds of all health-care costs are for treating chronic illnesses. Among health-care costs for older Americans, 95 percent are for chronic diseases. The cost of providing health care for one person aged 65 or older is three to five times higher than the cost for someone under age 65.

By 2030, health-care spending will increase by 25 percent, largely because the population will be older. This estimate does not take into account inflation and the higher costs of new technologies.

Ways to Promote and Preserve the Health of Older Adults and Reduce Costs

Death and decline associated with the leading chronic diseases are often preventable or can be delayed. Multiple opportunities exist to promote and preserve the health of older adults. The challenge is to more broadly apply what we already know about reducing the risk of chronic disease. Death is unavoidable, but the prevalence of chronic illnesses and the decline and disability commonly associated with them can be reduced.

Although the risk of developing chronic diseases increases as a person ages, the root causes of many of these diseases often begin early in life. Practicing healthy behaviors from an early age and getting recommended screenings can substantially reduce a person's risk of developing chronic diseases and associated disabilities. Research has shown that people who do not use tobacco, who get regular physical activity, and who eat a healthy diet significantly decrease their risk of developing heart disease, cancer, diabetes, and other chronic conditions.

Unfortunately, data on health-related behaviors among people aged 55–64 do not indicate a positive future for the health of older Americans. If a meaningful decline in chronic diseases among older adults is to occur, adults at younger ages, as well as our nation's children and adolescents, need to pursue health-promoting behaviors and get recommended preventive services. Communities can play a pivotal role in achieving this goal by making healthy choices easier and making changes to policies, systems, and environments that help Americans of all ages take charge of their health.[1]

---

[1] "The State of Aging & Health in America 2013," Centers for Disease Control and Prevention (CDC), July 9, 2013. Available online. URL: www.cdc.gov/aging/pdf/State-Aging-Health-in-America-2013.pdf. Accessed August 2, 2023.

HOW THE HEALTH-CARE TEAM CAN INVOLVE FAMILY MEMBERS IN CAREGIVING

Family members and other informal caregivers play a significant role in the lives of their loved ones. They may provide transportation and accompany an older adult to medical appointments. In many cases, they act as facilitators to help the patient express concerns and can reinforce the information you give. But, first, to protect and honor patient privacy, check with the patient by asking how they see the companion's role in the appointment.

It is important to keep the patients involved in their own health care and conversation. Whenever possible, try to sit so that you can address both the patient and companion face-to-face. Be mindful not to direct your remarks only to the companion.

You might ask the companion to step out of the exam room during part of the visit, so you can raise sensitive topics and provide the patient some private time if they wish to discuss personal matters. For example, if you are conducting a test of a patient's cognitive abilities, you might ask the companion to step out, so they cannot answer questions or cover for the patient's cognitive lapses.

Some patients may ask that you contact their long-distance caregivers to discuss conditions or treatment plans. Make sure these patients fill out any necessary paperwork giving permission for you to speak with specific family members or friends if they are not present at the appointment.

Families may want to make decisions for a loved one. Adult children especially may want to step in for a parent who has cognitive impairment. If a family member has been named the health-care agent or proxy, under some circumstances, they have the legal authority to make care decisions. However, without this authority, the patient is responsible for making their own choices. When necessary, set clear boundaries with family members and encourage others to respect them.

OBTAINING A THOROUGH HISTORY

Obtaining a complete medical history—including current and past concerns, lifestyle, and family history—is crucial to good health care.

You may need to be especially flexible when obtaining the medical history of older patients. When possible, have the patient tell their story only once, even if other health-care professionals in the office or home would typically assist in gathering the information. The process of providing their history to another staff member and then again to you can be tiring for patients.

Open-ended questions encourage a more comprehensive response, but yes-or-no or simple-choice questions may be helpful if the patient has trouble responding. Also, be sure to ask if anything in a person's health, medications, or lifestyle has changed since their last visit. You may want to get a detailed life and medical history as an ongoing part of older patients' office visits and use each visit to add to and update information.

The following are some strategies for obtaining a thorough history:

- **Gather preliminary data**. If feasible, request previous medical records or ask the patient or a family member to complete forms and worksheets at home or online prior to the appointment. Try to structure questionnaires for easy reading by using large type and providing enough space between items for thorough responses. Keep any questionnaires meant to be filled out in the waiting room as brief as possible.
- **Elicit current concerns**. Older patients tend to have multiple chronic conditions. You might start the session by asking your patient to talk about their main concern, for example, "What brings you in today?" or "What is bothering you the most?"
- **Ask prompting questions**. The main concern may not be the first one mentioned, especially if it is a sensitive topic. Asking, for example, "Is there anything else?" which you may have to ask more than once, helps get all of the patient's concerns on the table at the beginning of the visit. If there are too many concerns to address in one visit, plan with the patient to address some now and others next time. Encourage the patient (and their caregivers) to bring a written list of concerns and questions to a follow-up appointment.

- **Discuss medications**. Older people often take many medications prescribed by several different doctors, and some drug interactions can lead to major complications. Suggest that patients bring a list of all of their prescription medications, over-the-counter (OTC) drugs, vitamins, and dietary supplements, including the dosage and frequency of each. Or suggest that they bring everything with them in a bag. Check to ensure the patient is using each medication as directed.
- **Ask about family history**. The family history not only indicates the patient's likelihood of developing some diseases but also provides information about the health of relatives who care for the patient or who might do so in the future. Knowing the family structure will help you evaluate what support may be available from family members.
- **Ask about functional status**. The ability to perform basic ADLs reflects and affects a patient's health. There are standardized ADL assessments that can be done quickly in the office. Understanding an older patient's usual level of functioning and learning about any recent significant changes are fundamental to providing appropriate health care.
- **Consider a patient's life and social history**. Ask about where they live, who else lives in the home or nearby, neighborhood safety, their driving status, and access to transportation. Determine eating habits, assess their mood, and ask about tobacco, drug, and alcohol use. Factor in typical daily activities and work, education, and financial situations. Understanding a person's life and daily routine can help you understand how your patient's lifestyle might affect their health care and devise realistic, appropriate interventions.

DISCUSSING MEDICAL CONDITIONS AND TREATMENTS

Approximately 85 percent of older adults have at least one chronic health condition, and 60 percent have at least two chronic conditions. Clinicians can play an important role in educating patients and families about chronic health conditions and can connect them with appropriate community resources and services.

Most older patients want to understand their medical conditions and learn how to manage them. Likewise, family members and other caregivers can benefit from having this information. Physicians typically underestimate how much patients want to know and overestimate how long they spend giving information to patients. Devoting more attention to educating patients and their caregivers can improve patients' adherence to treatment, increase patients' well-being, and save you time in the long run.

Clear explanations of diagnoses are critical. Uncertainty about a health problem can be upsetting, and when patients do not understand their medical conditions, they are less likely to follow their treatment plans. It is helpful to begin by finding out what the patient understands about their condition, what they think will happen, and how much more they want to know. Based on the patient's responses, you can correct any misconceptions and provide appropriate information.

Treatment plans need to involve patients' input and consent. Ask about their goals and preferences for care and focus on what matters most to them. Check in with your patient about feasibility and acceptability throughout the process, thinking in terms of joint problem-solving and collaborative care. This approach can increase the patient's satisfaction while reducing demands on your time.

Treatment might involve lifestyle changes, such as a more nutritious diet and regular exercise, as well as medication. Tailor the plan to the patient's situation and lifestyle and try to reduce disruption to their routine. Keep medication plans as simple and straightforward as possible, indicating the purpose of each medication and when it should be taken. Tell the patient what to expect from the treatment.

The following tips may help discussions about medical conditions and treatment plans:

- A doctor's advice generally receives the greatest credence, so the doctor should introduce treatment plans. Other medical team members can help build on the doctor's original instructions.

- Let your patients know that you welcome questions. Tell them how to follow up if they think of any additional questions later.
- Some patients would not ask questions even if they wanted more information. Consider making information available even if it is not explicitly requested.
- Offer information through more than one channel. In addition to talking with the patient, you can use fact sheets, drawings, models, or videos. In many cases, referrals to websites and support groups can be helpful.
- Encourage the patient or caregiver to take notes. It is helpful to offer a pad and pencil. Active involvement in recording information may help your patient better retain information and adhere to the treatment plan.
- Repeat key points about the health problem and treatment plan at every office visit, provide oral and written instructions, and check that the patient and their caregiver understand the information.
- Provide encouragement and continued reinforcement for treatment or necessary lifestyle changes. Call attention to the patient's strengths and offer ideas for improvement.
- Make it clear that a referral to another doctor, if needed, does not mean you are abandoning the patient.

CONFUSION AND COGNITIVE PROBLEMS

A patient may still seem confused despite your best efforts to communicate clearly. In those instances, work to:

- support and reassure the patient, acknowledging when responses are correct or understood
- make it clear that the conversation is not a "test" but rather a search for information to help the patient
- consider having someone from your staff call the patient to follow up on instructions

Cognitive impairment, however, is more than general confusion or normal cognitive aging. If you observe changes in an older patient's cognition or memory, follow up with screening and diagnostic testing, as appropriate.

There are a variety of possible causes of cognitive problems, such as side effects from medications, metabolic and/or endocrine changes, delirium, or untreated depression. Some of these causes can be temporary and reversed with proper treatment. Other causes of cognitive problems, such as AD, are chronic conditions but may be treated with medications or nondrug therapies. Having an accurate diagnosis can also help families wanting to improve the person's QOL and better prepare for the future.[2]

---

[2] National Institute on Aging (NIA), "Talking with Your Older Patients," National Institutes of Health (NIH), January 25, 2023. Available online. URL: www.nia.nih.gov/health/talking-your-older-patients. Accessed August 2, 2023.

Part 2 | Managing End-of-Life Symptoms and Providing Comfort

Chapter 6 | Pain Management at the End of Life

Chapter Contents

Section 6.1 | Pain and Pain Management

ACUTE PAIN AND CHRONIC PAIN

The following are the two kinds of pain:
- **Acute pain.** This type of pain begins suddenly, lasts
  for a short time, and goes away as your body heals.
  You might feel acute pain after surgery or if you have a
  broken bone, infected tooth, or kidney stones.
- **Chronic pain.** Pain that lasts for three months or
  longer is called "chronic pain." This pain often affects
  older people. For some people, chronic pain is caused
  by a health condition such as arthritis. It may also
  follow acute pain from an injury, surgery, or other
  health issue that has been treated, such as postherpetic
  neuralgia (PHN) after shingles.

Living with any type of pain can be hard. It can cause many
other problems. For instance, pain can:
- get in the way of your daily activities
- disturb your sleep and eating habits
- make it difficult to continue working
- be related to depression or anxiety
- keep you from spending time with friends and family

DESCRIBING PAIN

Many people have a hard time describing pain. Think about the
following questions when you explain how the pain feels:
- Where does it hurt?
- When did the pain start? Does it come and go?
- What does it feel like? Is the pain sharp, dull, or
  burning? Would you use some other words to describe
  it?
- Do you have other symptoms?
- When do you feel the pain? In the morning? In the
  evening? After eating?
- Is there anything you do that makes the pain feel better
  or worse? For example, does using a heating pad or ice

pack help? Does changing your position from lying down to sitting up make it better?

- What medicines, including over-the-counter (OTC) medications, and nonmedicine therapies have you tried, and what was their effect?

Your doctor or nurse may ask you to rate your pain on a scale of 0–10, with 0 being no pain and 10 being the worst pain you can imagine. Or your doctor may ask if the pain is mild, moderate, or severe. Some doctors or nurses have pictures of faces that show different expressions of pain and ask you to point to the face that shows how you feel. Your doctor may ask you to keep a diary of when and what kind of pain you feel every day.

ATTITUDES ABOUT PAIN

Everyone reacts to pain differently. Some people feel they should be brave and not complain when they are hurt. Other people are quick to report pain and ask for help.

Worrying about pain is common. This worry can make you afraid to stay active, and it can separate you from your friends and family. Working with your doctor, you can find ways to continue to take part in physical and social activities despite having pain.

Some people put off going to the doctor because they think pain is part of aging and nothing can help. This is not true.

It is important to see a doctor if you have a new pain. Finding a way to manage pain is often easier if it is addressed early.

TREATING PAIN

Treating or managing chronic pain is important. Some treatments involve medications, and some do not. Your treatment plan should be specific to your needs.

Most treatment plans focus on both reducing pain and increasing ways to support daily function while living with pain.

Talk with your doctor about how long it may take before you feel better. Often, you have to stick with a treatment plan before you get relief. It is important to stay on a schedule. Sometimes, this is called "staying ahead" or "keeping on top" of your pain. Be sure to tell your doctor about any side effects. You might have to try different treatments until you find a plan that works for you. As your pain lessens, you can likely become more active and will see your mood lift and sleep improve.

MEDICINES TO TREAT PAIN

Your doctor may prescribe one or more of the following pain medications. Talk with your doctor about their safety and the right dose to take.

- **Acetaminophen.** This medication may help relieve all types of pain, especially mild-to-moderate pain. Acetaminophen is found in OTC and prescription medicines. People who have more than three drinks per day or who have liver disease should not take acetaminophen.
- **Nonsteroidal antiinflammatory drugs (NSAIDs).** NSAIDs include aspirin, naproxen, and ibuprofen. Long-term use of some NSAIDs can cause side effects, such as internal bleeding or kidney problems, which make them unsafe for many older adults. You may not be able to take ibuprofen if you have high blood pressure.
- **Narcotics (also called "opioids").** These medications are used for moderate-to-severe pain and require a doctor's prescription. They may be habit-forming. They can also be dangerous when taken with alcohol or certain other drugs. Examples of narcotics are codeine, morphine, and oxycodone.
- **Other medications.** Certain medications are sometimes used to treat pain. These include antidepressants, anticonvulsive medicines, local painkillers such as nerve blocks or patches, and ointments and creams.

As people age, they are at risk of developing more side effects from medications. It is important to take exactly the amount of pain medicine your doctor prescribes. Do not chew or crush your pills if they are supposed to be swallowed whole. Talk with your doctor or pharmacist if you are having trouble swallowing your pills.

Mixing any pain medication with alcohol or other drugs can be dangerous. Make sure your doctor knows all the medicines you take, including OTC drugs and dietary supplements, as well as the amount of alcohol you drink.

WHAT OTHER TREATMENTS HELP WITH PAIN

In addition to drugs, there are a variety of complementary and alternative approaches that may provide relief. Talk to your doctor about these treatments. It may take both medicine and other treatments to feel better.

- **Acupuncture**. This treatment uses hair-thin needles to stimulate specific points on the body to relieve pain.
- **Biofeedback**. This helps you learn to control your heart rate, blood pressure, muscle tension, and other body functions. This may help reduce your pain and stress level.
- **Cognitive behavioral therapy (CBT)**. CBT is a form of short-term counseling that may help reduce your reaction to pain.
- **Distraction**. This can help you cope with acute pain, taking your mind off your discomfort.
- **Electrical nerve stimulation**. This treatment uses electrical impulses to relieve pain.
- **Guided imagery**. This technique uses directed thoughts to create mental pictures that may help you relax, manage anxiety, sleep better, and have less pain.
- **Hypnosis**. This uses focused attention to help manage pain.
- **Massage therapy**. This therapy can release tension in tight muscles.
- **Mind-body stress reduction**. This treatment combines mindfulness meditation, body awareness, and yoga to increase relaxation and reduce pain.

- **Physical therapy.** This therapy uses a variety of techniques to help manage everyday activities with less pain and teaches you ways to improve flexibility and strength.

HELP YOURSELF FEEL BETTER

There are things you can do yourself that might help you feel better. Try to do the following:

- **Keep a healthy weight.** Putting on extra pounds can slow healing and make pain worse. A healthy weight might help with pain in the knees, back, hips, or feet.
- **Be physically active.** Pain might make you inactive, which can lead to more pain and loss of function. Activity can help.
- **Get enough sleep.** It can reduce pain sensitivity, help healing, and improve your mood.
- **Avoid tobacco, caffeine, and alcohol.** They can get in the way of treatment and increase pain.
- **Join a pain support group.** Sometimes, it can help talk to other people about how they deal with pain. You can share your thoughts while learning from others.

PAIN AT THE END OF LIFE

Not everyone who is dying is in pain. But, if a person has pain at the end of life, there are ways to help. Experts believe it is best to focus on making the person comfortable, without worrying about possible addiction or drug dependence.[1]

---

[1] National Institute on Aging (NIA), "Pain: You Can Get Help," National Institutes of Health (NIH), February 28, 2018. Available online. URL: www.nia.nih.gov/health/pain-you-can-get-help. Accessed August 7, 2023.

Section 6.2 | **Cancer Pain Control**

Cancer pain can range from mild to very severe. Some days, it can be worse than others. It can be caused by the cancer itself, the treatment, or both.

You may also have pain that has nothing to do with your cancer. Some people have other health issues or headaches and muscle strains. Always check with your doctor before taking any over-the-counter (OTC) medicine to relieve everyday aches and pains. This will help ensure that there will be no interactions with other drugs or safety concerns to know about.

DIFFERENT TYPES OF PAIN

Here are the common terms used to describe different types of pain:
- **Acute pain**. This type of pain ranges from mild to severe. It comes on quickly and lasts a short time.
- **Chronic pain**. This type of pain ranges from mild to severe and persists or progresses over a long period of time.
- **Breakthrough pain**. This type of pain is an intense rise in pain that occurs suddenly or is felt for a short time. It can occur by itself or in relation to a certain activity. It may happen several times a day, even when you are taking the right dose of medicine. For example, it may happen as the current dose of your medicine is wearing off.

WHAT CAUSES CANCER PAIN?

Cancer and its treatment cause most cancer pain. Major causes of pain include the following:
- **Pain from medical tests**. Some methods used to diagnose cancer or see how well treatment is working can be painful. Examples may be a biopsy, spinal tap, or bone marrow test. Do not let concerns about pain stop you from having tests done. Talk with your doctor ahead of time about the steps that will be taken to lessen any potential pain.

- **Pain from a tumor.** If the cancer grows bigger or spreads, it can cause pain by pressing on the tissues around it. For example, a tumor can cause pain if it presses on bones, nerves, the spinal cord, or body organs.
- **Pain from treatment.** Chemotherapy, radiation therapy, surgery, and other treatments may cause pain for some people. Some examples of pain from treatment are as follows:
  - **Neuropathic pain.** This is pain that may occur if treatment damages the nerves. The pain is often burning, sharp, or shooting. The cancer itself can also cause this kind of pain.
  - **Phantom pain.** You may still feel pain or other discomfort coming from a body part that has been removed by surgery. Doctors are not sure why this happens, but it is real.
  - **Joint pain (called "arthralgia").** This kind of pain is associated with the use of aromatase inhibitors, a type of hormonal therapy.

How much pain you feel depends on different things. These include the cause of the pain and how you experience it in your body. Everyone is different.

TALKING ABOUT YOUR PAIN

Pain control is part of the treatment. Talking openly is key. The most important member of the team is you. You are the only one who knows what your pain feels like. Talking about pain is important. It gives your health-care team the feedback they need to help you feel better.

Some people with cancer do not want to talk about their pain because they:

- think that they will distract their doctors from working on ways to help treat their cancer
- worry that they would not be seen as "good" patients
- worry that they would not be able to afford pain medicine

As a result, people sometimes get so used to living with their pain that they forget what it is like to live without it.

Tell your health-care team if you are:

- taking any medicine to treat other health problems
- taking more or less of the pain medicine than prescribed
- allergic to certain drugs
- using any OTC medicines, home remedies, or herbal or alternative therapies

This information could affect the pain-control plan your doctor suggests for you. If you feel uneasy talking about your pain, bring a family member or friend to speak for you. Or let your loved one take notes and ask questions. Remember, open communication between you, your loved ones, and your health-care team will lead to better pain control.

KNOW HOW TO DESCRIBE YOUR PAIN
Assess Pain Threshold

The first step in getting your pain under control is talking honestly about it. Try to talk with your health-care team and your loved ones about what you are feeling.

You will be asked to describe and rate your pain. This provides a way for your doctor to assess your pain threshold, which is the point at which a person becomes aware of pain. Knowing this will help measure how well your pain-control plan is working.

Your doctor may ask you to describe your pain in a number of ways. A pain scale is the most common way. The scale uses the numbers 0–10, where 0 is no pain and 10 is the worst. Some doctors show their patients a series of faces and ask them to point to the face that best describes how they feel. You will also need to talk about any new pain you feel.

This also means telling them:

- where you have pain
- what it feels like (sharp, dull, throbbing, constant, burning, or shooting)
- how strong your pain is

- how long it lasts
- what lessens your pain or makes it worse
- when it happens (what time of day, what you are doing, and what is going on)
- if it gets in the way of daily activities

Use a Pain Diary

Many patients have found it helpful to keep a record of their pain. Some people use a pain diary or journal. Others create a list or a computer spreadsheet. Choose the way that works best for you.

Your record could list the following:

- when you take pain medicine
- name and dose of the medicine you are taking
- any side effects you have
- how much the medicine lowers the pain level
- how long the pain medicine works
- other pain relief methods you use to control your pain
- any activity that is affected by pain or makes it better or worse
- things that you cannot do at all because of the pain

Share your record with your health-care team. It can help them figure out how helpful your pain medicines are or if they need to change your pain-control plan.

Share Your Beliefs about Medicines

Some people do not want to take medicine, even when it is prescribed by the doctor. Taking it may be against religious or cultural beliefs. Or there may be other personal reasons why someone would not take medicine.

If you feel any of these ways about pain medicine, it is important to share your views with your health-care team. If you prefer, ask a friend or family member to share them for you. Talking openly about your beliefs will help your health-care team find a plan that works best for you.

PAIN-CONTROL PLAN
Make Your Pain-Control Plan Work for You

Your pain-control plan will be designed for you and your body. Everyone has a different pain-control plan. Even if you have the same type of cancer as someone else, your plan may be different. ·

Take your pain medicine on schedule to keep the pain from starting or getting worse. This is one of the best ways to stay on top of your pain. Do not skip doses. Once you feel pain, it is harder to control and may take longer to get better.

Here are some other things you can do:

- Bring your list of medicines to each visit.
- Bring your pain record or diary.
- If you are seeing more than one doctor, make sure each one sees your list of medicines, especially if he or she is going to change or prescribe medicine.
- Do not wait for the pain to get worse.
- Never take someone else's medicine or share medicine. What helped a friend or relative may not help you.
- Do not get medicine from other countries or the Internet without telling your doctor.
- Ask your doctor to change your pain-control plan if it is not working.

Follow the Dose

The best way to control pain is to stop it before it starts or prevent it from getting worse. Do not wait until the pain gets bad or unbearable before taking your medicine. Pain is easier to control when it is mild. And you need to take pain medicine often enough to stay ahead of your pain. Follow the dose schedule your doctor gives you. Do not try to "hold off" between doses. If you wait:

- your pain could get worse
- it may take longer for the pain to get better or go away
- you may need larger doses to bring the pain under control

Keep a List of All Your Medicines

Make a list of all the medicines you are taking. If you need, ask a member of your family or health-care team to help you.

Your health-care team needs to know what you take and when. Tell them each drug you are taking, no matter how harmless you think it might be. Even OTC drugs, herbs, and supplements can interfere with cancer treatment. Or they could cause serious side effects or reactions.

Do Not Give Up Hope

Your pain can be managed. If you are still having pain that is hard to control, you may want to talk with your health-care team about seeing a pain or palliative care specialist. Whatever you do, do not give up. If one medicine does not work, there is almost always another one to try. And, unlike other medicines, there is no "right" dose for many pain medicines. Your dose may be more or less than someone else's. The right dose is the one that relieves your pain and makes you feel better.

HOW TO TELL WHEN YOU NEED A NEW PAIN-CONTROL PLAN

Here are a few things to watch out for and tell your health-care team about:
- Your pain is not getting better or going away.
- Your pain medicine does not work as long as your doctor said it would.
- You have breakthrough pain.
- You have side effects that do not go away.
- Pain interferes with things such as eating, sleeping, or working.
- The schedule or the way you take the medicine does not work for you.

MEDICINES TO TREAT CANCER PAIN

There is more than one way to treat pain. Your doctor prescribes medicine based on the kind of pain you have and how severe it is. In studies, these medicines have been shown to help control cancer pain. Doctors use three main groups of drugs for pain: OTC, prescription and nonopioid medicines, and opioids. You may also hear the term "analgesics" used for these pain relievers. Some are stronger than others. It helps know the different kinds of medicines, why and how they are used, how you take them, and what side effects you might expect.

Over-the-Counter Drugs for Mild-to-Moderate Pain

OTC drugs can be used to treat mild-to-moderate pain. On a scale of 0–10, an OTC drug may be used if you rate your pain from 1 to 4. These medicines are stronger than most people realize. In many cases, they are all you will need to relieve your pain. You just need to be sure to take them regularly.

You can buy most OTC drugs without a prescription. But you still need to talk with your doctor before taking them. Some of them may have things added to them that you need to know about. And they do have side effects. Common ones, such as nausea, itching, or drowsiness, usually go away after a few days. Do not take more than the label says unless your doctor tells you to do so.

ACETAMINOPHEN (TYLENOL®)

- Acetaminophen reduces pain. It is not helpful with inflammation. Most of the time, people do not have side effects from a normal dose of acetaminophen. However, it is important to know that regularly taking large doses can damage the liver.
- Drinking alcohol with this drug may cause liver damage.

Always tell the doctor if you are taking acetaminophen for the following reasons:
- Sometimes, it is used in other medicines, so you may be taking more than you should.
- Acetaminophen can lower a fever. If you are on chemotherapy, your doctor may not want you to take the medicine too often. It could cover up a fever, which would hide the fact you might have an infection.

NONSTEROIDAL ANTIINFLAMMATORY DRUGS

Nonsteroidal antiinflammatory drugs (NSAIDs), such as ibuprofen (which you may know as "Advil®" or "Motrin®") and aspirin, help control pain and inflammation. With NSAIDs, the most common side effect is stomach upset or indigestion, especially in older people. Eating food or drinking milk when you take these drugs may stop this from happening.

Other side effects NSAIDs may cause are as follows:
- bleeding of the stomach lining (especially if you drink alcohol)
- kidney problems, especially in the elderly or those with existing kidney problems
- heart problems, especially in those who already have heart disease (However, aspirin does not cause heart problems.)
- blood clotting problems, which means it is harder to stop bleeding after you have cut or hurt yourself

When taking NSAIDs, tell your doctor if:
- your stools become darker than normal
- you notice bleeding from your rectum
- you have an upset stomach
- you have heartburn symptoms
- you cough up blood

IMPORTANT TO REMEMBER WHEN TAKING NONSTEROIDAL ANTIINFLAMMATORY DRUGS

Some people have conditions that NSAIDs can make worse. In general, you should avoid these drugs if you:
- are allergic to aspirin
- are on steroid medicines
- have stomach ulcers or a history of ulcers, gout, or bleeding disorders
- are taking prescription medicines for arthritis
- have kidney problems
- have heart problems
- are planning surgery within a week

- are taking blood-thinning medicine (such as heparin or Coumadin®)

Talk to your health-care team before taking NSAIDs. As with acetaminophen, NSAIDs can lower fever. If you are on chemotherapy, your doctor may not want you to take them too often. The medicines can cover up a fever, hiding the fact that you might have an infection.

Other Prescription Medicines for Pain

Doctors also prescribe other types of medicine to relieve cancer pain. They can be used along with nonopioids and opioids. Some are as follows:

- **Antidepressants**. Some drugs can be used for more than one purpose. For example, antidepressants are used to treat depression, but they may also help relieve tingling and burning pain. Nerve damage from radiation, surgery, or chemotherapy can cause this type of pain.
- **Antiseizure medicines (anticonvulsants)**. Like antidepressants, anticonvulsants or antiseizure drugs can also be used to help control tingling or burning from nerve injury.
- **Steroids**. These drugs are mainly used to treat pain caused by swelling.

Opioids for Moderate-to-Severe Pain

If you are having moderate-to-severe pain, your doctor may recommend that you take stronger drugs called "opioids." Opioids are sometimes called "narcotics." You must have a doctor's prescription to take them.

Opioids may be long- or short-acting. Short-acting means that the drug begins working quickly and is prescribed as needed depending on your pain levels. Long-acting drugs are absorbed in the body more slowly, but they last longer and are taken regularly as prescribed. Short-acting is often prescribed in addition to long-acting to treat breakthrough pain.

Common short-acting opioids include:
- buprenorphine
- codeine
- diamorphine
- fentanyl®
- hydrocodone
- hydromorphone (e.g., Dilaudid®)
- methadone
- morphine®
- oxycodone®
- oxymorphone
- tapentadol
- tramadol

Long-acting opioids include:
- MS Contin®
- OxyContin®
- Duragesic®

GETTING RELIEF WITH OPIOIDS

Over time, people who take opioids for pain sometimes find that they need to take larger doses to get relief. This is caused by more pain, the cancer getting worse, or medicine tolerance. When a medicine does not give you enough pain relief, your doctor may increase the dose and how often you take it. He or she can also prescribe a stronger drug. Both methods are safe and effective under your doctor's care. Do not increase the dose of medicine on your own.

TOLERANCE, PHYSICAL DEPENDENCE, AND ADDICTION

People with cancer often need opioids for pain. When your health-care team discusses your options for taking opioids, you may hear the terms "tolerance," "physical dependence," and "addiction." It may be helpful to understand the difference between the three.

Some patients with cancer pain stop getting pain relief from opioids if they take them for a long time. This is called "tolerance."

The development of tolerance is not addiction. Larger amounts or a different opioid may be needed if your body stops responding to the original dose. Your health-care team will work with you to either increase your dose or change your medicine.

Physical dependence occurs when the body gets used to a certain level of the opioid and has withdrawal symptoms if the drug is suddenly stopped or taken in much smaller doses. Withdrawal consists of unpleasant physical or psychological symptoms, such as anxiety, sweating, nausea, and vomiting, to name a few. This is not the same as addiction though people with addiction will experience physical dependence. Physical dependence can happen with the chronic use of many drugs—including many prescription drugs, even if taken as instructed.

Addiction is a chronic disease characterized by:
- compulsive drug-seeking
- the inability to stop use despite harmful consequences
- failure to meet work, social, or family obligations
- sometimes tolerance and withdrawal

Although many patients who are prescribed opioids for cancer pain use them safely, some patients are at greater risk for addiction than others. It is very important for you to share any personal or family history of drug or alcohol abuse with your health-care team. Other factors in your life may also increase your risk of addiction. It is common for cancer patients to worry that they will become addicted to pain medicines. Your doctor will carefully prescribe and monitor your opioid doses so that you are treated for pain safely. Do not be afraid to take these medicines. Controlling your pain is one of the goals of your care.

MANAGING AND PREVENTING SIDE EFFECTS

Side effects vary with each person. It is important to talk to your doctor often about any side effects you are having. If needed, he or she can change your medicines or the doses you are taking. They can also add other medicines to your pain-control plan to help your side effects.

Do not let any side effects stop you from getting your pain managed. Your health-care team can talk with you about other ways to relieve them. There are solutions to getting your pain under control. Less common side effects include:

- dizziness
- confusion
- breathing problems (Call your doctor right away if this occurs.)
- itching
- trouble urinating
- altered sleep patterns (nightmares)

Constipation

Almost everyone taking opioids has some constipation. This happens because opioids cause the stool to move more slowly through your system, so your body takes more time to absorb water from the stool. The stool then becomes hard. Keep in mind that constipation will only go away if it is treated.

You can control or prevent constipation by taking the following steps:

- Ask your doctor about giving you laxatives and stool softeners (drugs to help you pass stool from your body) when you first start taking opioids. Taking these right when you start taking pain medicine may prevent the problem.
- Drink plenty of liquids. Drinking 8–10 glasses of liquid each day will help keep stools soft.
- Eat foods high in fiber, including raw fruits with the skin left on, vegetables, and whole-grain breads and cereals.
- Exercise as much as you are able. Any movement, such as light walking, will help.
- Call your doctor if you have not had a bowel movement in two days or more.

Drowsiness

Some opioids cause drowsiness. Or, if your pain has kept you from sleeping, you may sleep more at first when you begin taking opioids. The drowsiness could go away after a few days. If you are tired or drowsy:

- do not walk up and down stairs alone
- do not drive or use machines, equipment, or anything else that requires focus

Call your doctor if the drowsiness does not go away after a few days. He or she may adjust the dose you are taking or change drugs.

Nausea and Vomiting

Nausea and vomiting may go away after a few days of taking opioids. However, if your nausea or vomiting prevents you from taking your medicine or affects your ability to eat and drink, call your doctor right away. The following tips may help:

- Stay in bed for an hour or so after taking your medicine if you feel sick when walking around. This kind of nausea is like feeling seasick. Some OTC drugs may help, too. But be sure to check with your doctor before taking any other medicines.
- Your doctor may want to change or add medicines or prescribe anti-nausea drugs.
- Ask your doctor if something else could be making you feel sick. It might be related to your cancer or another medicine you are taking. Constipation can also add to nausea.

Starting a New Pain Medicine

Some pain medicines can make you feel sleepy when you first take them. This usually goes away within a few days. Also, some people get dizzy or feel confused. Tell your doctor if any of these symptoms persist. Changing your dose or the type of medicine can usually solve the problem.[2]

---

[2] "Support for People with Cancer—Cancer Pain Control," National Cancer Institute (NCI), January 2019. Available online. URL: www.cancer.gov/publications/patient-education/paincontrol.pdf. Accessed August 7, 2023.

Chapter 7 | Fatigue in End-of-Life Care

Chapter Contents

Section 7.1 | Understanding Fatigue and Its Impact

WHAT IS FATIGUE?

Fatigue is a feeling of weariness, tiredness, or lack of energy. It can be a normal response to physical activity, emotional stress, boredom, or lack of sleep, but it can also signal a more serious mental or physical condition.

Everyone feels tired now and then. If you feel tired continuously for multiple weeks, you may want to see your doctor who can help discover what is causing your fatigue and identify ways to relieve it.

WHAT CAUSES FATIGUE?

Sometimes, fatigue can be the first sign that something is wrong in your body. For example, people with rheumatoid arthritis (RA), a painful condition that affects the joints, often complain of fatigue. People with cancer may feel fatigued from the disease, treatments, or both.

Many medical problems and treatments can add to fatigue. These include:

- having medical treatments, such as chemotherapy and radiation, or recovering from major surgery
- infections
- chronic diseases such as diabetes, heart disease, kidney disease, liver disease, thyroid disease, and chronic obstructive pulmonary disease (COPD)
- untreated pain and diseases, such as fibromyalgia
- anemia
- sleep apnea and other sleep disorders
- recent stroke
- Parkinson disease (PD)
- taking certain medications, such as antidepressants, antihistamines, and medicines for nausea and pain

Talk with your doctor about any concerns you may have about fatigue and your health condition. Treating an underlying or known health problem may help reduce fatigue.

EMOTIONAL EXHAUSTION: CAN EMOTIONS CAUSE FATIGUE?

Do you worry about your health and who will take care of you? Have you recently lost a loved one? Or have you lost your mobility and independence? Emotional stresses like these can take a toll on your energy. Fatigue can be linked to many conditions, including:

- anxiety
- depression
- grief from the loss of family or friends
- stress from financial or personal problems
- feeling that you no longer have control over your life

Not getting enough sleep can also contribute to fatigue. Regular physical activity can improve your sleep, help reduce feelings of depression and stress, and boost your mood and overall well-being. Yoga, meditation, deep breathing, and stretching may help reduce stress and anxiety and help you get more rest. Therapy or certain medications may also help relieve anxiety and depression that may be contributing to fatigue.

Talk with your doctor if your mental health seems to be affecting your sleep or making you tired.

LIFESTYLE HABITS AND FATIGUE

Some lifestyle habits can make you feel tired, including the following:

- **Staying up too late**. A good night's sleep is important to feeling refreshed and energetic. Try going to bed and waking up at the same time every day.
- **Having too much caffeine**. Drinking caffeinated soda, tea, or coffee or even eating chocolate can keep you from getting a good night's sleep. Limit the amount of caffeine you have during the day and avoid it in the evening.
- **Drinking too much alcohol**. Alcohol is a central nervous system (CNS) depressant that changes the way you think and act. It may also interact negatively with certain medicines.

- **Getting too little or too much exercise**. Regular exercise can help boost your energy levels. Overdoing it without proper rest can cause stress and lead to fatigue.
- **Boredom**. If you were busy during your working years, you may feel lost about how to spend your time when you retire. Engaging in social and productive activities that you enjoy, such as volunteering in your community, can help maintain your well-being.

TIPS TO FEEL LESS TIRED

Making changes to your lifestyle may help you feel less tired. The following are a few examples:

- **Exercise regularly**. Almost anyone, at any age, can do some type of physical activity. If you have concerns about starting an exercise program, ask your doctor if there are any activities you should avoid. Moderate exercise may improve your appetite, energy, and outlook. Some people find that exercises combining balance and breathing (e.g., tai chi or yoga) improve their energy.
- **Try to avoid long naps (over 30 minutes) late in the day**. Long naps can leave you feeling groggy and may make it harder to fall asleep at night.
- **Stop smoking**. Smoking is linked to many diseases and disorders, such as cancer, heart disease, and breathing problems, all of which are associated with fatigue.
- **Ask for help if you feel swamped**. Some people have so much to do that just thinking about their schedules can make them feel tired. Working with others may help a job go faster and be more fun.
- **Participate in activities you enjoy**. Socializing with friends and family or volunteering in your community can help you feel more engaged and productive throughout the day.
- **Eat well and avoid alcohol**. Eating nutritious foods can give you energy throughout the day. Staying away

from alcoholic drinks can help you avoid negative interactions with medications.

- **Keep a fatigue diary**. This can help you find patterns throughout the day when you feel more or less tired. It can also help you plan out activities that may give you more energy.

WHEN SHOULD YOU SEE A DOCTOR FOR FATIGUE?

If you have been tired or been experiencing low energy for several weeks with no relief, call your health-care provider. They will ask questions about your sleep, daily activities, appetite, and exercise and likely provide a physical examination and order lab tests.

Your treatment will be based on your history and the results of your exam and lab tests. You may be prescribed medications to target underlying health problems, such as anemia or abnormal thyroid function. Health-care providers may also suggest therapy or certain medications to help reduce depression, anxiety, or other emotional contributors that are associated with fatigue. They may also advise that you eat a well-balanced diet and begin an exercise program.[1]

Section 7.2 | Managing Cancer-Related Fatigue

CANCER FATIGUE
Fatigue Is the Most Common Side Effect of Cancer Treatment

Cancer treatments such as chemotherapy, radiation therapy, hormone therapy, bone marrow transplantation, and immunotherapy can cause fatigue. Fatigue is also a common symptom of some types of cancer. People with cancer describe fatigue as feeling tired, weak, worn-out, heavy, and slow or that they have no energy or get-up-and-go. Fatigue in people with cancer may be called "cancer

---

[1] National Institute on Aging (NIA), "Fatigue in Older Adults," National Institutes of Health (NIH), March 27, 2023. Available online. URL: www.nia.nih.gov/health/fatigue-older-adults. Accessed July 27, 2023.

fatigue," "cancer-related fatigue," and "cancer-treatment-related fatigue."

Cancer Fatigue Is Different from Fatigue That Healthy People Feel

When a healthy person is tired from day-to-day activities, their fatigue can be relieved with sleep and rest. Cancer fatigue is different. People with cancer get tired after less activity than people who do not have cancer. Also, cancer fatigue is not completely relieved by sleep and rest, interferes with daily activities, and may last for a long time. Fatigue usually decreases after cancer treatment ends, but some people may still feel fatigue for months or years.

Fatigue Can Decrease Your Quality of Life

Cancer fatigue can affect all areas of your life by making you too tired to take part in daily activities, relationships, social events, and community activities. You might miss work or school, spend less time with family and friends, or spend more time sleeping. In some cases, physical fatigue leads to mental fatigue and mood changes. This can make it hard for you to pay attention, remember things, and think clearly. If you suffer from cancer fatigue, you may need to take leave from a job or stop working completely. Job loss can lead to money problems and the loss of health insurance. All these things can lessen your quality of life (QOL) and self-esteem.

CAUSES OF CANCER FATIGUE
Fatigue in People with Cancer May Have More than One Cause

Doctors do not know all the reasons people with cancer have fatigue. Many conditions may cause fatigue at the same time.

Fatigue in people with cancer may be caused by the following:
- cancer treatment
- receiving more than one type of treatment (e.g., both chemotherapy and radiation therapy)
- anemia (a lower-than-normal number of red blood cells (RBCs))
- hormone levels that are too low or too high

- trouble breathing or getting enough oxygen
- infection
- pain and other symptoms
- stress
- problems getting enough sleep
- loss of appetite or not getting enough calories and nutrients
- dehydration (loss of too much water from the body, such as from severe diarrhea or vomiting)
- changes in how well the body uses food for energy
- loss of weight, muscle, and/or strength
- medicines that cause drowsiness
- not being active
- being overweight
- tumors in certain parts of the body
- other medical conditions
- having fatigue before cancer treatment begins

Fatigue is common in people with advanced cancer who are not receiving cancer treatment.

It Is Not Clear How Cancer Treatments Cause Fatigue

It is unclear how cancer treatments such as surgery, chemotherapy, and radiation therapy cause fatigue.

When cancer treatment begins, many patients are already tired from medical tests, surgery, and the emotional stress of coping with the cancer diagnosis. Fatigue may get worse during treatment.

Different cancer treatments have different effects on a patient's energy level. The type and schedule of treatments can affect the amount of fatigue caused by cancer treatment. Some patients have more fatigue after cancer treatments than others do.

FATIGUE RELATED TO SURGERY

Fatigue is often a side effect of surgery, but patients usually feel better with time. However, fatigue related to surgery can be worse when the surgery is combined with other cancer treatments.

FATIGUE CAUSED BY CHEMOTHERAPY

Patients treated with chemotherapy usually feel the most fatigue in the days right after each treatment. Then the fatigue decreases until the next treatment. Some studies have shown that patients have the most severe fatigue about midway through all the cycles of chemotherapy. Fatigue decreases after chemotherapy is finished, but patients may not feel back to normal until a month or more after the last treatment.

Fatigue during chemotherapy may be increased by the following:

- pain
- depression
- anxiety
- anemia
- lack of sleep caused by some anticancer drugs

FATIGUE CAUSED BY RADIATION THERAPY

Many patients receiving radiation therapy have fatigue that keeps them from being as active as they want to be. After radiation therapy begins, fatigue usually increases until midway through the course of treatments and then stays about the same until treatment ends. For many patients, fatigue improves after radiation therapy stops. However, in some patients, fatigue will last months or years after treatment ends.

FATIGUE CAUSED BY HORMONE THERAPY

Women who are being treated with hormone therapy for breast cancer may have fatigue. Fatigue during hormone therapy may also be increased in breast cancer survivors who are younger than 55 years, are overweight, or have more pain and insomnia.

FATIGUE CAUSED BY IMMUNOTHERAPY

Immunotherapy often causes flu-like symptoms, such as fever, chills, headache, and muscle or body aches. Some patients may also have trouble thinking clearly. Fatigue symptoms depend on the type of immunotherapy used.

Anemia

Some types of chemotherapy stop the bone marrow from making enough new RBCs, causing anemia (too few RBCs to carry oxygen to the body). Anemia affects the patient's energy level and QOL. Anemia may be caused by the following:

- cancer
- cancer treatments
- a medical condition not related to the cancer

Nutrition

For many patients, the effects of cancer and cancer treatments make it hard to eat well. The body's energy comes from food. Fatigue may occur if the body does not take in enough food to give the body the energy it needs. In people with cancer, the following three major factors may affect nutrition:

- **A change in the way the body uses food**. A patient may eat the same amount as before having cancer, but the body may not be able to absorb and use all the nutrients from the food. This is caused by the cancer or its treatment.
- **An increase in the amount of energy needed by the body**. This is because of a growing tumor, infection, fever, or shortness of breath.
- **A decrease in the amount of food eaten**. This is because of low appetite, nausea, vomiting, diarrhea, or a blocked bowel.

Anxiety and Depression

The emotional stress of cancer can cause physical problems, including fatigue. It is common for you to have changes in moods and attitudes. You may feel anxiety and fear before and after a cancer diagnosis. These feelings may cause fatigue. The effect of the disease on your physical, mental, social, and financial well-being can increase emotional distress.

About 15–25 percent of people with cancer get depressed, which may increase fatigue caused by physical factors. Patients

who have depression before starting treatment are more likely to have depression during and after treatment. The following are signs of depression:
- lack of energy and mental alertness
- loss of interest in life
- problems thinking
- drowsiness
- feeling a loss of hope

Patients who have a history of stressful experiences in childhood, such as abuse and neglect, may have increased fatigue.

Fatigue and Memory
During and after cancer treatment, you may find that you cannot pay attention for very long and have a hard time trying to think, remember, and understand. This is called "attention fatigue." Sleep helps relieve attention fatigue, but sleep may not be enough when the fatigue is related to cancer. Take part in restful activities and spend time outdoors to help relieve attention fatigue.

Lack of Sleep
Some people with cancer are not able to get enough sleep. The following problems related to sleep may cause fatigue:
- waking up during the night
- going to sleep at different times every night
- sleeping more during the day and less at night
- being inactive during the day
- the time of day that cancer treatment is given

Poor sleep affects people in different ways. For example, the time of day that fatigue is worse may be different. Some people with cancer who have trouble sleeping may feel more fatigue in the morning. Others may have severe fatigue in both the morning and the evening. People with cancer who are inactive during the day have restless sleep or who are obese may have higher levels of fatigue.

Even in people with cancer who have poor sleep, fixing sleep problems does not always improve fatigue. A lack of sleep may not be the cause of the fatigue.

Medicines Other than Chemotherapy

Patients may take medicines for pain or conditions other than cancer that cause drowsiness. Opioids, antidepressants, and antihistamines have this side effect. If these medicines are taken at the same time, fatigue may be worse.

Taking opioids over time may lower the amount of sex hormones made in the testicles and ovaries. This can lead to fatigue as well as sexual problems and depression.

ASSESSMENT OF FATIGUE
Physical Exam and Health History

A physical exam will be done. This is an exam of the body to check general signs of health or anything that seems unusual. The doctor will check for problems such as trouble breathing or loss of muscle strength. Your walking, posture, and joint movements will be checked.

Blood tests will be done to check for anemia. The most common blood tests to check if the number of RBCs is normal are as follows:

- **Complete blood count (CBC) with differential**. This is a procedure in which a sample of blood is taken and checked for the following:
  - the number of RBCs and platelets
  - the number and type of white blood cells
  - the amount of hemoglobin (the protein that carries oxygen) in the RBCs
  - the portion of the blood sample made up of RBCs
- **Peripheral blood smear**. This is a procedure in which a sample of blood is checked for the number and kinds of white blood cells, the number of platelets, and changes in the shape of blood cells.
- **Other blood tests**. These may be done to check for other conditions that affect RBCs and include a bone

marrow aspiration and biopsy or a Coombs test. Blood tests to check the levels of vitamin B_{12}, iron, and erythropoietin may also be done.

The health-care team will take a health history by asking about the status of your cancer and cancer treatments. It is important that you and your family tell the health-care team if fatigue is a problem. You will be asked to describe the fatigue.

Other questions that you will be asked about include:

- the level of fatigue (You will be asked to rate the level of fatigue. The doctor may ask you to rate the fatigue on a scale from 0 to 10.)
- when the fatigue started, how long it lasts, and what makes it better or worse
- symptoms or side effects, such as hot flashes, that you are having from the cancer or the treatments
- medicines being taken
- sleeping and resting habits
- eating habits and changes in appetite or weight
- how the fatigue affects daily activities and lifestyle
- how fatigue affects being able to work
- whether you have depression, anxiety, or pain
- health habits and past illnesses and treatments

A fatigue assessment is repeated to see if there is a pattern for when fatigue starts or becomes worse. The same method of measuring fatigue is used at each assessment. This helps show changes in fatigue over time. The health-care team will check for other causes of fatigue that can be treated.

TREATMENT FOR FATIGUE
Treating the Conditions Related to Fatigue

Fatigue is often treated by relieving related conditions. Treatment for fatigue depends on the symptoms and whether the cause of fatigue is known. When the cause of fatigue is not known, treatment is usually given to relieve symptoms and teach you ways to cope with fatigue.

TREATMENT FOR ANEMIA

Anemia causes fatigue, so treating anemia when the cause of anemia is known helps decrease fatigue. When the cause is not known, treatment for anemia is supportive care and may include the following:

- **Change in diet**. Eat more foods rich in iron and vitamins combined with other treatments for anemia.
- **Transfusions of RBCs**. Transfusions work well to treat anemia. Even though problems from a transfusion are low, there are risks of an allergic reaction, infection, graft versus host disease, immune system changes, and too much iron in the blood.
- **Erythropoiesis-stimulating agents (ESAs)**. ESAs are drugs that cause the bone marrow to make more RBCs and may be used to treat anemia-related fatigue in terminal patients receiving chemotherapy. Since ESAs increase the risk of blood clots, a few patients are offered this treatment. The U.S. Food and Drug Administration (FDA) has not approved these drugs for the treatment of fatigue. Discuss the risks and benefits of these drugs with your doctor.

TREATMENT FOR PAIN AND DEPRESSION

If pain is making fatigue worse, your pain medicine may need to be changed. If too much pain medicine is making fatigue worse, the dose may be decreased, or the medicine might be changed to a different one. Fatigue in patients who have depression may be treated with antidepressant drugs.

Certain Drugs Are Being Studied for Cancer Fatigue

The following drugs are being studied for cancer fatigue:

- **Psychostimulants**. These drugs improve mood and help decrease fatigue and depression. Psychostimulant drugs may help some patients have more energy and a better mood and help them think and concentrate. The use of psychostimulants for treating fatigue is still being studied. The FDA has not approved psychostimulants for the treatment of fatigue.

- **Bupropion**. This is an antidepressant that is being studied to treat fatigue in patients with or without depression.
- **Steroids**. These drugs are being studied in patients with advanced cancer. Dexamethasone is a steroid that reduces inflammation but has unwanted side effects. In one clinical trial, patients who received dexamethasone reported less fatigue than the group that received a placebo.

Talk to your doctor about the risks and benefits of these drugs.

Dietary Supplements Are Being Studied for Cancer Fatigue

American ginseng in the form of capsules of ground gingerroot may be used to treat fatigue. In a clinical trial, people with fatigue who were being treated for cancer or who had finished cancer treatment received either ginseng or a placebo. The group receiving ginseng had less fatigue than the placebo group.

Other dietary supplements, such as coenzyme Q10 and L-carnitine, are also being studied in clinical trials. No positive results have been published.

Exercise Has a Positive Effect on Fatigue during and after Cancer Treatment

Exercise (including walking) may help people with cancer feel better and have more energy during and after treatment. The effect of exercise on fatigue in people with cancer is being studied. One study reported that breast cancer survivors who took part in enjoyable physical activity had less fatigue and pain and were better able to take part in daily activities. In clinical trials, some people with cancer reported the following benefits from exercise:

- more physical energy
- better appetite
- better memory

- more able to do the normal activities of daily living (ADL)
- better QOL
- more enjoyment with life
- a greater sense of well-being

Moderate activity for three to five hours a week may help with cancer fatigue. You are more likely to follow an exercise plan if you choose a type of exercise that you enjoy. Your health-care team can help you plan the best time and place for exercise and how often to exercise. You may need to start with light activity for short periods of time and build up to more exercise little by little. Studies have shown that exercise can be safely done during and after cancer treatment.

Mind and body exercises such as qigong, tai chi, and yoga may help relieve fatigue. These exercises combine activities such as movement, stretching, balance, and controlled breathing with spiritual activities such as meditation.

Cognitive Behavioral Therapy

Cognitive behavioral therapy (CBT) helps you change how you think and feel about certain things. Therapists use CBT and talk therapy to treat certain emotional or behavioral disorders. Talk therapy may help decrease your fatigue by working on problems related to cancer that make fatigue worse, such as:

- stress from coping with cancer
- fear that the cancer may come back
- feeling hopeless about fatigue
- lack of social support
- a pattern of sleep and activity that changes from day to day

Studies have shown that talk therapy can help control fatigue over long periods of time. CBT with hypnosis may also help decrease fatigue.

Other Ways to Manage Fatigue

You may feel that reporting fatigue is complaining and wait for your doctor to ask about it. Fatigue is a normal side effect that should be reported and treated.

Working with the health-care team and trying the following may help you cope with fatigue:

- Learn about possible medical causes of fatigue such as an electrolyte imbalance, breathing problems, or anemia.
- Maintain a healthy diet.
- Learn how patterns of rest and activity affect fatigue.
- Learn to avoid or change activities that cause fatigue.
- Identify things that help decrease fatigue.
- Schedule important daily activities during times of less fatigue. Give up less important activities.
- Plan activities that help you feel more alert but take less energy, such as watching a sunset, walking in a park, or bird-watching.
- Find exercise programs that you like.
- Ask if physical therapy is needed if you have nerve problems or muscle weakness.
- Ask if respiratory therapy is needed if you have trouble.
- Learn to tell if treatments for fatigue are working.
- Become familiar with the difference between fatigue and depression.

These changes will help you cope with fatigue and improve your QOL.[2]

Section 7.3 | Overcoming Fatigue after Cancer Treatment

Some cancer survivors report that they still feel tired or worn-out. In fact, fatigue is one of the most common complaints during the first year of recovery.

Rest or sleep does not cure the type of fatigue that you may have. Doctors do not know its exact causes. The causes of fatigue

---

[2] "Fatigue (PDQ®)—Patient Version," National Cancer Institute (NCI), August 20, 2021. Available online. URL: www.cancer.gov/about-cancer/treatment/side-effects/fatigue/fatigue-pdq. Accessed July 27, 2023.

are different for people who are receiving treatment than they are for those who have finished.

- Fatigue during treatment can be caused by cancer therapy. Other problems can also play a part in fatigue, such as anemia (having too few red blood cells (RBCs)) or having a weak immune system. Poor nutrition, not drinking enough liquids, and depression can also be causes. Pain can make fatigue worse.
- Researchers are still learning about what may cause fatigue after treatment.

How long will fatigue last? There is no normal pattern. For some, fatigue gets better over time. Some people, especially those who have had bone marrow transplants, may still feel energy loss years later.

Some people feel very frustrated when fatigue lasts longer than they think it should and when it gets in the way of their normal routine. They may also worry that their friends, family, and coworkers will get upset with them if they continue to show signs of fatigue.

GETTING HELP

Talk with your doctor or nurse about what may be causing your fatigue and what can be done about it. Ask about:

- how any medicines you are taking or other medical problems you have might affect your energy level
- how you can control your pain if pain is a problem for you
- exercise programs that might help, such as walking
- relaxation exercises
- changing your diet or drinking more fluids
- medicines or nutritional supplements that can help
- specialists who might help you, such as physical therapists, occupational therapists, nutritionists, or mental health-care providers

COPING WITH FATIGUE

Here are some ideas to cope with fatigue:

- Plan your day. Be active at the time of day when you feel most alert and energetic.
- Save your energy by changing how you do things. For example, sit on a stool while you cook or wash dishes.
- Take short naps or rest breaks between activities.
- Try to go to sleep and wake up at the same time every day.
- Do what you enjoy but do less of it. Focus on old or new interests that do not tire you out. For example, try to read something brief or listen to music.
- Let others help you. They might cook meals, run errands, or do the laundry. If no one offers, ask for what you need. Friends and family might be willing to help but may not know what to do.
- Choose how to spend your energy. Try to let go of things that do not matter as much now.
- Think about joining a support group. Talking about your fatigue with others who have had the same problem may help you find new ways to cope.[3]

[3] "Facing Forward—Life after Cancer Treatment," National Cancer Institute (NCI), March 2018. Available online. URL: www.cancer.gov/publications/patient-education/life-after-treatment.pdf. Accessed August 18, 2023.

Chapter 8 | The Essence of Palliative Care

Chapter Contents

Section 8.1 | Palliative Wound Care

Although typical medical treatment focuses on healing, the aim of palliative care is to treat symptoms and improve the quality of life (QOL) for terminally ill patients and their families. More than one-third of hospice patients and other individuals with serious illnesses suffer from issues such as pressure ulcers (bedsores), surgical wounds, and other skin problems as a result of the deterioration of the body and multi-organ systems failure. Palliative wound care is an effective method for relieving pain, treating infection, preventing new wounds from developing, and helping the patient and his or her family make the most of the remaining time they have together.

MANAGEMENT OF PALLIATIVE WOUND CARE

Palliative care takes a coordinated approach to treating wounds and lessening symptoms, with the ultimate goal of ensuring patient comfort and a sense of well-being. Generally, this means local wound care (treatment of the wound itself) and pain management.

Local Wound Care

Although healing is not always possible in palliative care, proper treatment of wounds can help prevent infection and improve the patient's state of mind. Wound care addresses the following issues:

- **Bleeding**. The repeated dressing and redressing of wounds often result in the tearing of tissue, which can lead to bleeding, increased discomfort, and infection. Topical vasoconstrictors are often used to stem blood flow, and a variety of sealants or barriers may be applied to the surface. Dressings with silicone adhesives may be used since they are less likely to cause trauma to the wound with repeated applications.
- **Exudates**. These are clear or pus-like liquids that ooze out of cuts or areas of inflammation. Normally, exudates are beneficial and central to the healing

83

process, but in the case of chronic wounds, they can cause problems such as infection of the wound or inflammation of the surrounding skin. The most common ways to manage exudates are through the use of the proper dressings and the application of topical steroids.

- **Infection**. Open wounds can easily become contaminated with bacteria, often leading to infection, which can spread and cause additional problems. And, in the case of chronically ill patients, who frequently have compromised immune systems, this can be particularly dangerous. The best practice is to prevent infection in the first place. This is accomplished by using wound dressings with antimicrobial agents, applying topical antibiotics, and cleansing and debriding (removing dead tissue) the area when changing dressings.
- **Odor**. Unpleasant odor is a common problem with wounds, particularly those in which infection has set in, and in addition to being a sign of physical issues, this has a tendency to negatively affect the patient's mental state. The first step in addressing or preventing odor is the proper cleansing of the wound, along with the application of topical antibiotics to treat infection and the use of specialized dressings.

Pain Management

Pressure ulcers and other skin problems can be especially painful, and unfortunately, they are extremely common among terminally ill patients and others requiring palliative care. Therefore, controlling pain is one of the most important components in palliative wound care and is perhaps the one with the most impact on the patient's well-being and QOL. Pain management may include the following:

- **Prevention**. The best way to manage pain is to prevent it as much as possible in the first place. This often means using special dressings that do not stick to wounds and training caregivers in the proper way to change dressings. Bedridden patients are usually turned frequently to prevent pressure ulcers, but in some cases, when certain wounds are present, this procedure can increase pain, so less frequent turning may be called for. Debridement, although necessary, can be extremely painful, so in some cases, medical professionals may need to administer a local anesthetic prior to the procedure.

- **Assessment**. Since pain is a subjective experience, assessing the degree to which it affects any given individual can be difficult. But, since palliative care includes involving the patient in decision-making, his or her own description of pain must be taken into account by caregivers. In addition, a variety of tools— numerical scales, charts, and drawings—are often used, as are physiological and behavior observations by medical professionals.
- **Topical anesthetics**. The application of pain-relief medication directly to the wound has the advantage of bypassing the circulatory system, thus avoiding many side effects and often allowing for lower doses. Common topical anesthetics include lidocaine, benzydamine, sucralfate, and morphine gel, sometimes with antibiotics added to help prevent infection. Dressings that contain slow-release pain-relief pain medication, such as ibuprofen, have also proven effective.
- **Systemic analgesics**. These medications can be administered orally, by injection, or through an IV and work by being absorbed into the bloodstream where they affect the body's pain receptors. Generally, the treatment of moderate pain will begin with medications such as acetaminophen and nonsteroidal anti-inflammatory drugs (NSAIDs). More severe pain often requires the use of opioid (narcotic) analgesics, such as morphine, meperidine, nalbuphine, butorphanol, and fentanyl. Although these medications relieve pain,

they tend to reduce the patient's mental status or, in large doses, make him or her sleep most of the time, so doctors need to balance their benefits against QOL.

- **Alternative methods**. A number of methods for controlling pain without medication—or with lower doses of medication—have proven effective in some cases. These include gentle massage, physical therapy, acupuncture, and relaxation techniques, such as biofeedback and hypnosis. Transcutaneous electrical nerve stimulation (TENS), which employs low-voltage electrical current for pain relief, has also been used with good results. And many patients respond well to pet therapy, as the presence of an animal and stoking its fur can have a very soothing effect.

LOCATIONS FOR PALLIATIVE WOUND CARE

Palliative wound care can take place in a hospital, an outpatient clinic (if the patient is ambulatory), at home, or in a hospice. In all cases, the palliative care team will typically consist of doctors, nurses, and social workers, as well as the patient and family members, who are integral parts of the management process. In some cases, other specialists, including massage therapists, pharmacists, and nutritionists, may be part of the team. Each location has its advantages and disadvantages, which depend on the illness, the severity of symptoms, the patient's preferences, and access to qualified caregivers.

- **Hospital care**. During the early stages of an illness, patients are generally treated in a hospital. And, even when treatment is completed or discontinued, many hospitals now have specialists on staff to provide palliative care although, unless the hospital has a hospice or other dedicated facility, this is usually only available for a limited time.
- **Outpatient palliative care**. If a patient is ambulatory, specialized wound care may be provided at a clinic that is outfitted and staffed for palliative care. The advantage of this type of care is that the patient and family

are able to maintain close to their normal routines, while the illness is managed as required by a team of professionals.

- **Palliative care at home.** Most patients prefer to live at home rather than in a care facility. And, with the many types of professional support available through a variety of hospital programs, government agencies, and private sources, many individuals with serious illnesses are able to do so. Generally, this means working with a team of visiting nurses, social workers, and other professionals—as well as the cooperation of family members—to ensure that adequate care is available as needed.

- **Hospice care.** When illnesses have progressed too far for home or outpatient care, palliative care in a hospice may be recommended. In most instances, hospices are for terminally ill patients who may have only months to live. Here, although the level of care is not as intense as in a hospital, the patient can be observed more closely, and professional help is generally more readily available. But, as with all palliative care, the emphasis is on patient comfort and QOL.

References

Graves, Marilyn L. and Sun, Virginia. "Providing Quality Wound Care at the End of Life," *Journal of Hospice & Palliative Nursing*, 15, no. 2 (2013): 66–74. http://dx.doi.org/10.1097/NJH.0b013e31827edcf0.

Hughes, Ronda G., et al. "Palliative Wound Care at the End of Life," Agency for Healthcare Research and Quality (AHRQ), U.S. Department of Health and Human Services (HHS), April 2005. Available online. URL: https://archive.ahrq.gov/professionals/systems/long-term-care/resources/coordination/wound/palliative-wound-care.pdf. Accessed September 14, 2023.

"Managing Pain Beyond Drugs," Web MD, August 14, 2015. Available online. URL: www.webmd.com/palliative-care/

managing-pain-beyond-drugs. Accessed September 14, 2023.

Tippett, Aletha W. "Palliative Wound Treatment Promotes Healing," Wounds, January 2015. Available online. URL: www.woundsresearch.com/article/palliative-wound-treatment-promotes-healing. Accessed September 14, 2023.

Woo, Kevin Y., et al. "Palliative Wound Care Management Strategies for Palliative Patients and Their Circles of Care," Lippincott® CMEConnection, March 2015. Available online. URL: http://cme.lww.com/files/PalliativeWoundCareManagementStrategiesfor PalliativePatientsandTheirCirclesofCare-1424293002666.pdf. Accessed September 14, 2023.

Section 8.2 | Palliative Care in Cancer

Palliative care may be provided at any point during cancer care, from diagnosis to the end of life. When a person receives palliative care, they may continue to receive cancer treatment.

HOW DOES SOMEONE ACCESS PALLIATIVE CARE?

The oncologist (or someone on the oncology care team) is the first person one should ask about palliative care. They may refer the patient to a palliative care specialist, depending on their physical and emotional needs. Some national organizations have databases for referrals.

WHAT ARE THE ISSUES ADDRESSED IN PALLIATIVE CARE?

The physical and emotional effects of cancer and its treatment may be very different from person to person. Palliative care can address a broad range of issues, integrating an individual's specific needs into care. A palliative care specialist will take the following issues into account for each patient:

- **Physical.** Common physical symptoms that can be addressed include pain, fatigue, loss of appetite, nausea, vomiting, shortness of breath, and insomnia.
- **Emotional and coping.** Palliative care specialists can provide resources to help patients and families deal with the emotions that come with a cancer diagnosis and cancer treatment. Depression, anxiety, and fear are only a few of the concerns that can be addressed through palliative care.
- **Spiritual.** With a cancer diagnosis, patients and families often look more deeply for meaning in their lives. Some find the disease brings them closer to their faith or spiritual beliefs, whereas others struggle to understand why cancer happened to them. An expert in palliative care can help people explore their beliefs and values so that they can find a sense of peace or reach a point of acceptance that is appropriate for their situation.
- **Caregiver needs.** Family members and friends are an important part of cancer care. Like the patient, they have changing needs. It is common for many caregivers to become overwhelmed by the extra responsibilities placed upon them. Many find it hard to care for their loved one who is sick while trying to handle other obligations, such as work, household duties, and taking care of their family. Uncertainty about how to help their loved one with medical situations, inadequate social support, and emotions such as worry and fear can also add to caregiver stress. These challenges can compromise caregivers' own health. Palliative care specialists can help families and friends cope and give them the support they need.
- **Practical needs.** Palliative care specialists can also assist with financial and legal worries, insurance questions, and employment concerns. Discussing

the goals of care is also an important component of palliative care. Such discussions can also include talking about advance directives and help guide communication among family members, caregivers, and members of the oncology care team.

WHAT IS THE DIFFERENCE BETWEEN PALLIATIVE CARE AND HOSPICE?

Whereas palliative care can begin at any point during cancer treatment, hospice care begins when curative treatment is no longer the goal of care and the sole focus is quality of life (QOL).

Palliative care can help patients and their loved ones make the transition from treatment meant to cure or control the disease to hospice care by:

- preparing them for physical changes that may occur near the end of life
- helping them cope with the different thoughts and emotional issues that arise
- providing support for family members and caregivers

WHO PAYS FOR PALLIATIVE CARE?

Private health insurance usually covers palliative care services. Medicare and Medicaid also pay for some kinds of palliative care. For example, Medicare Part B pays for some medical services that address symptom management. Medicaid coverage of some palliative care services varies by state. If patients do not have health insurance or are unsure about their coverage, they should check with a social worker or their hospital's financial counselor.

IS THERE ANY RESEARCH THAT SHOWS PALLIATIVE CARE IS BENEFICIAL?

Research shows that palliative care and its many components are beneficial to patient and family health and well-being. Some studies have shown that integrating palliative care into a patient's usual cancer care soon after a diagnosis of advanced cancer can improve their QOL and mood and may even prolong survival. The American Society of Clinical Oncology (ASCO) recommends that all patients with advanced cancer receive palliative care.[1]

---

[1] "Palliative Care in Cancer," National Cancer Institute (NCI), November 1, 2021. Available online. URL: www.cancer.gov/about-cancer/advanced-cancer/care-choices/palliative-care-fact-sheet. Accessed August 2, 2023.

Chapter 9 | **Artificial Hydration, Nutrition, and End-of-Life Care**

Patients suffering from life-threatening illnesses may, at some point, lose interest in food and fluids or may not be able to take them by mouth. Artificial hydration and nutrition is a treatment methodology that allows patients to receive food and fluids when they are no longer able to chew or swallow. This technique works not only for people at the end of their life but also for those who are recovering from surgery or suffering from temporary illnesses such as diarrhea, nausea, and vomiting.

TYPES OF ARTIFICIAL HYDRATION AND NUTRITION
There are different ways to provide artificial hydration and nutrition.

Intravenous Hydration
In intravenous (IV) hydration, fluids are injected directly into the patient's vein through a small needle that is hooked up to a plastic tube. This method involves only a few risks, such as:
- infection or bleeding at the site of insertion of the needle
- swelling and breathing problems due to an overload of fluid

Hypodermoclysis is a method similar to IV hydration by which the fluid is administered under the skin instead of in a vein.

Total Parenteral Nutrition
Total parenteral nutrition (TPN) is an IV nutrition. It involves the delivery of nutrition through a central line inserted in the armpit or neck and threaded through a vein. This method poses an increased risk of infection in the central line, which is highly dangerous to the patient.

Nasogastric Tubes
In this method, a thin tube is inserted into the nostril of the patient and made to pass to the stomach. A liquid formula delivered through the nasogastric (NG) tube provides artificial hydration and nutrition. The tube can be left in only for a short period of one to four weeks. This method has a higher risk of causing pneumonia and thereby reducing the survival rate of patients.

Gastrostomy Tubes
In this method, a gastrostomy (G) tube is placed into the wall of the stomach through surgery or percutaneously. This method is considered to be less risky than the other methods. However, there is a chance of developing pneumonia via this method, too.

ARTIFICIAL HYDRATION AND NUTRITION: AN OVERVIEW
Is Artificial Hydration and Nutrition Different from Normal Intake of Food and Fluids?
Yes, artificial hydration and nutrition medical treatment is completely different than eating and drinking. In artificial hydration and nutrition, the patient cannot feel the taste or texture of food and fluid. Moreover, it can be administered only by medical professionals, who ultimately decide what type and how much nutrition to be given and who monitor the side effects as well.

Can Artificial Hydration and Nutrition Save Lives?
Artificial hydration and nutrition can be effective for patients suffering from temporary illnesses such as dehydration, nausea, vomiting, diarrhea, and so on. It can also help patients recover faster

after surgery. However, it may not be beneficial to someone who is at the end of his or her life. In some cases, artificial hydration and nutrition may add to the discomfort of a dying person by causing bloating, irritation, swelling, diarrhea, and breathing problems.

Can a Patient Refuse to Take Artificial Hydration and Nutrition?

Legally, every patient has the right to decide to accept, refuse, or discontinue artificial hydration and nutrition. If the patient is able to communicate, he or she can directly convey this decision to the physician. When the patient is no longer able to talk, his or her advanced directives will be followed. However, when there is uncertainty about the decision of the patient, the treatment will usually be continued.

References

"Artificial Nutrition (Food) and Hydration (Fluids) at the End of Life," National Hospice and Palliative Care Organization (NHPCO), 2015. Available online. URL: www.nhpco.org/wp-content/uploads/2019/04/ ArtificialNutritionAndHydration.pdf. Accessed September 14, 2023.

Familydoctor.org, "Artificial Hydration and Nutrition," American Academy of Family Physicians (AAFP), January 15, 2018. Available online. URL: https:// familydoctor.org/artificial-hydration-and-nutrition. Accessed September 14, 2023.

Morrow, Angela. "Artificial Nutrition and Hydration," Verywell Health, May 12, 2019. Available online. URL: www.verywellhealth.com/artificial-nutrition-and- hydration-1132312. Accessed September 14, 2023.

Chapter 10 | **Nourishing Care for Cancer Patients**

NUTRITION IN CANCER CARE

Nutrition is a process in which food is taken in and used by the body for growth, to keep the body healthy, and to replace tissue. Good nutrition is important for good health. A healthy diet includes foods and liquids that have important nutrients (vitamins, minerals, protein, carbohydrates, fat, and water) the body needs.

Healthy Eating Habits during and after Cancer Treatment

A diet with a focus on plant-based foods along with regular exercise will help cancer patients keep a healthy body weight, maintain strength, and decrease side effects both during and after treatment.

Registered Dietitian Is an Important Part of the Health-Care Team

A registered dietitian (or nutritionist) is a part of a team of health professionals who help with cancer treatment and recovery. A dietitian will work with patients, their families, and the rest of the medical team to manage the patient's diet during and after cancer treatment.

Research has shown that including a registered dietitian in a patient's cancer care can help the patient live longer.

Cancer and Cancer Treatments May Cause Side Effects That Affect Nutrition

Nutrition problems are likely when tumors involve the head, neck, esophagus, stomach, intestines, pancreas, or liver.

For many patients, the effects of cancer treatments make it hard to eat well. Cancer treatments that affect nutrition include:

- chemotherapy
- hormone therapy
- radiation therapy
- surgery
- immunotherapy
- stem cell transplant

Cancer and Cancer Treatments May Cause Malnutrition

Cancer and cancer treatments may affect taste, smell, appetite, and the ability to eat enough food or absorb the nutrients from food. This can cause malnutrition, which is a condition caused by a lack of key nutrients. Alcohol abuse and obesity may increase the risk of malnutrition.

Malnutrition can cause the patient to be weak, tired, and unable to fight infection or finish cancer treatment. As a result, malnutrition can decrease the patient's quality of life (QOL) and become life-threatening. Malnutrition may be made worse if the cancer grows or spreads.

Eating the right amount of protein and calories is important for healing, fighting infection, and having enough energy.

Anorexia and Cachexia Are Common Causes of Malnutrition in Cancer Patients

Anorexia is the loss of appetite or desire to eat. It is a common symptom in patients with cancer. Anorexia may occur early in the disease or later if the cancer grows or spreads. Some patients already have anorexia when they are diagnosed with cancer. Most patients who have advanced cancer will have anorexia. Anorexia is the most common cause of malnutrition in cancer patients.

Cachexia is a condition marked by weakness, weight loss, and fat and muscle loss. It is common in patients with tumors that affect eating and digestion. It can occur in cancer patients who are eating well but are not storing fat and muscle because of tumor growth.

Some tumors change the way the body uses certain nutrients. The body's use of protein, carbohydrates, and fat may change when tumors are in the stomach, intestines, or head and neck. A patient may seem to be eating enough, but the body may not be able to absorb all the nutrients from the food.

Cancer patients may have anorexia and cachexia at the same time.

EFFECTS OF CANCER TREATMENT ON NUTRITION
Chemotherapy and Hormone Therapy

Chemotherapy and hormone therapy affect nutrition in different ways. Chemotherapy affects cells all through the body. Chemotherapy uses drugs to stop the growth of cancer cells, either by killing the cells or by stopping them from dividing. Healthy cells that normally grow and divide quickly may also be killed. These include cells in the mouth and digestive tract.

Hormone therapy adds, blocks, or removes hormones. It may be used to slow or stop the growth of certain cancers. Some types of hormone therapy may cause weight gain.

Chemotherapy and hormone therapy cause different nutrition problems. Side effects from chemotherapy may cause problems with eating and digestion. When more than one chemotherapy drug is given, each drug may cause different side effects, or when drugs cause the same side effect, the side effect may be more severe.

The following side effects are common:
- loss of appetite
- nausea
- vomiting
- dry mouth
- sores in the mouth or throat
- changes in the way food tastes
- trouble swallowing
- feeling full after eating a small amount of food
- constipation
- diarrhea

Patients who receive hormone therapy may need changes in their diet to prevent weight gain.

Radiation Therapy

Radiation therapy kills cancer cells and healthy cells in the treatment area. How severe the side effects are depends on the following:

- the part of the body that is treated
- the total dose of radiation and how it is given

Radiation therapy to any part of the digestive system has side effects that cause nutrition problems. Most of the side effects begin two to three weeks after radiation therapy begins and go away a few weeks after it is finished. Some side effects can continue for months or years after treatment ends.

The following are some of the more common side effects:

- for radiation therapy to the brain or head and neck:
  - loss of appetite
  - nausea
  - vomiting
  - dry mouth or thick saliva (Medication may be given to treat a dry mouth.)
  - sore mouth and gums
  - changes in the way food tastes
  - trouble swallowing
  - pain when swallowing
  - being unable to fully open the mouth
- for radiation therapy to the chest:
  - loss of appetite
  - nausea
  - vomiting
  - trouble swallowing
  - pain when swallowing
  - choking or breathing problems caused by changes in the upper esophagus
- for radiation therapy to the abdomen, pelvis, or rectum:
  - nausea
  - vomiting
  - bowel obstruction
  - colitis
  - diarrhea

Radiation therapy may also cause tiredness, which can lead to a decrease in appetite.

Surgery

Surgery increases the body's need for nutrients and energy. The body needs extra energy and nutrients to heal wounds, fight infection, and recover from surgery. If the patient is malnourished before surgery, it may cause problems during recovery, such as poor healing or infection. For these patients, nutrition care may begin before surgery.

Surgery to the head, neck, esophagus, stomach, or intestines may affect nutrition. Most cancer patients are treated with surgery. Surgery that removes all or part of certain organs can affect a patient's ability to eat and digest food.

The following are nutrition problems caused by surgery:

- loss of appetite
- trouble chewing
- trouble swallowing
- feeling full after eating a small amount of food

Immunotherapy

Immunotherapy may affect nutrition. The side effects of immunotherapy are different for each patient and the type of immunotherapy drug given.

The following nutrition problems are common:

- tiredness
- fever
- nausea
- vomiting
- diarrhea

Stem Cell Transplant

Patients who receive a stem cell transplant have special nutrition needs. Chemotherapy, radiation therapy, and other medicines used before or during a stem cell transplant may cause side effects that keep a patient from eating and digesting food as usual.

Common side effects include the following:
- mouth and throat sores
- diarrhea

Patients who receive a stem cell transplant have a high risk of infection. Chemotherapy or radiation therapy given before the transplant decreases the number of white blood cells (WBCs), which fight infection. It is important that these patients learn about safe food handling and avoid foods that may cause infection.

After a stem cell transplant, patients are at risk for acute or chronic graft versus host disease (GVHD). GVHD may affect the gastrointestinal tract or liver and change the patient's ability to eat or absorb nutrients from food.

NUTRITION ASSESSMENT IN CANCER CARE

The health-care team may ask questions about diet and weight history.

Screening is used to look for health problems that affect the risk of poor nutrition. This can help find out if the patient is likely to become malnourished and if nutrition therapy is needed.

The health-care team may ask questions about the following:
- weight changes over the past year
- changes in the amount and type of food eaten
- problems that have affected eating, such as loss of appetite, nausea, vomiting, diarrhea, constipation, mouth sores, dry mouth, changes in taste and smell, or pain
- ability to walk and do other activities of daily living (dressing, getting into or out of a bed or chair, taking a bath or shower, and using the toilet)

A physical exam is done to check the body for general health and signs of disease. The patient is checked for signs of loss of weight, fat, and muscle and for fluid buildup in the body.

Counseling and diet changes are made to improve the patient's nutrition.

A registered dietitian can work with patients and their families to counsel them on ways to improve the patient's nutrition. The registered dietitian gives care based on the patient's nutrition and diet needs. Changes to the diet are made to help decrease symptoms from cancer or cancer treatment. These changes may be in the types and amount of food, how often a patient eats, and how food is eaten (e.g., at a certain temperature or taken with a straw).

A registered dietitian works with other members of the health-care team to check the patient's nutritional health during cancer treatment and recovery. In addition to the dietitian, the health-care team may include the following:

- physician
- nurse
- social worker
- psychologist

The goal of nutrition therapy for patients who have advanced cancer depends on the overall plan of care (POC).

The goal of nutrition therapy in patients with advanced cancer is to give patients the best possible QOL and control symptoms that cause distress.

Patients with advanced cancer may be treated with anticancer therapy and palliative care, or palliative care alone, or maybe in hospice care. Nutrition goals will be different for each patient. Some types of treatment may be stopped if they are not helping the patient.

As the focus of care goes from cancer treatment to hospice or end-of-life care, nutrition goals may become less aggressive, and a change to care is meant to keep the patient as comfortable as possible.

TREATMENT OF SYMPTOMS

When side effects of cancer or cancer treatment affect normal eating, changes can be made to help the patient get the nutrients they need. Eating foods that are high in calories, protein, vitamins, and minerals is important. Meals should be planned to meet the patient's nutrition needs and tastes in food.

The following are some of the more common symptoms caused by cancer and cancer treatment and ways to treat or control them.

Anorexia

The following may help cancer patients who have anorexia (loss of appetite or desire to eat):

- Eat foods that are high in protein and calories. The following are high-protein food choices:
  - beans
  - chicken
  - fish
  - meat
  - yogurt
  - eggs
- Add extra protein and calories to food, such as using protein-fortified milk.
- Eat high-protein foods first in your meal when your appetite is strongest.
- Sip only small amounts of liquids during meals.
- Drink milkshakes, smoothies, juices, or soups if you do not feel like eating solid foods.
- Eat foods that smell good.
- Try new foods and new recipes.
- Try blenderized drinks that are high in nutrients (check with your doctor or registered dietitian first).
- Eat small meals and healthy snacks often throughout the day.
- Eat larger meals when you feel well and are rested.
- Eat your largest meal when you feel hungriest, whether at breakfast, lunch, or dinner.
- Make and store small amounts of favorite foods, so they are ready to eat when you are hungry.
- Be as active as possible so that you will have a good appetite.
- Brush your teeth and rinse your mouth to relieve symptoms and aftertaste.
- Talk to your doctor or registered dietitian if you have eating problems such as nausea, vomiting, or changes in how foods taste and smell.

If these diet changes do not help with the anorexia, tube feedings may be needed so that you will get enough nutrients each day. Medicines may be given to increase appetite.

Nausea

The following may help cancer patients control nausea:
- Choose foods that appeal to you. Do not force yourself to eat food that makes you feel sick. Do not eat your favorite foods to avoid linking them to being sick.
- Eat foods that are bland, soft, and easy to digest, rather than heavy meals.
- Eat dry foods such as crackers, breadsticks, or toast throughout the day.
- Eat foods that are easy on your stomach, such as white toast, plain yogurt, and clear broth.
- Eat dry toast or crackers before getting out of bed if you have nausea in the morning.
- Eat foods and drink liquids at room temperature (not too hot or too cold).
- Slowly sip liquids throughout the day.
- Suck on hard candies such as peppermints or lemon drops if your mouth has a bad taste.
- Stay away from food and drink with strong smells.
- Eat five or six small meals every day instead of three large meals.
- Sip on only small amounts of liquid during meals to avoid feeling full or bloated.
- Do not skip meals and snacks. An empty stomach may make your nausea worse.
- Rinse your mouth before and after eating.
- Do not eat in a room that has cooking odors or that is very warm. Keep the living space at a comfortable temperature and well-ventilated.
- Sit up or lie with your head raised for one hour after eating.
- Plan the best times for you to eat and drink.
- Relax before each cancer treatment.

- Wear clothes that are loose and comfortable.
- Keep a record of when you feel nausea and why.
- Talk with your doctor about using anti-nausea medicine.

Vomiting

The following may help cancer patients control vomiting:
- Do not eat or drink anything until the vomiting stops.
- Drink small amounts of clear liquids after the vomiting stops.
- After you are able to drink clear liquids without vomiting, drink liquids such as strained soups or milkshakes that are easy on your stomach.
- Eat five or six small meals every day instead of three large meals.
- Sit upright and bend forward after vomiting.
- Ask your doctor to order medicine to prevent or control vomiting.

Dry Mouth

The following may help cancer patients with a dry mouth:
- Eat foods that are easy to swallow.
- Moisten food with sauce, gravy, or salad dressing.
- Eat foods and drinks that are very sweet or tart, such as lemonade, to help make more saliva.
- Chew gum or suck on hard candy, ice pops, or ice chips.
- Sip water throughout the day.
- Do not drink any type of alcohol, beer, or wine.
- Do not eat foods that can hurt your mouth (such as spicy, sour, salty, hard, or crunchy foods).
- Keep your lips moist with lip balm.
- Rinse your mouth every one to two hours. Do not use mouthwash that contains alcohol.
- Do not use tobacco products and avoid secondhand smoke.

- Ask your doctor or dentist about using artificial saliva or similar products to coat, protect, and moisten your mouth and throat.

Mouth Sores

The following can help patients who have mouth sores:
- Eat soft foods that are easy to chew, such as milkshakes, scrambled eggs, and custard.
- Cook foods until soft and tender.
- Cut food into small pieces. Use a blender or food processor to make food smooth.
- Suck on ice chips to numb and soothe your mouth.
- Eat foods cold or at room temperature. Hot foods can hurt your mouth.
- Drink with a straw to move liquid past the painful parts of your mouth.
- Use a small spoon to help you take smaller bites, which are easier to chew.
- Stay away from the following:
  - citrus foods, such as oranges, lemons, and limes
  - spicy foods
  - tomatoes and ketchup
  - salty foods
  - raw vegetables
  - sharp and crunchy foods
  - drinks with alcohol
- Do not use tobacco products.
- Visit a dentist at least two weeks before starting immunotherapy, chemotherapy, or radiation therapy to the head and neck.
- Check your mouth each day for sores, white patches, or puffy and red areas.
- Rinse your mouth three to four times a day. Mix ¼ teaspoon baking soda, ⅛ teaspoon salt, and one cup warm water for a mouth rinse. Do not use mouthwash that contains alcohol.
- Do not use toothpicks or other sharp objects.

Taste Changes

The following may help cancer patients who have taste changes:

- Eat poultry, fish, eggs, and cheese instead of red meat.
- Add spices and sauces to foods (marinate foods).
- Eat meat with something sweet, such as cranberry sauce, jelly, or applesauce.
- Try tart foods and drinks.
- Use sugar-free lemon drops, gum, or mints if there is a metallic or bitter taste in your mouth.
- Use plastic utensils and do not drink directly from metal containers if foods have a metallic taste.
- Try to eat your favorite foods if you are not nauseated. Try new foods when feeling your best.
- Try recipes for high-protein, vegetarian dishes.
- Chew food longer to allow more contact with taste buds if food tastes dull but not unpleasant.
- Keep foods and drinks covered, drink through a straw, turn a kitchen fan on when cooking, or cook outdoors if smells bother you.
- Brush your teeth and take care of your mouth. Visit your dentist for checkups.

Sore Throat and Trouble Swallowing

The following may help cancer patients who have a sore throat or trouble swallowing:

- Eat soft foods that are easy to chew and swallow, such as milkshakes, scrambled eggs, oatmeal, or other cooked cereals.
- Eat foods and drinks that are high in protein and calories.
- Moisten food with gravy, sauces, broth, or yogurt.
- Stay away from the following foods and drinks that can burn or scratch your throat:
  - hot foods and drinks
  - spicy foods
  - foods and juices that are high in acid

- sharp or crunchy foods
- drinks with alcohol
- Cook foods until soft and tender.
- Cut food into small pieces. Use a blender or food processor to make food smooth.
- Drink with a straw.
- Eat five or six small meals every day instead of three large meals.
- Sit upright and bend your head slightly forward when you eat or drink and stay upright for at least 30 minutes after eating.
- Do not use tobacco.
- Talk to your doctor about tube feeding if you cannot eat enough to stay strong.

Lactose Intolerance

The following may help patients who have symptoms of lactose intolerance:

- Use lactose-free or low-lactose milk products. Most grocery stores carry food (such as milk and ice cream) labeled "lactose free" or "low lactose."
- Choose milk products that are low in lactose, such as hard cheeses (such as cheddar) and yogurt.
- Try products made with soy or rice (such as soy and rice milk and frozen desserts). These products do not contain lactose.
- Avoid only the dairy products that give you problems. Eat small portions of dairy products, such as milk, yogurt, or cheese, if you can.
- Try nondairy drinks and foods with calcium added.
- Eat calcium-rich vegetables, such as broccoli and greens.
- Take lactase tablets when eating or drinking dairy products. Lactase breaks down lactose, so it is easier to digest.
- Prepare your own low-lactose or lactose-free foods.

Weight Gain

The following may help cancer patients prevent weight gain:

- Eat a lot of fruits and vegetables.
- Eat foods that are high in fiber, such as whole-grain breads, cereals, and pasta.
- Choose lean meats, such as lean beef, pork trimmed of fat, and poultry (such as chicken or turkey) without skin.
- Choose low-fat milk products.
- Eat less fat (eat only small amounts of butter, mayonnaise, desserts, and fried foods).
- Cook with low-fat methods, such as broiling, steaming, grilling, or roasting.
- Eat less salt.
- Eat foods that you enjoy, so you feel satisfied.
- Eat only when hungry. Consider counseling or medicine if you eat because of stress, fear, or depression. If you eat because you are bored, find activities you enjoy.
- Eat smaller amounts of food at meals.
- Exercise daily.
- Talk with your doctor before going on a diet to lose weight.

TYPES OF NUTRITION SUPPORT
Nutrition Support Helps Patients Who Cannot Eat or Digest Food Normally

It is best to take in food by mouth whenever possible. Some patients may not be able to take in enough food by mouth because of problems from cancer or cancer treatment.

Nutrition Support Can Be Given in Different Ways

In addition to counseling by a dietitian and changes to the diet, nutrition therapy includes nutritional supplement drinks and enteral and parenteral nutrition support. Nutritional supplement drinks help cancer patients get the nutrients they need. They provide energy, protein, fat, carbohydrates, fiber, vitamins, and minerals. They are not meant to be the patient's only source of nutrition.

A patient who is not able to take in the right amount of calories and nutrients by mouth may be fed using the following:

- **Enteral nutrition**. Nutrients are given through a tube inserted into the stomach or intestines.
- **Parenteral nutrition**. Nutrients are infused into the bloodstream.

Nutrition support can improve a patient's QOL during cancer treatment but may cause problems that should be considered before making the decision to use it. The patient and health-care team should discuss the harms and benefits of each type of nutrition support.

Enteral Nutrition

Enteral nutrition is also called "tube feeding." Enteral nutrition gives the patient nutrients in liquid form (formula) through a tube that is placed into the stomach or small intestine. The following types of feeding tubes may be used:

- **Nasogastric (NG) tube**. This tube is inserted through the nose and down the throat into the stomach or small intestine. This is used when enteral nutrition is only needed for a few weeks.
- **Gastrostomy and jejunostomy tubes**. A gastrostomy tube is inserted into the stomach, and a jejunostomy tube is inserted into the small intestine through an opening made on the outside of the abdomen. This is usually used for long-term enteral feeding or for patients who cannot use a tube in the nose and throat.

The type of formula used is based on the specific needs of the patient. There are formulas for patients who have special health conditions, such as diabetes, or other needs, such as religious or cultural diets.

Parenteral Nutrition

Parenteral nutrition carries nutrients directly into the bloodstream. Parenteral nutrition is used when the patient cannot take food by mouth or by enteral feeding. Parenteral feeding does not use the stomach or intestines to digest food. Nutrients are given to the patient directly into the blood through a catheter inserted into a vein. These nutrients include proteins, fats, vitamins, and minerals.

The catheter may be placed into a vein in the chest or in the arm. A central venous access catheter is placed beneath the skin and into a large vein in the upper chest. The catheter is put in place by a surgeon. This type of catheter is used for long-term parenteral feeding.

A peripheral venous catheter is placed into a vein in the arm and is put in place by trained medical staff. This type of catheter is usually used for short-term parenteral feeding for patients who do not have a central venous access catheter.

The patient is checked often for infection or bleeding at the place where the catheter enters the body.

MEDICINES TO TREAT LOSS OF APPETITE AND WEIGHT LOSS
Medicine and Nutrition Therapy to Treat Loss of Appetite and Weight Loss

It is important that cancer symptoms and side effects that affect eating and cause weight loss are treated early. Both nutrition therapy and medicine can help lessen the effects that cancer and its treatment have on weight loss.

Different Types of Medicine May Be Used to Treat Loss of Appetite and Weight Loss

Medicines that improve appetite and cause weight gain, such as prednisone and megestrol, may be used to treat loss of appetite and weight loss. Studies have shown that the effect of these medicines may not last long or there may be no effect. Treatment with a combination of medicines may work better than treatment with one medicine. Patients who are treated with a combination of medicines may have more side effects.

NUTRITION NEEDS AT THE END OF LIFE

For patients at the end of life, the goals of nutrition therapy are focused on relieving symptoms rather than getting enough nutrients.

Common symptoms that can occur at the end of life include the following:

- anorexia (loss of appetite)
- dry mouth
- swallowing problems
- nausea
- vomiting

Patients who have problems swallowing may find it easier to swallow thick liquids than thin liquids.

Patients often do not feel much hunger at all and may want very little food. Sips of water, ice chips, and mouth care can decrease thirst in the last few days of life. Good communication with the health-care team is important to understand the patient's changes in nutrition needs.

How Much Nutrition and Fluids Will Be Given at the End of Life?

Cancer patients and their caregivers have the right to make informed decisions. The patient's religious and cultural preferences may affect their decisions. The health-care team may work with the patient's religious and cultural leaders when making decisions. The health-care team and a registered dietitian can explain the benefits and risks of using nutrition support for patients at the end of life. In most cases, there are more harms than benefits if the patient is not expected to live longer than a month.

Possible benefits of nutrition support for patients expected to live longer than a month include the following:

- improved QOL
- less risk of death due to malnutrition
- fewer physical, mental, and psychological problems

The risks of nutrition support at the end of life include the following:

- sepsis (bacteria or their toxins in the blood or tissues) with the use of parenteral nutrition
- aspiration (the accidental breathing in of food or fluid into the lungs) with the use of enteral nutrition

- sores and breakdown of the skin where the enteral feeding tube is inserted
- diarrhea with the use of enteral and parenteral nutrition
- complications caused by fluid overload (a condition where there is too much fluid in the blood) with the use of enteral and parenteral nutrition

NUTRITION TRENDS IN CANCER
Special Diets to Improve Prognosis

Cancer patients may try special diets to make their treatment work better, prevent side effects from treatment, or treat the cancer itself. However, for most of these special diets, there is no evidence that shows they work.

VEGETARIAN OR VEGAN DIET

It is not known if following a vegetarian or vegan diet can help side effects from cancer treatment or the patient's prognosis. If the patient already follows a vegetarian or vegan diet, there is no evidence that shows they should switch to a different diet.

MACROBIOTIC DIET

A macrobiotic diet is a high-carbohydrate, low-fat, plant-based diet. No studies have shown that this diet will help cancer patients.

KETOGENIC DIET

A ketogenic diet limits carbohydrates and increases fat intake. The purpose of the diet is to decrease the amount of glucose (sugar) the tumor cells can use to grow and reproduce. It is a hard diet to follow because exact amounts of fats, carbohydrates, and proteins are needed. However, the diet is safe.

Several clinical trials are recruiting glioblastoma patients to study whether a ketogenic diet affects glioblastoma tumor activity. Patients with glioblastoma who want to start a ketogenic diet should talk to their doctor and work with a registered dietitian.

However, it is not yet known how the diet will affect the tumor or its symptoms.

Similarly, a study comparing the ketogenic diet to a high-fiber, low-fat diet in women with ovarian cancer or endometrial cancer found that the ketogenic diet was safe and acceptable. There is not enough evidence to know how the ketogenic diet will affect ovarian or endometrial tumors or their symptoms.

Benefits of Dietary Supplements

A dietary supplement is a product that is added to the diet. It is usually taken by mouth and usually has one or more dietary ingredients. Cancer patients may take dietary supplements to improve their symptoms or treat their cancer.

VITAMIN C

Vitamin C is a nutrient that the body needs in small amounts to function and stay healthy. It helps fight infection, heal wounds, and keep tissues healthy. Vitamin C is found in fruits and vegetables. It can also be taken as a dietary supplement.

PROBIOTICS

Probiotics are live microorganisms used as dietary supplements to help with digestion and normal bowel function. They may also help keep the gastrointestinal tract healthy.

Studies have shown that taking probiotics during radiation therapy and chemotherapy can help prevent diarrhea caused by those treatments. This is true for patients who receive radiation therapy to the abdomen. Cancer patients who are receiving radiation therapy to the abdomen or chemotherapy that is known to cause diarrhea may be helped by probiotics. Similarly, studies are looking at the potential benefits of taking probiotics for cancer patients who are receiving immunotherapy.

MELATONIN

Melatonin is a hormone made by the pineal gland (a tiny organ near the center of the brain). Melatonin helps control the body's sleep cycle. It can also be made in a laboratory and taken as a dietary supplement.

Several small studies have shown that taking a melatonin supplement with chemotherapy and/or radiation therapy for treatment of solid tumors may be helpful. It may help reduce the side effects of treatment. Melatonin does not appear to have side effects.

ORAL GLUTAMINE

Oral glutamine is an amino acid that is being studied for the treatment of diarrhea and mucositis (inflammation of the lining of the digestive system, often seen as mouth sores) caused by chemotherapy or radiation therapy. Oral glutamine may help prevent mucositis or make it less severe.

Cancer patients who are receiving radiation therapy to the abdomen may benefit from oral glutamine. Oral glutamine may reduce the severity of diarrhea. This can help the patients continue with their treatment plan.[1]

[1] "Nutrition in Cancer Care (PDQ®)—Patient Version," National Cancer Institute (NCI), December 9, 2022. Available online. URL: www.cancer.gov/about-cancer/treatment/side-effects/appetite-loss/nutrition-pdq. Accessed August 3, 2023.

Part 3 | Medical Decisions and End-of-Life Care

Chapter 11 | Advance Care Planning: Preferences for Care at the End of Life

PATIENTS WITH CHRONIC ILLNESS NEED ADVANCE PLANNING

People with terminal cancer generally follow an expected course, or "trajectory," of dying. Many maintain their activities of daily living (ADL) until about two months prior to death, after which most functional disability occurs.

In contrast, people with chronic diseases such as heart disease or chronic obstructive pulmonary disease (COPD) go through periods of slowly declining health marked by sudden severe episodes of illness requiring hospitalization, from which the patient recovers. This pattern may repeat itself over and over, with the patient's overall health steadily declining, until the patient dies. For these individuals, there is considerable uncertainty about when death is likely to occur.

Patients who suffer from chronic conditions, such as stroke, dementia, or the frailty of old age, go through a third trajectory of dying, marked by a steady decline in mental and physical ability that finally results in death. Patients are not often told that their chronic disease is terminal, and estimating a time of death for people suffering from chronic conditions is much more difficult than it is for those dying of cancer.

When patients are hospitalized for health crises resulting from their chronic incurable disease, medical treatment cannot cure the underlying illness, but it is still effective in resolving the immediate emergency and thus possibly extending the patient's life. At any one of these crises, the patient may be close to death, yet there is

119

often no clearly recognizable threshold between being very ill and actually dying. Patients may become too incapacitated to speak for themselves, and decisions about which treatments to provide or withhold are usually made jointly between the patient's physician and family or surrogate.

PATIENTS VALUE ADVANCE CARE PLANNING DISCUSSIONS

According to patients who are dying and their families who survive them, lack of communication with physicians and other health-care providers causes confusion about medical treatments, conditions and prognoses, and the choices that patients and their families need to make. One study by the Agency for Healthcare Research and Quality (AHRQ) indicated that about one-third of patients would discuss advance care planning if the physician brought up the subject and about one-fourth of patients had been under the impression that advance care planning was only for people who were very ill or very old. Only 5 percent of patients stated that they found discussions about advance care planning too difficult.

Many AHRQ-funded studies have shown that discussing advance care planning and directives with their doctor increased patient satisfaction among patients aged 65 and over. Patients who talked with their families or physicians about their preferences for end-of-life care:

- experienced less fear and anxiety
- felt they had more ability to influence and direct their medical care
- believed that their physicians had a better understanding of their wishes
- indicated a greater understanding and comfort level than they had before the discussion

Compared to surrogates of patients who did not have an advance directive, surrogates of patients with an advance directive who had discussed its content with the patient reported greater understanding, better confidence in their ability to predict the patient's preferences, and a stronger belief in the importance of having an advance directive.

Finally, patients who had advance planning discussions with their physicians continued to discuss and talk about these concerns with their families. Such discussions enabled patients and families to reconcile their differences in end-of-life care and could help the family and physician come to an agreement if they should need to make decisions for the patient.

OPPORTUNITIES EXIST FOR ADVANCE PLANNING DISCUSSIONS

Many AHRQ studies indicate that physicians can conduct advance care planning discussions with some patients during routine out-patient office visits. Hospitalization for a serious and progressive illness offers another opportunity. The Patient Self-Determination Act (PSDA) requires facilities such as hospitals that accept Medicare and Medicaid money to provide written information to all patients concerning their rights under state law to refuse or accept treatment and to complete advance directives.

Patients often send cues to their physicians that they are ready to discuss end-of-life care by talking about wanting to die or asking about hospice. Certain situations, such as approaching death or discussions about prognoses or treatment options that have poor outcomes, also lend themselves to advance care planning discussions. Predicting when patients are near death is difficult, but providers can ask themselves the question: "Are the patients sick enough today that it would not be surprising to find that they had died within the next year (or a few months or six months)?"

A STRUCTURED PROCESS FOR DISCUSSIONS IS HELPFUL

Researchers sponsored by the AHRQ have suggested the following five-part process that physicians can use to structure discussions on end-of-life care:

- **Initiate a guided discussion**. During this discussion, the physicians should share their medical knowledge of hypothetical scenarios and treatments applicable to a patient's particular situation and find out the patient's preferences for providing or withholding treatments under certain situations. The hypothetical scenarios should cover a range of possible prognoses and any disability that could result from treatment. By presenting various hypothetical scenarios and probable treatments and noting when the patient's preferences change from "treat" to "do not treat," the physician can begin to identify the patient's personal preferences and values.

The physician can also determine if the patient has an adequate understanding of the scenario, the treatment, and possible outcomes. One AHRQ-funded study indicated that elderly patients have enough knowledge about advance directives, cardiopulmonary resuscitation (CPR), and artificial nutrition/hydration on which to base decisions for treatment at the end of life, but they do not always understand their realistic chances for a positive outcome. Other research indicates that patients significantly overestimate their probability of survival after receiving CPR and have little or no understanding of mechanical ventilation. In one study, after patients were told their probability of survival, over half changed their treatment preference from wanting CPR to refusing CPR. Patients may not know of the risks associated with the use of mechanical ventilation that a physician is aware of, such as neurological impairment or cardiac arrest.

- **Introduce the subject of advance care planning and offer information**. Patients should be encouraged to complete both an advance directive and durable power of attorney. The patient should understand that when no advance directive or durable power of attorney exists, patients essentially leave treatment decisions to their physicians and family members. Physicians can provide this information themselves; refer the patient to other educational sources, including brochures or videos; and recommend that the patient talk with the clergy or a social worker to answer questions or address concerns.

- **Prepare and complete advance care planning documents**. Advance care planning documents should contain specific instructions. AHRQ studies indicate that the standard language contained in advance directives often is not specific enough to be effective in directing care. Many times, instructions do not state the cutoff point of the patient's illness that should be used to discontinue treatment and allow the person to die. Terms such as "no advanced life support" are too vague to offer guidance on specific treatments. If a patient does not want to be on a ventilator, the physician should ask the patient if this is true under all circumstances or only specific circumstances. One AHRQ-funded study found that because patient preferences were not clear in advance directives, life-sustaining treatment was discontinued only when it was clearly medically futile.

- **Review the patient's preferences on a regular basis and update documentation**. Patients should be reminded that advance directives can be revised at any time. Although AHRQ studies show that patients' preferences were stable over time when considering hypothetical situations, other research indicates that patients often changed their minds when confronted with the actual situation or as their health status changed. Some patients who stated that they would rather die than endure a certain condition did not choose death once that condition occurred. Other research shows that patients who had an advance directive maintained stable treatment preferences 86 percent of the time over a two-year period, while patients who did not have an advance directive changed their preferences 59 percent of the time. Both patients with and patients without a living will be more likely to change their preferences and desire increased treatment once they become hospitalized, suffer an accident, become depressed, or lose functional ability or social activity. Another study linked changes in depression to changes in preferences for CPR. Increased depression was associated with patients' changing their initial preference for CPR to a refusal of CPR, while less depression was associated with patients' changing their preference from refusal of CPR to acceptance of CPR. It is difficult for people to fully imagine what a prospective health state might be like. Once they experience that health state, they may find it more or less tolerable than they imagined. During reviews of advance directives, physicians should note which preferences stay the same and which change. Preferences that change indicate that the physician needs to investigate the basis for the change.

- **Apply the patient's desires to actual circumstances**. Conflicts sometimes arise during discussions about end-of-life decision-making. AHRQ-sponsored research indicates that if patients desired nonbeneficial treatments or refused beneficial treatments, most physicians stated that they would negotiate with them, trying to educate and convince them to either forgo a nonbeneficial treatment or accept a beneficial treatment. If the treatment was not harmful, expensive, or complicated, about one-third of physicians would allow the patient to receive a nonbeneficial treatment. Physicians stated that they would also enlist the family's help or seek a second opinion from another physician. Many patients do not lose their decision-making capacity at the end of life. Physicians and family members can continue discussing treatment preferences with these patients as their condition changes. However, physicians and families may encounter the difficulty of knowing when an advance directive should become applicable to patients who are extremely sick and have lost their decision-making capacity but are not necessarily dying. There is no easy answer to this dilemma. One AHRQ study found that advance directives were invoked only once patients had crossed a threshold to be "absolutely, hopelessly ill." The patients' physicians and surrogates determined that boundary on an individual basis. AHRQ studies have shown that patients' treatment was generally consistent with their preferences if those preferences were clearly stated in an advance directive and the physician was aware that they had an advance directive.

Even if patients require a decision for a situation that was not anticipated and addressed in their advance directive, physicians and surrogates can still make an educated determination based on the knowledge they have about the patients' values, goals, and thresholds for treatment. AHRQ research indicates that patients choose a treatment based on the quality of the prospective health state, the invasiveness and length of treatment, and possible outcomes.

PATIENTS HAVE PREFERENCE PATTERNS FOR HYPOTHETICAL SITUATIONS

Many AHRQ-funded studies indicate that patients are more likely to accept treatment for conditions they consider better than death and to refuse treatment for conditions they consider worse than death. Results from the study conducted on health states considered worse than death. Patients were also more likely to accept treatments that were less invasive, such as CPR, than invasive treatments, such as mechanical ventilation. Patients were more likely to accept short-term or simple treatments, such as antibiotics, than long-term invasive treatments, such as permanent tube-feeding.

PATIENT PREFERENCE PATTERNS CAN PREDICT OTHER CHOICES

Acceptance or refusal of invasive and noninvasive treatments under certain circumstances can predict what other choices the patient would make under the same or different circumstances. According to AHRQ research, patients' refusal of noninvasive treatments was predictive of their refusal of invasive treatments, and accepting invasive treatments predicted their acceptance of noninvasive treatments. Refusal of noninvasive treatments, such as antibiotics, strongly predicted that invasive treatments, such as major surgery, would also be refused. Decisions with the strongest predictive ability were refusing antibiotics or simple tests and accepting major surgery or dialysis.

An AHRQ research also reveals that patients were more likely to refuse treatment under hypothetical conditions as their prognosis became worse. For example, more adults would refuse both invasive and noninvasive treatments for a scenario of dementia with a terminal illness than for dementia only. Adults were also more likely to refuse treatment for a scenario of a persistent vegetative state than for a coma with a chance of recovery. More patients preferred treatment if there was even a slight chance of recovery from a coma or a stroke. Fewer patients would want complicated and invasive treatments if they had a terminal illness. Finally, patients were more likely to want treatment if they would remain cognitively intact rather than impaired.[1]

---

[1] Agency for Healthcare Research and Quality (AHRQ), "Advance Care Planning, Preferences for Care at the End of Life," U.S. Department of Health and Human Services (HHS), March 2003. Available online. URL: https://archive. ahrq.gov/research/findings/factsheets/aging/endliferia/endria.html. Accessed August 14, 2023.

Chapter 12 | End-of-Life Care for Individuals with Dementia

People often live for years with dementia. While it can be difficult to think of these diseases as terminal, they do eventually lead to death. Caregivers often experience special challenges surrounding the end of life of someone with dementia in part because the disease progression is so unpredictable. The following are some considerations for end-of-life care for people with dementia.

MAKING MEDICAL DECISIONS FOR PEOPLE WITH DEMENTIA

Even with dementia, a person's body may continue to be physically healthy. However, dementia causes a gradual loss of thinking, remembering, and reasoning abilities, which means that people with dementia at the end of life may no longer be able to make or communicate choices about their health care. If there are no advance care planning documents in place and the family does not know the person's wishes, caregivers may need to make difficult decisions on behalf of their loved one about care and treatment approaches.

When making health-care decisions for someone with dementia, it is important to consider the person's quality of life (QOL). For example, medications are available that may delay or keep symptoms from getting worse for a limited time. Medications may also help control some behavioral symptoms in people with mild-to-moderate Alzheimer or related dementia. However, some caregivers might not want drugs prescribed for people in the later stages of these diseases if the side effects outweigh the benefits.

It is important to consider the goals of care and weigh the benefits, risks, and side effects of any treatment. You may need to make a treatment decision based on the person's comfort rather than trying to extend their life or maintain their abilities for longer.

Questions to Ask about End-of-Life Care for a Person with Dementia

As a caregiver, you will want to understand how the available medical options presented by the health-care team fit with the needs of both the family and the person with dementia. You might ask the health-care team the following questions:

- Who can help me with end-of-life care for my loved one living with dementia?
- How will your suggested approaches affect their quality of life (QOL)?
- What are my options if I can no longer manage the care of my loved one at home?
- How can I best decide when a visit to the doctor or hospital is necessary?
- Should I consider hospice at home, and if so, does the hospice team have experience working with people living with dementia?

BEING THERE FOR A PERSON WITH DEMENTIA AT THE END OF LIFE

As dementia progresses, caregivers may find it hard to provide emotional or spiritual comfort to a person who has severe memory loss. However, even in the advanced stages of dementia, a person may benefit from such connections.

Sensory connections—targeting someone's senses, including hearing, touch, or sight—may also bring comfort. Being touched or massaged can be soothing. Listening to music, white noise, or sounds from nature seems to relax some people and lessen agitation. Just being present can be calming to the person.

Palliative or hospice care teams may be helpful in suggesting ways for people with dementia and their families to connect at the end of life. They may also be able to help identify when someone with dementia is in the last days or weeks of life.

Signs of the final stages of dementia include some of the following:

- being unable to move around on one's own
- being unable to speak or make oneself understood
- having eating problems such as difficulty swallowing

Though palliative and hospice care experts have unique experiences with what happens at the end of life and may be able to give a sense of timing, it is hard to predict exactly how much time a person has left.

SUPPORTING DEMENTIA CAREGIVERS AT THE END OF LIFE

Caring for people with Alzheimer or other dementia at the end of life can be demanding and stressful for the family caregiver. Depression and fatigue are common problems for caregivers because many feel they are always on call. Family caregivers may have to cut back on work hours or leave work altogether because of their caregiving responsibilities.

It is not uncommon for those who take care of a person with advanced dementia to feel a sense of relief when death happens. It is important to realize such feelings are normal. Hospice care experts can provide support to family caregivers near the end of life as well as help with their grief.

If you are a caregiver, ask for help when you need it and learn about respite care at www.nia.nih.gov/health/what-respite-care.

Importance of Advance Care Planning for People with Dementia and Their Caregivers

Someone newly diagnosed with dementia might not be able to imagine the later stages of the disease. But, when a person is first diagnosed with Alzheimer or another dementia, it is important to make plans for the end of life before the person with the disease can no longer complete advance directives and other important legal documents. End-of-life care decisions are more complicated for caregivers if the dying person has not expressed the kind of care they would prefer.[1]

[1] National Institute on Aging (NIA), "End-of-Life Care for People with Dementia," National Institutes of Health (NIH), January 31, 2022. Available online. URL: www.nia.nih.gov/health/end-life-care-people-dementia. Accessed July 27, 2023.

Chapter 13 | End-of-Life Care for Young Cancer Patients

It is extremely difficult for anyone, especially young people in their 20s and 30s, to be told that their treatment(s) have not worked. If the cancer you have continues to progress despite treatment, it may be called "end-stage cancer." As you process this information and make choices about the end-of-life care you would like to receive, know that your voice and views matter. In fact, they are what is most important.

TALKING ABOUT END-OF-LIFE ISSUES

You may have many questions about how you may feel in the coming weeks and months. You might want to know about how long people with your type of end-stage cancer often live. Learning about choices for physical and emotional care at the end of life and sharing your personal preferences will help you receive the care that is best for you. As a young person, you may choose to look ahead and make the most of the time that remains, in comparison to older adults who often look back on their lives.

Until now, you and your health-care team have been focused on stopping the spread of cancer. Therefore, it may be challenging to shift gears and talk about end-of-life care. Your health-care team may look to you for cues about how much medical information you want, what emotional support you need, and what is most important to you in the time ahead. Keep in mind that you should be at the center of all decision-making.

Having conversations about issues surrounding life and death does not mean that you or your health-care team are giving up. It takes courage to reflect on, talk about, and accept that it is no longer possible to keep the cancer from advancing. Your health-care team will provide you with care and medicines that focus on the best quality of life (QOL) possible. Hope will be redirected toward things that are most important to you, in the coming weeks and months.

THINKING ABOUT PRIORITIES: YOUNG PEOPLE WITH END-STAGE CANCER

As you think about things you want to do and the people you want to be with, here are some questions that may be helpful to reflect on and answer.

Who and What Are Most Important to You?

If you are like many young people, it is hard to process what is happening, much less talk about it. You may find yourself busy providing support to parents, spouses or partners, and young children. You may try to keep difficult thoughts and feelings to yourself—although sharing your feelings with the people you are closest to will help you feel less isolated and fearful. Counseling and bereavement support services are available at most hospitals for young people and their families. While you may want to protect people around you from feeling sad, it is both okay and important to let people know how you are feeling.

Sharing and Making Memories

Spending meaningful time with friends and family may be especially important. Tell your health-care team about the things you would like to do. Reach out to people you want to see and make plans as you are interested and able. You may choose to write notes for friends and family for them to read now or later. Some young people enjoy creating a memory box or book that includes objects, poems, quotes, and other things that have special meaning. Memory boxes and books can also bring comfort to your family and friends.

MAKING END-OF-LIFE CARE DECISIONS

Talking about your preferences for end-of-life care will help you receive the care and treatment that feels right and best to you.

Commonly Asked Questions from Young People with Cancer

Some people on your health-care team are easier to talk with than others. Close personal bonds may make it easier to open up and have honest conversations.

As you think about questions to ask your health-care team, consider adding the following to your list:
- Are there treatments that are not curative but might slow my cancer?
- What are my choices to control pain and other symptoms?
- What are my choices for where to receive end-of-life care? What services are provided if I choose to receive end-of-life care at home?
- Do you have suggestions to help me start conversations with friends? Will you help me and be there with me when I talk with my family?
- What resources could help me learn more about end-of-life care choices?

Young people who make decisions earlier, rather than later, say that it frees them to focus on living and lowers their levels of stress and anxiety.

Planning Guides for Young People

Voicing My Choices™ (https://paliativo.org.br/wp-content/uploads/download-manager-files/voicingmychoices.pdf) is a guide designed to help adolescents and young adults make end-of-life choices that might otherwise be delayed or avoided. Resources such as this one may be used at your hospital to help you, your health-care team, and your family talk about how you want to be comforted and supported—both emotionally and physically—medical treatment(s) you do and do not want to receive, the place you would like to be when you are at the end of your life, who you want to make decisions for you if you are not able to make them yourself, and how you wish to be remembered. While not everyone wants to participate in planning their memorial service, documents such as Voicing My Choices allow you to voice your preferences—such as specific readings, music, photos, attendees, and food.

Learning More about End-of-Life Care

The Choices for Care When Treatment May Not Be an Option web page (www.cancer.gov/about-cancer/advanced-cancer/care-choices) can help you and your family navigate through key questions you may have, including the following:

- **Where is end-of-life care given?** Hospice care is end-of-life care that is given at your home, in the hospital, or at a respite or hospice center. Young people often choose to receive their end-of-life care at home, where they can be in a familiar environment, close to family and friends around the clock.
- **What kind of care and support are given?** Palliative care (also called "comfort care," "supportive care," or "symptom management") is an approach that addresses you as a whole person, not just your disease.
- **How do I communicate what I would like?** An advance directive is a legal document in which you select the type of medical care you would like to receive if you are no longer able to make medical decisions for yourself. Developing an advance directive is a process, not a one-time conversation, especially for young people.

Leaving Memories and a Legacy

Some young people choose to think about ways they will be remembered. You may want to plant a tree or flowers, make a collage with friends, create art that can be saved or shared in a public space, or set up a scholarship or small legacy fund in your name.[1]

---

[1] "Young People Facing End-of-Life Care Decisions," National Cancer Institute (NCI), September 23, 2020. Available online. URL: www.cancer.gov/types/aya/end-of-life. Accessed July 31, 2023.

Chapter 14 | Cancer and End-of-Life Concerns

WHAT DOES END-OF-LIFE CARE MEAN FOR PEOPLE WHO HAVE CANCER?

When a person's health-care team determines that the cancer can no longer be controlled, medical testing and cancer treatment often stop. However, people's care continues with an emphasis on improving their quality of life (QOL) and that of their loved ones and making them comfortable for the following weeks or months.

Medicines and treatments people receive at the end of life can control pain and other symptoms, such as constipation, nausea, and shortness of breath. Some people remain at home while receiving these treatments, whereas others enter a hospital or other facility. Either way, services are available to help patients and their families with the medical, psychological, social, and spiritual issues around dying. Hospice programs are the most comprehensive and coordinated providers of these services.

The period at the end of life is different for each person. The signs and symptoms people have may vary as their illness continues, and each person has unique needs for information and support. Questions and concerns that family members have about end of life should be discussed with each other, as well as with the health-care team, as they arise.

Communication about end-of-life care and decision-making during the final months of a person's life is very important. Research has shown that if people who have advanced cancer discuss their options for care with a doctor early on, those people's level of stress decreases and their ability to cope with illness increases. Studies also show that patients prefer an open and honest conversation with their doctor about choices for end-of-life care early in the course of their disease and are more satisfied when they have this talk.

Experts strongly encourage patients to complete advance directives, which are documents stating a person's wishes for care. They also designate who the patients choose as the decision-maker for their care when they are unable to decide. It is important for people with cancer to have these decisions made before they become too sick to make them. However, if people do become too sick before they have completed an advance directive, it is helpful for family caregivers to know what type of care their loved one would want to receive.[1]

QUALITY CARE AT THE END OF LIFE
Decide What Quality Care at the End of Life Means for You

Your care continues even after all treatments have stopped. End-of-life care is more than what happens moments before dying. Care is needed in the days, weeks, and sometimes even months before death. During this time, many patients feel it is important to:

- have their pain and symptoms controlled
- avoid the long process of dying
- feel a sense of control over what is happening to them
- cause less emotional and financial burden on the family
- become closer to loved ones

Your doctors and family need to know the kind of end-of-life care you want.

Make End-of-Life Care Decisions Early

You may be able to think about your options more clearly if you talk about them before the decisions need to be made. It is a good idea to let your doctors, family, and caregivers know your wishes before there is an emergency.

---

[1] "End-of-Life Care for People Who Have Cancer," National Cancer Institute (NCI), June 28, 2021. Available online. URL: www.cancer.gov/about-cancer/advanced-cancer/care-choices/care-fact-sheet. Accessed August 3, 2023.

END-OF-LIFE CARE DECISIONS TO BE MADE

Care decisions for the last stages of cancer can be about treatments and procedures, pain control, place of care, and spiritual issues.

Chemotherapy

Some patients choose to begin new chemotherapy treatment in the end stages of cancer. Others wish to let the disease take its course when a cure is not expected. In the end stages of cancer, chemotherapy usually does not help you live longer, and it may lower the quality of the time that remains. Each person and each cancer are different. Talking with your doctor about the effects of treatment and your QOL can help you make a decision. You can ask if the treatment will make you comfortable or if it will help you live longer.

Pain and Symptom Control

Controlling pain and other symptoms can help you have a better QOL in the end stages of cancer. Pain and symptom control can be part of your care in any place of care, such as the hospital, home, and hospice.

Cardiopulmonary Resuscitation

It is important to decide if you want to have cardiopulmonary resuscitation (CPR). CPR is a procedure used to try to restart the heart and breathing when it stops. In advanced cancer, the heart, lungs, and other organs begin to fail, and it is harder to restart them with CPR. Your doctor can help you understand how CPR works and talk with you about whether CPR is likely to work for you.

People who are near the end of life may choose not to have CPR done. Your decision about having CPR is personal. Your own spiritual or religious views about death and dying may help you decide. If you decide you do not want CPR, you can ask your doctor to write a do-not-resuscitate (DNR) order. This tells other health-care professionals not to perform CPR if your heart or breathing stops. You can remove the DNR order at any time.

Talk with your doctors and other caregivers about CPR as early as possible (e.g., when being admitted to the hospital) in case you are not able to make the decision later. If you do choose to have your doctor write a DNR, it is important to tell all your family members and caregivers about it.

In the United States, if there is no DNR order, you will be given CPR to keep you alive.

Ventilator Use

A ventilator is a machine used to help you breathe and keep you alive after normal breathing stops. It does not treat a disease or condition. It is used only for life support. You can tell doctors whether you would want to be put on a ventilator if your lungs stop working or if you cannot breathe on your own after CPR. If your goal of care is to live longer, you may choose to have a ventilator used. Or you may choose to have a ventilator for only a certain length of time. It is important to tell your family and health-care providers what you want before you have trouble breathing.

Religious and Spiritual Support

Your religious or spiritual beliefs may help you with end-of-life decisions. You can also talk with a member of your church, a social worker, or even other people who have cancer.

TALKING WITH YOUR DOCTOR ABOUT END-OF-LIFE CARE
How to Start the Conversation

Some doctors do not ask patients about end-of-life issues. If you want to make choices about these issues, talk with your doctors so that your wishes can be carried out. Open communication can help you and your doctors make decisions together and create a plan of care (POC) that meets your goals and wishes. If your doctor is not comfortable talking about end-of-life plans, you can talk to other specialists for help.

End-of-Life Concerns: Consult with Your Doctor
UNDERSTAND YOUR PROGNOSIS

Having a good understanding of your prognosis is important when making decisions about your care and treatment during advanced cancer. You will probably want to know how long you have to live. That is a hard question for doctors to answer. It can be different for each person and depends on the type of cancer, where it has spread, and whether you have other illnesses. Treatments can work differently for each person. Your doctor can talk about the treatment options with you and your family and explain the effects they may have on your cancer and your QOL. Knowing the benefits and risks of available treatments can help you decide on your goals of care for the last stages of the cancer.

DECIDE ON YOUR CARE GOALS
Your care goals for advanced cancer depend in part on whether QOL or length of life is more important to you. Your goals of care may change as your condition changes or if new treatments become available. Tell your doctor what your goals of care are even if you are not asked. It is important that you and your doctor are working toward the same goals.

TAKE PART IN MAKING DECISIONS
Do you want to take part in making the decisions about your care? Or would you rather have your family and your doctors make those decisions? This is a personal choice, and your family and doctors need to know what you want.

Early Communication and Being Prepared for End-of-Life Issues
Many patients who start talking with their doctors early about end-of-life issues report feeling better prepared. Better communication with your doctors may make it easier to deal with concerns about being older, living alone, relieving symptoms, spiritual well-being, and how your family will cope in the future.

Ways to Improve Communication with Your Doctors
Tell your doctor how you and your family wish to receive information and the type of information you want. Also, ask how you can get information at times when you cannot meet face-to-face.

Remembering what your doctor said and even remembering what you want to ask can be hard to do. Some of the following may help communication and help you remember what was said:

- Have a family member go with you when you meet your doctor.
- Make a list of the questions you want to ask the doctor during your visit.
- Get the information in writing.
- Record the discussion with tape recorders, smartphones, or on video.
- Ask if your doctor or clinic offers any of the following:
  - a cancer consultation preparation package, which includes aids such as a question idea sheet, booklets on decision-making and patient rights, and information about the clinic
  - a talk with a psychologist about advance planning and end-of-life issues
  - an end-of-life preference interview, which includes a list of questions that can help you explain your wishes about the end of life

SUPPORTIVE CARE

Supportive care is given to prevent or treat, as early as possible, the symptoms of the cancer, side effects caused by treatments, and psychological, social, and spiritual problems related to the cancer or its treatment. During active treatment to cure the cancer, supportive care helps you stay healthy and comfortable enough to continue receiving the cancer treatments. In the last stages of cancer, when a cure is no longer the goal, supportive care is used for side effects that continue.

PALLIATIVE CARE

Palliative care is specialized medical care for people with serious or life-threatening illnesses. The focus of palliative care is relief from pain and other symptoms both during active treatment and when treatment has been stopped. Palliative care is offered in some hospitals, outpatient centers, and the home.

Palliative care helps improve your QOL by preventing and relieving suffering. When you are more comfortable, your family's QOL may also be better. Palliative care includes treating physical symptoms such as pain and helping you and your family with emotional, social, and spiritual concerns. When palliative treatment is given at the end of life, the focus is on relieving symptoms and distress caused by the process of dying and making sure your goals of care are followed.

HOSPICE

When treatment is no longer helping, you may choose hospice. Hospice is a program that gives care to people who are near the end of life and have stopped treatment to cure or control their cancer. Hospice care focuses on QOL rather than length of life. The hospice team offers physical, emotional, and spiritual support for patients who are expected to live no longer than six months. The goal of hospice is to help patients live each day to the fullest by making them comfortable and relieving their symptoms. This may include supportive and palliative care to control pain and other symptoms, so you can be as alert and comfortable as possible. Services to help with the emotional, social, and spiritual needs of you and your family are also an important part of hospice care.

Hospice programs are designed to keep the patient at home with family and friends, but hospice care may also be given in hospice centers and in some hospitals and nursing homes. The hospice team includes doctors, nurses, spiritual advisors, social workers, nutritionists, and volunteers. Team members are specially trained on issues that occur at the end of life. The hospice program continues to give help, including grief counseling, to the family after their loved one dies. Ask your doctor for information if you wish to receive hospice care.

ADVANCE PLANNING
Making Decisions about End-of-Life Care and Reducing Stress

There may come a time when you cannot tell the health-care team what you want. When that happens, would you prefer to have your doctor and family make decisions? Or would you rather make decisions early, so your wishes will be known and can be followed when the time comes? If not planned far ahead of time, the end-of-life decisions must be made by someone other than you.

Planning ahead for end-of-life care helps with the following:

- Make sure your doctors and family know what your wishes are.
- Allow you to refuse the use of treatments.
- Decrease the emotional stress on your family, who would have to make decisions if you are not able to.
- Reduce the cost of care if you choose not to receive life-saving procedures.
- Ease your mind to have these decisions already made.

You can make your wishes known with an advance directive.

Advance Directive

Advance directive is the general term for different types of documents that state what your wishes are for certain medical treatments when you can no longer tell those wishes to your caregivers. In addition to decisions about relieving symptoms at the end of life, it is also helpful to decide if and when you want certain treatments to stop. Advance directives make sure your wishes about treatments and life-saving procedures to keep you alive are known ahead of time. Without knowing your wishes, doctors will do everything medically possible to keep you alive, such as CPR and the use of a ventilator (breathing machine).

Each state has its own laws for advance directives. Make sure your advance directives follow the laws of the state where you live and are being treated. State-specific advance directives can be downloaded from the CaringInfo website (www.caringinfo.org/planning/advance-directives/by-state) of the National Hospice and Palliative Care Organization.

The following are types of documents that communicate your wishes in advance:

- **Living will.** A legal document that states whether you want certain life-saving medical treatments to be used or not used under certain circumstances. Some of the treatments covered by a living will include CPR, the use of a ventilator (breathing machine), and tube-feeding.

- **Health care proxy (HCP)**. A document in which you choose a person (called a "proxy") to make medical decisions if you become unable to do so. It is important that your proxy knows your values and wishes so that he or she can make the decisions you would make if you are able. You do not have to state specific decisions about individual treatments in the document, just state that the proxy will make medical decisions for you. HCP is also known as "durable power of attorney for health care" (DPOAHC) or "medical power of attorney" (MPOA).

- **DNR order**. A document that tells medical staff in the hospital not to do CPR if your heart or breathing stops. A DNR order is a decision only about CPR. It does not affect other treatments that may be used to keep you alive, such as medicine or food.

- **Out-of-hospital DNR order**. A document that tells emergency medical workers outside a hospital that you do not wish to have CPR or other types of resuscitation. Each state has its own rules for a legal out-of-hospital DNR order, but it is usually signed by the patient, a witness, and the doctor. It is best to have several copies, so one can quickly be given to emergency medical workers when needed.

- **Do-not-intubate (DNI) order**. A document that tells medical staff in a hospital or nursing facility that you do not wish to have a breathing tube inserted and to be put on a ventilator (breathing machine).

- **Physician orders for life-sustaining treatment (POLST)**. A form that states what kind of medical treatment you want toward the end of your life. It is signed by you and your doctor.

- **Medical orders for life-sustaining treatment (MOLST)**. A form that states the care you would like to receive if you are not able to communicate. This care includes CPR, intubation (breathing tubes), and other life-saving procedures. Under current law, the information in an MOLST form must be followed both in the home and hospital by all medical staff, including emergency medical workers.

Caregivers Need to Have Copies of Your Advance Directives

Give copies of your advance directives to your doctors, caregivers, and family members. Advance directives need to move with you. If your doctors or your place of care changes, copies of your advance directives need to be given to your new caregivers. This will make sure that your wishes are known through all cancer stages and places of care. You can change or cancel an advance directive at any time.

TRANSITION TO END-OF-LIFE CARE

The word transition can mean a passage from one place to another. The transition or change from looking toward recovery to receiving end-of-life care is not an easy one, and there are important decisions to be made. If you become too sick before you have made your wishes known, others will make care and treatment decisions for you without knowing what you would have wanted. It may be less stressful for everyone if you, your family, and your health-care providers have planned ahead for this time.

The goal of end-of-life care is to prevent suffering and relieve symptoms. The right time to transition to end-of-life care is when this supports your changing condition and changing goals of care.

There are certain times when you may think about stopping treatment and transitioning to comfort care. These include the following:

- finding out that the cancer is not responding to treatment and that more treatment is not likely to help
- having poor QOL due to the side effects or complications of treatment
- being unable to carry out daily activities when the disease progresses

Cancer and End-of-Life Concerns

Together with your doctor, you and your family members can share an understanding of treatment choices and when the transition to end-of-life care is the best choice. When you make the decisions and plans, doctors and family members can be sure they are doing what you want.[2]

---

[2] "Planning the Transition to End-of-Life Care in Advanced Cancer (PDQ®)—Patient Version," National Cancer Institute (NCI), July 22, 2020. Available online. URL: www.cancer.gov/about-cancer/advanced-cancer/planning/end-of-life-pdq. Accessed August 3, 2023.

Chapter 15 | **HIV/AIDS and End-of-Life Concerns**

Palliative care is not curative care but is supportive, symptom-oriented care. It may be needed at any point in the course of disease progression to relieve patients' suffering and promote quality of life (QOL). Palliative care is important for patients with any medical condition, even if they are not actively in hospice. It may be used in conjunction with disease-specific care or as the sole approach to care. Palliative care includes the following:

- management of symptoms (e.g., fatigue and pain)
- treatment of adverse effects (e.g., nausea and vomiting)
- psychosocial support (e.g., depression and advance care planning)
- end-of-life care

The U.S. Health Resources and Services Administration (HRSA) Human Immunodeficiency Virus/Acquired Immunodeficiency Syndrome (HIV/AIDS) Bureau (HAB) Working Group on Palliative Care in HIV has provided the following working definition of palliative care:

Palliative care is patient- and family-centered care. It optimizes QOL by active anticipation, prevention, and treatment of suffering. It emphasizes the use of an inter-disciplinary team approach throughout the continuum of illness, placing critical importance on the building of respectful and trusting relationships. Palliative care addresses physical, intellectual, emotional, social, and spiritual needs. It facilitates patient autonomy, access to information, and choice.

Palliative care for patients with HIV infection comprises a continuum of treatment consisting of therapy directed at AIDS-related illnesses (e.g., infection or malignancy) and treatments focused on providing comfort and symptom control throughout the life span. This care may involve multidimensional and multi-disciplinary services, including HIV medicine, nursing, pharmacy, social work, complementary or alternative medicine (CAM), and physical therapy.

PALLIATIVE CARE IN THE ERA OF ANTIRETROVIRAL THERAPY

With advances in HIV-specific therapy and care, HIV infection is no longer a rapidly fatal illness. Instead, patients who are able to tolerate antiretroviral therapy (ART) usually experience a manageable chronic illness.

The death rate from AIDS, however, continues to be significant: approximately 15,000 deaths per year in the United States. In many parts of the world, patients are still not able to obtain specific treatments for HIV or opportunistic illnesses, and supportive or palliative care may be the primary mode of care available to patients with advanced AIDS. Regardless of access to disease-specific treatment, people living with HIV continue to experience symptoms from HIV disease and its comorbid conditions, and those taking ART may experience adverse effects. Integrating palliative care and disease-specific care is important for treating patients with HIV in order to promote QOL and relieve suffering.

Subjective

The patient with advanced HIV disease complains of one or more of the following:

- agitation
- anorexia
- chronic pain
- constipation
- cough

- decubitus ulcers or pressure sores
- delirium
- dementia
- depression
- diarrhea
- dry mouth
- dry skin
- dyspnea
- fatigue
- fever
- hiccups
- increased secretions ("death-rattle")
- nausea
- pruritus
- sleep disturbance
- sweats
- vomiting
- weakness
- weight loss

Objective
Conduct a complete symptom-directed physical examination.

Assessment and Plan Treatment
Common symptoms of people with late-stage HIV infection and their possible causes are listed in Table 15.1. Also, disease-specific treatments and palliative interventions are included. Depending on the situation, either or both of these types of treatments may be appropriate. Consider the patient's disease stage and symptom burden, the risks and benefits of therapies, and the patient's wishes. When assessing each of the patient's symptoms, include the psychiatric review of symptoms (depression, anxiety, and psychosis) and consider the following aspects of each symptom:
- onset, progression, frequency, and severity
- degree of distress and impact on function
- aggravating and alleviating factors

Table 15.1. Common Symptoms in Patients with AIDS and Possible Disease-Specific and Palliative Interventions

Symptom	Possible Causes	Disease-Specific or Curative Treatment	Palliative Treatment
Constitutional			
Fatigue and weakness	• AIDS • Opportunistic infection (OI) • Anemia • Hypoandrogenism	• ART • Treating specific infections • Erythropoietin, transfusion • Testosterone/androgens in men with concomitant hypogonadism (For women, androgens are investigational and not approved by the U.S. Food and Drug Administration (FDA) for this use.)	• Psychostimulants (give in the morning; also useful as a treatment for depression and sedation owing to opioids; avoid in patients with anxiety and agitation (e.g., methylphenidate, dextroamphetamine, and modafinil; pemoline is not first-line because of hepatotoxicity risk)) • Corticosteroids (prednisone and dexamethasone)
Weight loss/ anorexia	• HIV • Malignancy	• ART • Specific treatment of malignancy • Nutritional support	• Testosterone/androgens in men with hypogonadism • Oxandrolone for two- to four-week courses (An anabolic steroid that may be a useful adjunct can help increase lean body mass but also has virilizing effects.) • Megestrol acetate that can improve appetite and fatigue but has not been shown to improve nutritional status (Possible adverse effects include deep vein thrombosis (DVT), glucose intolerance, and hypoandrogenism in men.)

Table 15.1. Continued

Symptom	Possible Causes	Disease-Specific or Curative Treatment	Palliative Treatment
Weight loss/ anorexia			• Dronabinol, a cannabinol derivative, that helps increase appetite but over the long term (greater than or equal to 12 months) does not significantly increase weight • Recombinant human growth hormone that can improve lean body mass but is associated with significant side effects (headache, edema, and myalgias) and is expensive (Consider for patients with severe wasting if no other therapies are effective.) • Corticosteroids that can help increase appetite in the short term but not increase weight (The duration of effect is short-lived.)
Fevers and sweats	• Disseminated *Mycobacterium avium* complex and other infections (opportunistic or other) • Lymphoma and other malignancies • Immune reconstitution inflammatory syndrome (IRIS) • Medication reaction	• Specific treatment of OI or malignancy • ART • Discontinue causative medication (if drug reaction)	• Acetaminophen • NSAIDs (ibuprofen, naproxen, and indomethacin) • Anticholinergics that can be useful for sweats (hyoscyamine and glycopyrrolate) • H₂ antagonists that can be useful for sweats (ranitidine and famotidine; dose at least 12 hours apart from atazanavir or rilpivirine; note that cimetidine should be avoided in patients taking fosamprenavir or delavirdine because of drug interactions)

Table 15.1. Continued

Symptom	Possible Causes	Disease-Specific or Curative Treatment	Palliative Treatment
Pain			
Nociceptive, somatic, and visceral	• OIs • HIV-related malignancies, nonspecific	• Specific treatment of disease entities	• NSAIDs and opioids (Refer to the World Health Organization (WHO) analgesic ladder.) • Corticosteroids that can be useful for treating inflammatory-mediated pain, often as an adjunct to opioids (may worsen some conditions) • Benzodiazepines or muscle relaxants for muscle spasms (clonazepam, diazepam, and baclofen) • Nonpharmacologic therapies (e.g., massage and physical therapy)

Neuropathic	• HIV-related peripheral neuropathy
	• Cytomegalovirus (CMV)
	• Varicella-zoster virus (VZV)
	• Medications (e.g., stavudine, isoniazid, and vincristine)
		• ART
		• Discontinue offending medication
		• Change antiretroviral (ARV) or other regimen
			• NSAIDs and opioids (Refer to the WHO analgesic ladder.)
			• Neuropathic pain medications:
			  • Tricyclics (nortriptyline and imipramine)
			  • Anticonvulsants (gabapentin, pregabalin, and lamotrigine)
			  • Muscle relaxants (e.g., baclofen)
			  • Benzodiazepines that can be useful adjuncts (clonazepam and diazepam)
			• Corticosteroids that can be useful for treating inflammatory-mediated pain, often as an adjunct to opioids (that may worsen some conditions) acupuncture

Table 15.1. Continued

Symptom	Possible Causes	Disease-Specific or Curative Treatment	Palliative Treatment
Gastrointestinal			
Nausea and vomiting	• ARV medications • Esophageal candidiasis • CMV esophagitis	• Specific treatment of disease entities • Change ARV regimen	• Dopamine antagonists (prochlorperazine and haloperidol) • Prokinetic agents (metoclopramide) • Serotonin antagonists (granisetron, ondansetron, and dolasetron) • Antihistamines (diphenhydramine, promethazine, and meclizine) • Anticholinergics (hyoscyamine and scopolamine) • Somatostatin analogs in patients with bowel obstruction to reduce gut motility (can be used with anticholinergics (octreotide)) • Benzodiazepines (lorazepam) • Marijuana, dronabinol that can help increase appetite

Table 15.1. Continued

Symptom	Possible Causes	Disease-Specific or Curative Treatment	Palliative Treatment
Gastrointestinal			
Diarrhea	• *M. avium* complex • Cryptosporidiosis • CMV colitis • Microsporidiosis • Other intestinal infections • Malabsorption • Medications (e.g., protease inhibitors (PIs))	• Specific treatment of disease entities • Discontinue offending medication	• Bismuth and methylcellulose • Psyllium • Kaolin • Diphenoxylate with atropine • Loperamide • Calcium carbonate • Ferrous sulfate • Tincture of opium for severe chronic diarrhea unresponsive to other therapies • Crofelemer for ARV-related diarrhea • Octreotide for profuse, refractory watery diarrhea (expensive and needs subcutaneous administration)

Constipation	• Dehydration
	• Malignancy
	• Anticholinergic medications
	• Opioids
	• Reduced activity
		• Hydration
		• Radiation and chemotherapy
		• Medication adjustment
			• Activity/diet modification
			• Prophylaxis for patients taking opioids with docusate with senna
			• Peristalsis stimulating agents:
			  • Anthracenes (senna)
			  • Polyphenolics (bisacodyl)
			  • Softening agents:
			    • Surfactant laxatives (docusate)
			    • Bulk-forming agents (bran, methylcellulose)
			    • Osmotic laxatives (lactulose, sorbitol)
			    • Saline laxatives (magnesium hydroxide)

Table 15.1. Continued

Symptom	Possible Causes	Disease-Specific or Curative Treatment	Palliative Treatment
Respiratory			
Dyspnea	• *Pneumocystis jiroveci* pneumonia • Bacterial pneumonia • Anemia • Pleural effusion, mass, or obstruction • Decreased respiratory muscle function	• Specific treatment of disease entities • Erythropoietin, transfusion • Drainage, radiation, or surgery	• Use of a fan and open windows • Relaxation techniques, massage, and guided imagery • Oxygen supplement titrated to comfort if the patient is hypoxic • Bronchodilators (albuterol, ipratropium, and inhaled steroids) if there is bronchospasm • Opioids, particularly morphine, to decrease the sense of air hunger and respiratory rate • Benzodiazepines (e.g., lorazepam) to reduce the anxiety that often accompanies dyspnea
Cough	• *P. jiroveci* pneumonia • Bacterial pneumonia • Tuberculosis (TB) • Acid reflux • Postnasal drip	• Specific treatment of disease entities	• Cough suppressants (dextromethorphan, codeine, hydrocodone, morphine, and aerosolized lidocaine) • Bronchodilators (albuterol, ipratropium, and inhaled steroids) if there is bronchospasm • H_2 blockers or proton pump inhibitors (PPIs; ranitidine, omeprazole) if there is acid reflux (caution: interactions with atazanavir, rilpivirine)

Table 15.1. Continued

Symptom	Possible Causes	Disease-Specific or Curative Treatment	Palliative Treatment
Respiratory			
Cough			• Decongestants (pseudoephedrine, phenylephrine, and steroid nasal sprays) for postnasal drip
Increased secretions ("death-rattle")	• Fluid shifts • Ineffective cough • Sepsis • Pneumonia	• Antibiotics as indicated	• Atropine, hyoscyamine, transdermal scopolamine, and glycopyrrolate • Fluid restriction, discontinuing intravenous fluids
Hiccups	• Aerophagia (swallowing air) • *Candida* and other causes of esophagitis, including GERD • Vagus and phrenic nerve irritation • CNS mass lesions • Uremia • Alcohol intoxication • Anesthesia	• treatment of underlying etiology (e.g., antifungals for *Candida* esophagitis and acid reducers for GERD)	• Metoclopramide that can promote gastric emptying • Chlorpromazine (antipsychotic) that can reduce the CNS response (Start at a low dosage to reduce the risk of dystonia and drowsiness.) • Baclofen that can reduce the CNS response
Dermatologic			
Dry skin	• Dehydration • End-stage renal disease • End-stage liver disease • Malnutrition medications (e.g., indinavir)	• Hydration • Dialysis • Nutritional support • Discontinue offending medication	• No soaps, most of which dry the skin further • Emollients with or without salicylates • Emollients with urea (e.g., Ultra Mide 25) • Emollients with lactate (e.g., Lac-Hydrin) • Lubricating ointments or creams (e.g., petrolatum, Eucerin)

Table 15.1. Continued

Symptom	Possible Causes	Disease-Specific or Curative Treatment	Palliative Treatment
Dermatologic			
Pruritus	• Fungal infection • End-stage renal disease • End-stage liver disease • Dehydration and dry skin • Eosinophilic folliculitis • Opioid side effect	• Antifungal agents (e.g., itraconazole for eosinophilic folliculitis) • Dialysis • Hydration • Topical corticosteroids	• No soaps and hot baths/showers • Warm compresses • Treatments for dry skin • Topical agents (menthol, phenol (e.g., Sarna lotion), calamine, doxepin, and capsaicin) • Antihistamines (hydroxyzine, doxepin, and diphenhydramine) • Corticosteroids (topical or systemic) • Opioid antagonists (naloxone and naltrexone) that can be useful for treating uremic and biliary-associated pruritus • Antidepressants • Anxiolytics • Thalidomide in intractable pruritus, but beware of side effects, including neuropathy
Decubitus ulcers and pressure sores	• Poor nutrition • Decreased mobility and prolonged bed rest	• Increasing mobility • Enhancing nutrition	• Prevention (nutrition, mobility, and skin integrity) • Wound protection (semipermeable film and hydrocolloid dressing) • Debridement (normal saline, enzymatic agents, and alginates)

Table 15.1. Continued

Symptom	Possible Causes	Disease-Specific or Curative Treatment	Palliative Treatment
Neuropsychiatric			
Delirium/ agitation	• Electrolyte imbalances and glucose abnormalities • Dehydration • Hypoxia • Toxoplasmosis • Cryptococcal meningitis • CNS masses and metastases • Sepsis • Medication adverse effects (e.g., benzodiazepines, opioids, efavirenz, and corticosteroids) • Intoxication or withdrawal	• Correct imbalances • Hydration • Oxygen supplementation • Specific treatment of disease entities • Discontinuing offending medications	• Neuroleptics (haloperidol, risperidone, and chlorpromazine) to induce sedation in severe agitation • Benzodiazepines (e.g., lorazepam, diazepam, and midazolam) in the "terminal restlessness" of the last few days of life to relieve myoclonus, seizures, and restlessness (Note: In some patients, these may have adverse effects.)
Dementia	• HIV-associated dementia • Other dementia (e.g., Alzheimer dementia, Parkinson dementia, and multi-infarct dementia)	• ART	• Psychostimulants (methylphenidate) • Memantine (NMDA antagonist) that has been used in patients with Alzheimer dementia but has unclear benefits for patients with HIV-associated dementia • Low-dose neuroleptics (haloperidol, chlorpromazine) that can be useful in psychotic delirium

Table 15.1. Continued

Symptom	Possible Causes	Disease-Specific or Curative Treatment	Palliative Treatment
Neuropsychiatric			
Depression	• Chronic illness • Reactive depression and major depression	• Antidepressants	• Antidepressants that are useful when the patient has a life expectancy of several months or more: SSRIs, SNRIs, mirtazapine (useful in the lowest dosages for insomnia), and bupropion though beware of lowering the seizure threshold (Note that tricyclic antidepressants are not considered first- or second-line therapy owing to side effects, though they may be useful for treating refractory melancholic or delusional depression.) • Psychostimulants that are useful for patients who have urgent, severe depression or are weeks from death (methylphenidate, pemoline, dextroamphetamine, and modafinil)

Abbreviations: ART = antiretroviral therapy; CNS = central nervous system; GERD = gastroesophageal reflux disease; NMDA = N-methyl-D-aspartate; NSAID = nonsteroidal anti-inflammatory drug; SNRI = serotonin norepinephrine reuptake inhibitor; SSRI = selective serotonin reuptake inhibitor.

- previous treatments and their efficacy
- what the patient believes is causing the symptom
- coping strategies and supports
- the patient's personal goals of care with this particular symptom

Practitioners should note that some of the palliative treatments may have substantial long-term adverse effects and should be used to alleviate symptoms only in late-stage or dying patients.

PATIENT EDUCATION

- Discuss advance care planning and the option of hospice care, if appropriate, with patients.
- Provide patients and their family members with detailed information so that they understand the illness and associated treatments.
- Instruct patients to discuss their pain or other bothersome symptoms with their health-care provider.
- Encourage patients to talk with their health-care provider if they are feeling anxious, depressed, or fearful.
- Discuss with patients what their death might be like. Some patients may feel relieved to be able to talk openly about their last days. Assure them that their pain will be controlled and that their health-care provider will be there to help them.[1]

---

[1] "Guide for HIV/AIDS Clinical Care," Health Resources and Services Administration (HRSA), April 2014. Available online. URL: https://ryanwhite.hrsa.gov/sites/default/files/ryanwhite/grants/2014-guide.pdf. Accessed August 17, 2023.

Chapter 16 | **Ethics and Legal Considerations in End-of-Life Care**

Doctors and nurses deal with various ethical and legal issues regarding end-of-life care. Health-care providers should discuss the treatment options, potential outcomes, and the negative consequences that might outweigh the longevity of life with the patient and their family members. They must also stay up to date with the changes in legislation and follow moral principles and professional ethics regarding palliative care. Based on their approval, doctors must proceed while adhering to all related laws and professional guidelines.

ETHICAL PRINCIPLES OF END-OF-LIFE CARE

Ethics in end-of-life care are based on the following four important principles that must be carried out with honesty, dignity, and responsibility:

- **Autonomy**. Patients must make their own decisions about the mode of treatment or whether they want to be treated further or not.
- **Justice**. Health resources must be fairly distributed with equality.
- **Beneficence**. Health-care professionals should make decisions that are beneficial to the patient.
- **Non-maleficence**. Health-care professionals must ensure that they do not harm patients.

ETHICAL ISSUES IN END-OF-LIFE CARE

Some of the key ethical challenges faced in end-of-life care are as follows:

- **Communication with the patient**. End-of-life conversations are difficult for everyone, including nurses, family members, and patients. It is essential to inform the patient about all the possible harmful effects of the available treatment options. The patient decides the type of treatment they prefer or whether they wish to undergo treatment at all.

- **Symptom management**. Making decisions regarding managing symptoms for patients in palliative care is highly challenging because the benefits of treatment must outweigh the possible negative side effects. Health-care professionals must balance and prioritize the patient's best interests.

- **Patient's final decisions**. Keeping track of patients' decisions while handling end-of-life care is essential. When the patient is able, health-care professionals should encourage them to talk to family members regarding their desired decisions, making it easy for health-care providers when the patient loses consciousness.

- **Ethics committee in decision-making**. There are cases in which the patient's family does not accept decisions made by doctors and nurses. In such situations, doctors should follow the decisions of the ethics committee or the laws of the country.

- **Terminal sedation**. This is the last option when patients do not respond to any treatment method. It is not done to hasten death but to ease their pain and suffering.

- **Assisted dying**. A lethal substance or drug is given to the patient to hasten death when the patient desires to end their life to stop further suffering. There are two types of assisted dying: assisted suicide and euthanasia. Assisted suicide refers to a situation when the patient carries out the act of ending their own life with the necessary means provided by the physician. Euthanasia is when the physician carries out the act of ending the patient's life.

LEGAL CONSIDERATIONS IN END-OF-LIFE CARE

Health-care providers must consider the patient's legal documents in which they communicate their advanced directives and medical care preferences.

Two important advanced directives are as follows:

- **Living will.** This legal document details how the patient prefers to be treated during end-of-life care.
- **Durable power of attorney for health care (DPOAHC).** This document names the person responsible for handling the patient's affairs when they are unable to communicate. The representative should be aware of the patient's desires and must share the patient's treatment preferences with doctors in critical situations.

Some of the medical care preferences are as follows:

- **Do Not Attempt Resuscitation (DNAR).** If a patient orders DNAR, it means that cardiopulmonary resuscitation (CPR) should not be performed on the patient.
- **Allow Natural Death (AND).** This order is followed when the patient wants to die naturally without any life support. However, symptoms may be managed to keep them pain-free until their natural death occurs.
- **Physician Order to Life-Sustaining Treatment (POLST).** This order communicates a patient's wishes and directions for care through a medical directive. POLST allows the patient to choose the mode of treatment.

Patients under palliative care must be comfortable and empowered to make choices about their care and treatment based on their preferences and values. Health-care providers must make decisions that prioritize the patient and align with legal rights and ethical values.

References

Akdeniz, Melahat; Yardımcı, Bülent; and Kavukcu, Ethem. "Ethical Considerations at the End-of-Life Care," National Center for Biotechnology Information (NCBI), March 12, 2021. Available online. URL: www.ncbi.nlm.nih.gov/pmc/articles/PMC7958189. Accessed August 16, 2023.

Cobbs, Elizabeth L.; Blackstone, Karen; and Lynn, Joanne. "Legal and Ethical Concerns at the End of Life," MSD Manual, September 2022. Available online. URL: www.msdmanuals.com/en-in/home/fundamentals/death-and-dying/legal-and-ethical-concerns-at-the-end-of-life. Accessed August 14, 2023.

Lowey, Susan E. "Ethical Concerns in End-of-Life Care," Milne Publishing, December 15, 2015. Available online. URL: https://milnepublishing.geneseo.edu/nursingcare/chapter/ethical-concerns-in-end-of-life-care. Accessed August 16, 2023.

National Institute on Aging, "Advance Care Planning: Advance Directives for Health Care," National Institutes of Health (NIH), October 31, 2022. Available online. URL: www.nia.nih.gov/health/advance-care-planning-advance-directives-health-care. Accessed August 17, 2023.

Chapter 17 | Life-Sustaining Treatments and Their Impact on the Final Days

MAKING DECISIONS ABOUT TREATMENTS

Decisions about whether to use life-sustaining treatments that may extend life in the final weeks or days cause a great deal of confusion and anxiety. Some of these treatments are ventilator use, parenteral nutrition, and dialysis.

People near death may be guided by their doctor, but they have the right to make their own choices about life-sustaining treatments. The following are some of the questions to discuss:

- What are the person's goals of care?
- How would the possible benefits of life-sustaining treatments help reach the person's goals of care, and how likely is the desired outcome?
- How would the possible harms of life-sustaining treatments affect the person's goals of care? Is the possible benefit worth the possible harm?
- Besides possible benefits and harms of life-sustaining treatments, what else can affect the decision?
- Are there other resources, such as palliative care, a chaplain, or a medical ethicist, that could help the person or family make decisions about life-sustaining treatments?

CHOICES ABOUT CARE AND TREATMENT

A person may wish to receive all possible treatments, only some treatments, or no treatment at all in the last days of life. These decisions may be written down ahead of time in an advance directive, such as a living will. An advance directive is a general term for different types of legal documents that describe the treatment or care a patient wishes to receive or not receive when he or she is no longer able to speak their wishes.

Studies have shown that people with cancer who have end-of-life discussions with their doctors choose to have fewer procedures, such as resuscitation or the use of a ventilator. They are also less likely to be in intensive care, and the cost of their health care is lower during their final week of life. Reports from their caregivers show that these people live just as long as those who choose to have more procedures and have a better quality of life (QOL) in their last days.

SPIRITUAL ASSESSMENT

A spiritual assessment is a method or tool used by doctors to understand the role that religious and spiritual beliefs have in a person's life. This may help the doctor understand how these beliefs affect the way the person copes with cancer and makes decisions about cancer treatment.

Serious illnesses such as cancer may cause people or family caregivers to have doubts about their beliefs or religious values and cause spiritual distress. Some studies show that people with cancer may feel anger at God or may have a loss of faith after being diagnosed. Other people may have feelings of spiritual distress when coping with cancer. Spiritual distress may affect end-of-life decisions and increase depression.

Doctors and nurses, together with social workers and psychologists, may be able to offer care that supports a person's spiritual health. They may encourage the person to meet with their spiritual or religious leaders or join a spiritual support group. This may improve a person's QOL and ability to cope. When people with advanced cancer receive spiritual support from the medical team, they are more likely to choose hospice care and less aggressive treatment at the end of life.

FLUIDS

The goals of giving fluids at the end of life should be discussed by the patient, family, and doctors.

Fluids may be given when the person can no longer eat or drink normally. Fluids may be given with an intravenous (IV) catheter or through a needle under the skin.

Decisions about giving fluids should be based on the person's goals of care. Giving fluids has not been shown to help patients live longer or improve their QOL. However, the harms are minor, and the family may feel there are benefits if the person is less fatigued and more alert.

The family may also be able to give the person sips of water or ice chips or swab the mouth and lips to keep them moist.

NUTRITION SUPPORT

Nutrition support can improve health and boost healing during cancer treatment. The goals of nutrition therapy for people during the last days of life are different from the goals for people in active cancer treatment and recovery. In the final days of life, people often lose the desire to eat or drink and may not want food or fluids that are offered to them. Also, procedures used to put in feeding tubes may be hard on them.

Making Plans for Nutrition Support

The goal of end-of-life care is to prevent suffering and relieve symptoms. If nutrition support causes the person more discomfort than help, then nutrition support near the end of life may be stopped. The needs and best interests of each person guide the decision to give nutrition support. When decisions and plans about nutrition support are made by the person near death, doctors and family members can be sure they are doing what the person wants.

Types of Nutrition Support

If the person cannot swallow, the following two types of nutrition support are commonly used:
- **Enteral nutrition.** It uses a tube inserted into the stomach or intestine.

167

- **Parenteral nutrition.** It uses an IV catheter inserted into a vein.

Each type of nutrition support has benefits and risks.

ANTIBIOTICS

The benefits of using antibiotics in the last days of life are unclear. The use of antibiotics and other treatments for infection is common in people in the last days of life, but it is hard to tell how well they work. It is also hard to tell if there are any benefits of using antibiotics at the end of life.

Overall, doctors want to make the person comfortable in the last days of life rather than give treatments that may not help them live longer.

TRANSFUSIONS

Many people with advanced cancer have anemia. People with advanced blood cancers may have thrombocytopenia (a condition in which there is a lower-than-normal number of platelets in the blood). Deciding whether to use blood transfusions for these conditions is based on the following:

- goals of care
- how long the person is expected to live
- the benefits and risks of the transfusion

The decision can be hard to make because people usually need to receive transfusions in a medical setting rather than at home.

Many people with cancer are used to receiving blood transfusions during active treatment or supportive care and may want to continue transfusions to feel better. However, studies have not shown that transfusions are safe and effective at the end of life.

RESUSCITATION

People should decide whether or not they want cardiopulmonary resuscitation (CPR). It is an important decision for a person near death to make whether to have CPR (trying to restart the heart and breathing when it stops). It is best if people talk with their family, doctors, and caregivers about their wishes for CPR as early as possible (e.g., when being admitted to the hospital or when active cancer treatment is stopped). A do-not-resuscitate (DNR) order is written by a doctor to tell other health professionals not to perform CPR at the moment of death so that the natural process of dying occurs. If the person wishes, he or she can ask the doctor to write a DNR order. The person can ask that the DNR order be changed or removed at any time.

LAST DAYS IN THE HOSPITAL OR INTENSIVE CARE UNIT
Choices for Intensive Care Unit Use

Near the end of life, people with advanced cancer may be admitted to a hospital or intensive care unit (ICU) if they have not made other choices for their care. In the ICU, patients or family members have to make hard decisions about whether to start, continue, or stop aggressive treatments that may make the person live longer but harm their QOL. Families may be unsure of their feelings or have trouble deciding whether to limit or avoid treatments.

Sometimes, treatments such as dialysis or blood transfusions may be tried for a short time. However, at any time, patients or families may talk with doctors about whether they want to continue with ICU care. They may choose instead to change over to comfort care in the final days.

Ventilator Use

A ventilator is a machine that helps people breathe. Sometimes, using a ventilator will not improve the person's condition but will keep them alive longer. If the goal of care is to help the person live longer, a ventilator may be used according to the person's wishes. If ventilator support stops helping or is no longer what the person wants, the person, their family, and the health-care team may decide to turn the ventilator off.

Family members will be given information about how the person may respond when the ventilator is removed and about pain relief or sedation to keep the person comfortable. Family members will be given time to contact other loved ones who wish to be there. Chaplains or social workers may be called to support the family.

SUFFERING AND PALLIATIVE SEDATION AT THE END OF LIFE

The emotions of patients and caregivers are closely connected. Patients and caregivers share the distress of cancer, with the caregiver's distress sometimes being greater than the patient's distress. Since the caregiver's suffering can affect the person's well-being and the caregiver's adjustment to loss, early and constant support of the caregiver is very important.

Palliative sedation lowers the level of consciousness and relieves extreme pain and suffering. It uses drugs called "sedatives" to relieve extreme suffering by making a person calm and unaware.

The decision about whether to sedate a person at the end of life is a hard one. Sedation may be considered for a person's comfort or for a physical condition such as uncontrolled pain. Palliative sedation may be given on and off or until death. A person's thoughts and feelings about end-of-life sedation may depend greatly on his or her own culture and beliefs. Some people who become anxious facing the end of life may want to be sedated. Some people and their families may wish to have a level of sedation that allows them to communicate with each other. Other people may wish to have no procedures, including sedation, just before death.

Studies have not shown that palliative sedation shortens life when used in the last days.

It is important for the person to tell family members and health-care providers of his or her wishes about sedation at the end of life. When a person makes his or her wishes about sedation known ahead of time, doctors and family members can be sure they are doing what the person wants. Families may need support from the health-care team and mental health counselors while palliative sedation is used.[1]

---

[1] "Last Days of Life (PDQ®)—Patient Version," National Cancer Institute (NCI), March 27, 2023. Available online. URL: www.cancer.gov/about-cancer/advanced-cancer/caregivers/planning/last-days-pdq. Accessed August 4, 2023.

Chapter 18 | Organ Donation and Transplantation

WHAT IS ORGAN DONATION?

Organ donation involves taking healthy organs and tissues from one person and transplanting them to another person. Experts say that the organs from one donor can save or help as many as 50 people. The following are the organs you can donate:

- internal organs: kidneys, heart, liver, pancreas, intestines, and lungs
- skin
- bone and bone marrow
- cornea

Most organ and tissue donations occur after the donor has died. But some organs and tissues can be donated while the donor is alive.

People of all ages and backgrounds can be organ donors. If you are under the age of 18, your parent or guardian must give you permission to become a donor. If you are aged 18 or older, you can show you want to be a donor by signing a donor card. You should also let your family know your wishes.[1]

[1] MedlinePlus, "Organ Donation," National Institutes of Health (NIH), November 17, 2017. Available online. URL: https://medlineplus.gov/organdonation.html. Accessed August 23, 2023.

WHAT IS ORGAN TRANSPLANTATION?

You may need an organ transplant if one of your organs has failed. This can happen because of illness or injury. When you have an organ transplant, doctors remove an organ from another person and place it in your body. The organ may come from a living donor or a donor who has died.

The following are the organs that can be transplanted:

- heart
- intestine
- kidney
- liver
- lung
- pancreas

You often have to wait a long time for an organ transplant. Doctors must match donors to recipients to reduce the risk of transplant rejection. Rejection happens when your immune system attacks the new organ. If you have a transplant, you must take drugs for the rest of your life to help keep your body from rejecting the new organ.[2]

WHO CAN BE A DONOR?
How Old Do You Have to Be to Sign Up?

All adults in the United States—and in some states, people under the age of 18—can sign up to be organ donors. Doctors decide at the time of death if someone is a good fit. Often, a parent or guardian needs to give permission to allow someone under the age of 18 to donate.

Is There Any Age Limit?

There is no age limit for organ donation. Newborns and older adults have been organ donors. The health of your organs is more important than your age. The transplant team will decide at the time of death if donation is possible.

---

[2] MedlinePlus, "Organ Transplantation," National Institutes of Health (NIH), April 1, 2016. Available online. URL: https://medlineplus.gov/organtransplantation.html. Accessed August 23, 2023.

Do You Have to Be a U.S. Citizen to Donate or Receive Organs in the United States?

No. You can donate and receive organs in the United States even if you do not live in the country or are not a U.S. citizen. Doctors give organs to people based on medical needs, not citizenship.

If You Have an Illness, Can You Still Donate?

You may be a donor even if you have an illness. When you die, doctors will decide if donation is possible.

Can You Be an Organ and Tissue Donor and Donate Your Body to Medical Science?

Total body donation is often not an option if you choose to be an organ and tissue donor. You may still be an eye donor. Some medical schools and research groups may accept an organ donor for research.

If you wish to donate your entire body, arrange that with the medical school of your choice.

HOW SIGN-UP WORKS
Can You Sign Up as an Organ Donor?

Anyone over the age of 18 can sign up. In many states, people under the age of 18 can sign up as well. The following are a few ways to sign up:

- Sign up online now in your state. It is quick and easy.
- Visit your state motor vehicle office to sign up.

Let your family know about your decision. If the time comes, they will not feel surprised and can help carry out your wishes. The transplant team may ask them for information.

What Happens When You Sign Up in Your State?

When you sign up in your state, you are giving permission to donate your organs when you die. Usually, that means dying in a hospital and on artificial support. You will stay on your state's registry unless you remove yourself.

You Have an Organ Donor Card. Is That Enough?

No. You may not have the card with you, or it may get missed in the event of your death. If you wish to be a donor, sign up in your state registry.

You Have Your Organ Donor Status on Your Driver's License. Is That Enough?

That is an important step. It is also important to share your wishes with your family. Most families want to carry out the wishes of their loved ones. Be sure to tell them how you feel.

Can You Choose What You Want to Donate?

Most states give you the option to choose which organs and tissues you want to donate or to donate everything usable. Check with your state registry.

Can You Remove Yourself from the Registered Donors List?

Yes. You can change your donor status at any time. Look for an option such as "updating your status" on your state's site.

If you have a donor mark on your driver's license, removing yourself from the registry will not change that. So, unless your state uses a removable sticker on the license to identify donors, you will need to change your license at your local motor vehicle office.

If You Sign Up as a Donor, Will Doctors Carry Out Your Wishes?

If you are over the age of 18 and signed up as an organ donor in your state registry, you have legally given permission for your donation. No one can change your consent. If you are under the age of 18, your parents or legal guardian must give permission for your donation.

HOW DONATION WORKS
What Organs and Tissues Can You Donate?

- eight vital organs: heart, kidneys (two), pancreas, lungs (two), liver, intestines, hands, and face

- tissues, cornea, skin, heart valves, bone, blood vessels, and connective tissue
- bone marrow and stem cells, umbilical cord blood, and peripheral blood stem cells (PBSCs)

If You Are a Registered Donor, Will It Affect the Medical Care You Receive at the Hospital?

No. When you go to a hospital, saving your life comes first. Donation does not become a possibility until all lifesaving methods have failed. The medical team trying to save your life is separate from the transplant team.

Will Donation Damage Your Body? Can You Have an Open-Casket Funeral?

Hospital workers treat your body with care and respect during the donation process. You can donate your organs, eyes, and tissues and still have an open-casket funeral.

Will Your Family Pay for Donation?

No. Your family pays for your medical care and funeral costs. They do not pay to donate your organs. Insurance or the people who receive the organ donation pay those costs.

Can You Sell Your Organs?

No. You may not sell your organs. It is against U.S. federal law to buy or sell organs. People who buy or sell organs may face prison sentences and fines.

One reason Congress made this law was to make sure rich people do not unfairly receive donated organs and tissues.

HOW THE ORGAN MATCHING PROCESS WORKS
Can People of Different Races and Ethnicities Match Each Other?

Yes. People of different ethnicities match each other.

How Does a Donor Organ Match to Someone Who Needs It?

A national computer system matches donated organs to people who need them.

It bases matching decisions on things such as blood type, time spent waiting, and geographic location.

You Would Like to Donate a Kidney to Someone. How Can You Find Out If You Are a Match?

In the United States, you can donate a kidney to a family member, friend, or anyone on the waiting list while you are alive. They will test to see if you are a match and if you are healthy enough to have surgery.

Remember that there is a lot to do before they can consider you a living donor. Get a list of the living donation steps you need to take.

THE NEED FOR TRANSPLANTS
How Many People Are Waiting for Organs?

The number of people waiting for organs changes every day. As of October 2022, the number was over 105,500. Every 10 minutes, another person is added to the waiting list.

You can find the recent data from the Organ Procurement and Transplantation Network (OPTN). The number of people who need a lifesaving transplant continues to go up faster than the number of available organs.

Why Do Minorities Have a Higher Need for Transplants?

More than half of all people on the transplant waiting list are from a racial or ethnic minority group. Some diseases that cause end-stage organ failure are more common in these groups of people.

For example, African Americans, Asians, Native Hawaiians and Pacific Islanders, and Hispanics/Latinos are three times more likely than Whites to suffer from end-stage renal (kidney) disease, often as the result of high blood pressure (HBP).

Native Americans are four times more likely than Whites to suffer from diabetes. An organ transplant is sometimes the best—or only—option for saving a life.[3]

DONATION AFTER LIFE
How to Register as a Donor
First, decide to donate your organs, eyes, or tissues. Next, register as a donor in your state. Signing up does not mean you will be able to donate your organs, eyes, or tissues. Registering usually takes place many years before donation becomes possible. But it is the first step to being eligible to save lives.

Medical Care Provided to Potential Donors
Doctors treat all patients the same. The medical team will do everything possible to save your life. A doctor may put you on life support. This keeps blood flowing to the organs.

Doctors Test for Brain Death
Doctors run tests to find out if there is brain death. A patient with brain death has no brain activity, cannot breathe on their own, and cannot recover.

Doctors confirm brain death and note the time of death. Then organ donation is possible.

Organ Procurement Organization
If you are near death or die, the hospital tells the local organ procurement organization (OPO). This follows federal rules. The hospital will tell the OPO about you. The OPO decides if you are a possible donor. If so, someone from the OPO travels to the hospital.

---

[3] Organdonor.gov, "Organ Donation FAQ," Health Resources and Services Administration (HRSA), March 2022. Available online. URL: www.organdonor.gov/learn/faq. Accessed August 23, 2023.

Authorizing Donation

The OPO needs your legal consent. They will review your state's registry. If you are in it, that is legal consent for donation. If you are not, they may check your driver's license or another legal form. The OPO may ask your closest blood relative (next of kin) for approval.

Once they have approval, they do a medical evaluation. This is your complete medical and social history. They get this from your family.

How Donors Are Matched to Recipients

If the evaluation allows you to donate, the OPO contacts the OPTN.

The OPTN is a national database. It has all patients in the United States waiting for a transplant. The OPO enters information about a donor into the system, and the search begins.

The system creates a list of patients who match the donor (by organ). The system offers each available organ to the transplant team of the best-matched patient.

The transplant surgeon makes the final decision. They decide whether the organ is good for their patient. They may refuse the organ if their patient is too sick or they cannot reach them in time.

Most organs go to patients in the area where doctors recovered the organs. Other organs may go to patients in other parts of the country.

What Happens When Doctors Remove and Transplant Organs?

Doctors will keep your organs on artificial support. Machines keep oxygen going to the organs. The medical team and OPO official will check the condition of each organ.

A transplant surgical team will replace the medical team that treated the donors before they died (the medical team trying to save your life and the transplant team are never the same).

The surgical team will remove the donor's organs and tissues. They remove the organs; then they remove approved tissues such as bone, cornea, and skin. They close all cuts. Organ donation does not prevent open-casket funerals.

Organs only stay healthy for a short period of time after removal. Minutes count. The OPO official plans for the moving of the organs. The organs go to the hospitals where the patient(s) who need them. Organs may go by ambulance, helicopter, or commercial airplane.

How Surgeons Transplant Organs

The operation takes place after the transport team arrives at the hospital with the new organ. The person getting the organ is at the hospital. They may be in the operating room waiting for the organ.

Surgical teams work to transplant the new organs into the waiting patient.[4]

---

[4] Organdonor.gov, "Donation after Life," Health Resources and Services Administration (HRSA), September 2021. Available online. URL: www.organdonor.gov/learn/process/donation-after-life. Accessed August 23, 2023.

Chapter 19 | **Euthanasia, Assisted Suicide, and Ethical Dilemmas**

Every patient longs for a life free of suffering. When suffering is prolonged, a patient sometimes reaches the point of being unwilling to go on. Patients in extreme duress and unremitting pain and those aware of the ongoing medical costs associated with continuing a treatment that will not end in a cure but will likely leave surviving family members in considerable debt may come to decide that death is preferable to life and continued treatment. Physician-assisted suicide (PAS) is suicide undertaken with the aid of a physician or other health-care provider. PAS can be accomplished in two ways. In the first method, the physician provides the patient with information and a humane means to end his or her life. In the second method, the physician not only provides the information and means to end life but also takes co-responsibility to ensure the safe and effective execution of the act.

In recent years, "physician-assisted suicide" or "PAS" has replaced the term "physician-assisted death." PAS differs from "euthanasia," which refers to the act of assisting people to end their lives without the approval of a controlling legal authority.

UNDERSTANDING EUTHANASIA AND PALLIATIVE SEDATION
Euthanasia, also called "mercy killing," is generally defined as a deliberate intervention undertaken at a patient's request to end his or her life to relieve intractable suffering. While both euthanasia

and palliative sedation address extreme suffering associated with painful terminal illnesses, euthanasia may have slightly different connotations in different countries. In euthanasia, the physician administers appropriate medication in the required lethal amount to ensure that the patient loses consciousness and ceases to breathe. This is followed by cardiac arrest and death. The patient's death signifies that the intervention was successful.

Palliative sedation, also called "terminal sedation," is defined as the administration of nonopioid drugs as an intervention to treat unremitting, refractory pain or other clinical symptoms that have failed to respond to symptom-specific palliative care. The practice aims to sedate a terminally ill patient to a lowered state of consciousness that limits the patient's awareness of suffering and pain. Interventions for safely achieving sedation are used in other medical contexts, such as surgery, and do not have a detrimental effect on life, nor do they hasten the end-of-life process.

Often used as a last resort, palliative sedation is not considered an isolated intervention but rather a symptom-control strategy within the continuum of palliative care. That being said, death may or may not occur on achieving symptom control. Palliative sedation differs from euthanasia in three aspects: the intervention itself, the intention, and the act. While euthanasia involves an explicit intention to aid the patient in ending life, palliative sedation involves providing relief from otherwise unmanageable symptoms.

CORE ETHICAL ISSUES AND ATTITUDES REGARDING PHYSICIAN-ASSISTED SUICIDE AND EUTHANASIA

The ethical debate over personal control at life's end has generated serious discussion concerning the pros and cons of legalizing PAS and euthanasia. Mounting concern about the potential harm or abuse of legalizing the practices remains a huge deterrent to the legalization of these practices. One argument against PAS asserts that while the practice may seem compatible with patient autonomy and self-determination, the manner in which the practice is applied in a medical setting would actually undermine patient autonomy.

Some argue that mental disorders such as major depression can prevent patients from making a rational choice and thereby raise serious concerns regarding the role of patient self-determination in the practice of PAS. Detractors also point out that a lack of viable alternatives for medical treatment or personal support can compel patients to choose PAS as a means of ending suffering, pain, and further medical expenses associated with end-of-life medical treatment. This lack of viable alternatives, they argue, also requires serious consideration of the rationale behind these practices.

The debate about PAS and euthanasia also raises complex questions about the goals of the medical profession and the duties of physicians. While some hold that PAS may be considered ethically legitimate in exceptional cases, they also advocate that professional standards are necessary and that the legal system should not authorize such practices. Others advocate legalizing PAS, euthanasia, or both for the terminally ill patient.

OPPOSITION TO PHYSICIAN-ASSISTED SUICIDE

Some argue that the physician's role as a healer and obligation to respect human life are deeply established in the code of medical ethics and that the Hippocratic Oath is in total variance with PAS and euthanasia. Opponents of PAS also argue that the practice goes against the deep belief in the right to life.

Studies say that religion and spirituality deeply influence end-of-life decisions. Religious doctrines defend the sacredness of life, recognize a supreme being as the "giver" of life, and bestow on this supreme being the right to judge when life should end. Both PAS and euthanasia are perceived as moral transgressions by most religious belief systems. Most religious systems, on the other hand, approve the use of palliative care to manage pain when it is administered alongside spiritual care, which includes creative, narrative, and ritualistic work. Such practices have been widely used to improve quality of life (QOL) in the short term while helping to manage both physical and spiritual suffering during the end of life.

References

"Physician-Assisted Suicide," American Medical Association (AMA), n.d. Available online. URL: www.ama-assn.

org/delivering-care/ethics/physician-assisted-suicide.
Accessed September 14, 2023.
"The Physician's Role in Physician-Assisted Suicide," National
Center for Biotechnology Information (NCBI), August 8,
2012. Available online. URL: www.ncbi.nlm.nih.gov/pmc/
articles/PMC5774652. Accessed September 14, 2023.

Part 4 | **End-of-Life Care Facilities**

Chapter 20 | Home Care for Critical Illnesses

Chapter Contents

Section 20.1 | Home Health Care for Critical and Elderly Patients

Home health care helps older adults live independently for as long as possible, even with an illness or injury. It covers a wide range of services and can often delay the need for long-term nursing home care.

Home health care may include occupational and physical therapy, speech therapy, and skilled nursing. It may involve helping older adults with activities of daily living (ADL), such as bathing, dressing, and eating. It can also include assistance with cooking, cleaning, other housekeeping, and monitoring one's medication regimen.

It is important to understand the difference between home health-care and home care services. Although home health care may include some home care services, it is medical in nature. Home care services include chores and housecleaning, whereas home health care usually involves helping someone to recover from an illness or injury. Home health-care professionals are often licensed practical nurses, therapists, or home health aides. Most of them work for home health agencies, hospitals, or public health departments licensed by the state.

ENSURING QUALITY CARE

As with any important purchase, it is wise to talk with friends, neighbors, and your local area agency on aging (AAA) to learn more about the home health-care agencies in your community. Consider using the following questions to guide your search:

- How long has the agency served this community?
- Does the agency have a brochure describing services and costs? (If so, take or download it.)
- Is the agency an approved Medicare provider?
- Does a national accrediting body, such as the Joint Commission for the Accreditation of Healthcare Organizations (JCAHO), certify the quality of care?
- Does the agency have a current license to practice (if required by the state)?

- Does the agency offer a "bill of rights" that describes the rights and responsibilities of both the agency and the person receiving care?
- Does the agency prepare a care plan for the patient (with input from the patient, his or her doctor, and family members)? Will the agency update the plan as necessary?
- How closely do supervisors oversee care to ensure quality?
- Are agency staff members available around the clock, seven days a week, if necessary?
- Does the agency have a nursing supervisor available for on-call assistance at all times?
- Whom does the agency call if the home health-care worker cannot come when scheduled?
- How does the agency ensure patient confidentiality?
- How are agency caregivers hired and trained?
- How does the agency screen prospective employees?
- Will the agency provide a list of references for its caregivers?
- What is the procedure for resolving problems if they occur? Whom can I call with questions or complaints?
- Is there a sliding fee schedule based on the ability to pay, and is financial assistance available to pay for services?

When purchasing home health care directly from an individual provider (instead of an agency), it is even more important to conduct thorough screening. This should include an interview with the home health caregiver. You should also request references. Prepare for the interview by making a list of the older adult's special needs. For example, the patient may require help getting into or out of a wheelchair. If so, the caregiver must be able to provide appropriate assistance.

Whether you arrange for home health care through an agency or hire an independent aide, it helps spend time preparing the person who will provide care. Ideally, you will spend a day with the caregiver, before the job formally begins, to discuss what is involved in the daily routine. At a minimum, inform the caregiver (verbally and in writing) of the following things that he or she should know:

- health conditions, including illnesses and injuries
- signs of an emergency medical situation
- general likes and dislikes
- medication, including how and when each must be taken
- need for dentures, eyeglasses, canes, walkers, hearing aids, and so on
- possible behavior problems and how best to handle them
- mobility issues (trouble walking, getting into or out of a wheelchair, etc.)
- allergies, special diets, or other nutritional needs
- therapeutic exercises with detailed instructions

A WORD OF CAUTION

Although most states require home health-care agencies to perform criminal background checks on their workers and carefully screen applicants, actual regulations will vary depending on where you live. Therefore, before contacting a home health-care agency, you may want to call your local AAA or the Department of Public Health to learn what laws apply in your state.

PAYING FOR CARE

The cost of home health care varies across and within states. In addition, costs will fluctuate based on the type of health-care professional required. Home care services can be paid directly by patients and their families or through a variety of public and private sources. Sources for home health-care funding include Medicare, Medicaid, the Older Americans Act (OAA), the Veterans Administration, and private insurance.[1]

---

[1] Eldercare Locator, "Home Healthcare," Administration for Community Living (ACL), December 2, 2017. Available online. URL: https://eldercare.acl.gov/Public/Resources/Factsheets/Home_Health_Care.aspx. Accessed August 22, 2023.

Section 20.2 | Home Care for Cancer Patients

ROLES OF INFORMAL CAREGIVERS

Caregivers help people with cancer during and after treatment.

An informal caregiver, often a family member or friend, gives care to someone they have a personal relationship with, usually without payment. They may or may not live in the same home or geographic area as the person they are caring for.

Caregivers help with the daily needs of another person by:
- helping with personal needs, such as bathing, dressing, and mobility
- doing or arranging housework, such as cleaning, shopping, and cooking
- managing finances
- planning for care and services such as making appointments, providing transportation, and reporting problems
- visiting often
- providing emotional support

Formal caregivers are trained professionals who are paid to provide care for a patient.

NEEDS OF INFORMAL CAREGIVERS

Caregivers may have questions about treatment and side effects, how to find helpful resources, and ways to practice self-care.

If you are a caregiver, your information needs will change as the person with cancer's needs change during and after treatment. As a member of the care team, you may play an important role in coordinating your loved one's care, giving drugs and managing side effects, and keeping family members informed.

You may have questions for the health-care provider about the following:
- **Cancer**. What can you tell me about the type of cancer my family member or friend has?
- **Risks and benefits**. What are the risks and benefits of treatment?

- **Side effects**. How do I care for my family member or friend when they are having side effects from treatment while at home?
- **Medical and nursing tasks**. How do I give an injection? How do I set up the tube feedings?
- **Recovery**. How long will it take for my family member or friend to recover?
- **Complementary and alternative therapies**. Do I need to check with you before my family member or friend uses complementary and alternative (CAM) therapy? What CAM therapies are useful?
- **Care for yourself**. What are the best ways I can maintain my health and well-being while caregiving?
- **Emotions felt by patients and caregivers**. What are some ways we can deal with what we are feeling?
- **Local, community-based resources**. What are some local resources I can turn to?

Caregivers also have emotional, social, and financial needs.

It is easy to become overwhelmed as a caregiver. And it is normal to worry about what the future holds for your loved one. You may need support for yourself to:

- manage fears about your loved one's condition and future
- balance the time needed for your job and the time needed for caregiving
- find time for your friends
- pay your bills

People with cancer also worry about these things, but their top concern and the top concern of caregivers may not be the same, which may cause added stress.

Caregivers may have different needs after their loved one completes treatment.

When people with cancer complete treatment, the needs of caregivers decrease, but some caregivers may continue to worry about:

- the cancer coming back
- how to reduce stress in the survivor's life
- how to understand the survivor's experience

Caregiver distress increases when the person with cancer is at the end of life.

Caregivers of people who are nearing the end of life often have a low mental and physical quality of life (QOL). Caregiver distress and the need for additional support increase as the person with cancer nears the end of life.

Hospice care can provide much-needed support to people with cancer and their caregivers. Caregivers are often relieved by the hospice care team's ability to honor their loved one's care goals and provide high-quality end-of-life care.

BENEFITS OF BEING AN INFORMAL CAREGIVER

Some caregivers report positive experiences from caregiving that often lead to personal growth in the following areas:

- **Acceptance**. Adjusting to things that cannot change.
- **Family**. Feeling a closer bond with family.
- **Appreciation**. Being aware of love and support and having a greater joy of life.
- **Reprioritization**. Arranging life priorities in a new order of importance.
- **Increased faith**. Having a greater sense of closeness to God and renewed spiritual practices.
- **Empathy**. Understanding and feeling what others feel.
- **Positive self-view**. Feeling good about oneself.
- **Better health habits**. Eating a healthy diet, getting more exercise, and keeping up with medical checkups.

BURDENS OF BEING AN INFORMAL CAREGIVER

Caregivers may feel burdened when caring for people with cancer.

You may find it hard to cope with the emotional and physical aspects of caring for someone with cancer. This may lead to caregiver burden.

Caregiver burden is the stress or strain felt by the person who cares for the family member or friend who needs help during treatment or an illness. A burden is felt when the demands of caregiving are greater than the resources available to them. These demands can lead to negative effects of caregiving such as:

- anxiety
- depression
- posttraumatic stress disorder (PTSD)
- decline in QOL

Caregiver burden may be increased by certain factors, such as gender and age.

The following factors may increase caregiver burden:

- **Female gender**. Women, especially those who work, are more likely to have caregiver burden.
- **Age**. Caregiver burden can occur at any age.
  - **Older caregivers**. These caregivers are at risk of caregiver burden because their health, social, or financial situations may make it hard for them to care for others. As a result, they are more likely to have depression, poor health, and a higher risk of death than noncaregivers in the same age group. Older caregivers are at risk of caregiver burden when they have the following conditions:
    - health problems of their own that they neglect
    - fixed incomes
    - small social support networks
    - less time to exercise
    - trouble remembering to take their own medicines
    - fatigue from lack of sleep
  - **Middle-aged caregivers**. These caregivers may worry about being able to balance their caregiving and work responsibilities. They may worry about missing workdays, being less productive at work, and needing to take a leave of absence.
  - **Younger caregivers**. These caregivers often juggle work and their own family duties. They may also have to give up a part of their social lives to be a caregiver.

- **Culture**. There are cultural perspectives on caregiving that may increase the risk of caregiver burden. For example, some cultures have strong family ties, leading caregivers to use fewer support services, including counseling and support groups, home care, long-term care, and hospice services. Additionally, different cultures may have beliefs about death and dying that make discussions with the health-care team about prognosis and care difficult. Being unable to have these discussions can add to a caregiver's sense of burden and duty.
- **Socioeconomic status**. This is the social standing of someone that is measured by a person's education, income, and job. People with a lower socioeconomic status may have less access to resources and financial help. Lower incomes and limited financial options may cause patients and their families to make treatment-related choices that are not the same as their doctor prescribed.
- **Employment**. Caregivers may need to take time off from their job or make changes in the hours they work or the duties they perform. Work progress may suffer when a caregiver is not focused and can lead to anxiety and depression.
- **Role strain**. A caregiver may have many roles. They may also be a spouse, parent, child, friend, employee, or student. Role strain happens when the rights, duties, and behaviors of one role conflict with a different role. Sometimes, having more than one role can increase stress for a caregiver, but sometimes, it reduces stress by allowing them to step away from the caregiver role for a while. For example, when a caregiver goes to work, they may benefit from the support of their employer and coworkers and from the time away from caregiving.
- **Site of care**. Caregivers have more burden when the person with cancer leaves the hospital and

comes home. The caregiver now must help manage the person's symptoms and may be unsure about the prognosis or if the cancer can spread. Visits by home health nurses can help reduce this burden. Sudden changes in the site of care, such as going back to the hospital, also increase caregiver burden.

- **Patient characteristics**. Caregivers may have more burden when the person with cancer has poor physical and mental health, such as anxiety and depression. If the person has a poor QOL, this may also increase caregiver burden.

PARENTS AS CAREGIVERS

Caring for a child with cancer is a stressful time for parents.

Being told that your child has cancer is extremely distressing. Many parents say they feel shocked, overwhelmed, and confused. Parents must manage the same needs and burdens as other caregivers while remaining strong for their sick child and their other children.

Parents caring for children with cancer may report symptoms of traumatic stress during and after their child's diagnosis. Symptoms include:

- repeated, unwanted thoughts
- avoiding difficult thoughts, feelings, and situations
- increased heart rate and blood pressure

Although stress levels decrease for most parents after their child finishes treatment, some parents report long-term traumatic stress symptoms after treatment ends.

The stress levels of parents may be affected by several factors.

The following factors may reduce stress in parents caring for children with cancer:

- social support from family and friends
- support from health-care team members
- maintaining a positive view of the child's QOL
- believing that treatments will have a positive outcome
- being employed

WAYS TO REDUCE CAREGIVER BURDEN

There are many ways to help you decrease caregiver burden.

The following therapies or skills may prevent or reduce caregiver burden:

- **Cognitive behavioral therapy (CBT)**. CBT helps change the way a caregiver thinks and feels about certain things.
- **Complementary and/or alternative therapies**. Many options, such as guided imagery, massage therapy, or healing touch, help caregivers manage stress and anxiety.
- **Family/couples therapy**. Counseling helps families work through problems in a way that makes the family stronger.
- **Interpersonal therapy**. One-on-one counseling focuses on your relationships with other people to reduce caregiver burden.
- **Problem-solving/skill building**. This helps the caregiver develop the following skills:
  - ability to assess and manage the patient's symptoms
  - identifying solutions to caregiving problems
  - enhancing the caregiver's ability to cope with cancer caregiving roles and duties
- **Psychoeducational**. This helps caregivers cope by providing them with information about:
  - diagnosis
  - prognosis
  - self-care/home care
  - impact on partners and family
  - hospital care
  - follow-up and recovery
- **Palliative care**. Using palliative care improves the loved one's QOL. When their QOL is improved, the caregiver often feels less burdened.
- **Supportive therapy**. This is a type of therapy that addresses the emotional needs of caregivers.[2]

---

[2] "Informal Caregivers in Cancer (PDQ®)—Patient Version," National Cancer Institute (NCI), August 16, 2023. Available online. URL: www.cancer.gov/about-cancer/coping/family-friends/family-caregivers-pdq. Accessed August 22, 2023.

Section 20.3 | **Assistive Devices and Rehabilitation for Chronic Conditions**

ASSISTIVE DEVICES AND THEIR USE

Some examples of assistive technologies are as follows:

- mobility aids, such as wheelchairs, scooters, walkers, canes, crutches, prosthetic devices, and orthotic devices
- hearing aids to help people hear or hear more clearly
- cognitive aids, including computer or electrical assistive devices, to help people with memory, attention, or other challenges in their thinking skills
- computer software and hardware, such as voice recognition programs, screen readers, and screen enlargement applications, to help people with mobility and sensory impairments use computers and mobile devices
- tools, such as automatic page-turners, bookholders, and adapted pencil grips, to help learners with disabilities participate in educational activities
- closed captioning to allow people with hearing problems to watch movies, television programs, and other digital media
- physical modifications in the built environment, including ramps, grab bars, and wider doorways to enable access to buildings, businesses, and workplaces
- lightweight, high-performance mobility devices that enable persons with disabilities to play sports and be physically active
- adaptive switches and utensils to allow those with limited motor skills to eat, play games, and accomplish other activities
- devices and features of devices to help perform tasks, such as cooking, dressing, and grooming; specialized handles and grips; devices that extend reach; and lights on telephones and doorbells are a few examples[3]

---

[3] "What Are Some Types of Assistive Devices and How Are They Used?" *Eunice Kennedy Shriver* National Institute of Child Health and Human Development (NICHD), October 24, 2018. Available online. URL: www.nichd.nih.gov/health/topics/rehabtech/conditioninfo/device. Accessed August 23, 2023.

REHABILITATIVE TECHNOLOGIES AND THEIR USE

Rehabilitative technologies and techniques help people recover or improve function after injury or illness. The following are a few examples:

- **Robotics.** Specialized robots help people regain and improve function in their arms or legs after a stroke.
- **Virtual reality.** People who are recovering from injury can retrain themselves to perform motions within a virtual environment.
- **Musculoskeletal modeling and simulations.** These computer simulations of the human body can pinpoint underlying mechanical problems in a person with a movement-related disability. This technique can help improve assistive aids or physical therapies.
- **Transcranial magnetic stimulation (TMS).** TMS sends magnetic impulses through the skull to stimulate the brain. This system can help people who have had a stroke recover movement and brain function.
- **Transcranial direct current stimulation (tDCS).** In tDCS, a mild electrical current travels through the skull and stimulates the brain. This can help recover movement in patients recovering from stroke or other conditions.
- **Motion analysis.** Motion analysis captures video of human motion with specialized computer software that analyzes the motion in detail. The technique gives health-care providers a detailed picture of a person's specific movement challenges to guide them with proper therapy.

Some devices incorporate multiple types of technologies and techniques to help users regain or improve function. For example, the BrainGate project, which was partially funded by the *Eunice Kennedy Shriver* National Institute of Child Health and Human Development (NICHD) through the National Center for Medical

Rehabilitation Research (NCMRR), relied on tiny sensors being implanted in the brain. The user could then think about moving their arm, and a robotic arm would carry out the thought.[4]

[4] "What Are Some Types of Rehabilitative Technologies?" *Eunice Kennedy Shriver* National Institute of Child Health and Human Development (NICHD), October 24, 2018. Available online. URL: www.nichd.nih.gov/health/topics/rehabtech/conditioninfo/use. Accessed August 23, 2023.

Chapter 21 | Long-Term Care and Quality End-of-Life Support

WHAT IS LONG-TERM CARE?

Long-term care involves a variety of services designed to meet a person's health or personal care needs during a short or long period of time. These services help people live as independently and safely as possible when they can no longer perform everyday activities on their own.

Long-term care is provided in different places by different caregivers, depending on a person's needs. Most long-term care is provided at home by unpaid family members and friends. It can also be given in a facility such as a nursing home or in the community, for example, in an adult day care center.

The most common type of long-term care is personal care—help with everyday activities, also called "activities of daily living" (ADL). These activities include bathing, dressing, grooming, using the toilet, eating, and moving around—for example, getting out of bed and moving to a chair.

Long-term care also includes community services such as meals, adult day care, and transportation services. These services may be provided free or for a fee.

People often need long-term care when they have a serious, ongoing health condition or disability. The need for long-term care can arise suddenly, such as after a heart attack or stroke. Most often, however, it develops gradually, as people get older and frailer or as an illness or disability gets worse.

WHAT ARE THE DIFFERENT TYPES OF HOME-BASED LONG-TERM CARE SERVICES?

Home-based long-term care includes health, personal, and support services to help people stay at home and live as independently as possible. Most long-term care is provided either in the home of the person receiving services or at a family member's home. In-home services may be short-term—for someone who is recovering from an operation, for example—or long-term—for people who need ongoing help. Most home-based services involve personal care, such as help with bathing, dressing, and taking medications, and supervision to make sure a person is safe. Unpaid family members, partners, friends, and neighbors provide most of this type of care.

Home-based long-term care services can also be provided by paid caregivers, including caregivers found informally, and health-care professionals, such as nurses, home health-care aides, therapists, and homemakers, who are hired through home health-care agencies. These services include home health care, homemaker services, friendly visitor/companion services, and emergency response systems.

Home Health Care

Home health care involves part-time medical services ordered by a physician for a specific condition. These services may include nursing care to help a person recover from surgery, an accident, or illness. Home health care may also include physical, occupational, or speech therapy and temporary home health aide services. These services are provided by home health-care agencies approved by Medicare, a government insurance program for people over the age of 65.

Homemaker and Personal Care Services

Home health agencies offer homemaker and personal care services that can be purchased without a physician's order. Homemaker services include help with meal preparation and household chores. Personal care includes help with bathing and dressing. Agencies do not have to be approved by Medicare to provide these kinds of services.

Friendly Visitor and Senior Companion Services

Friendly visitor/companion services are usually staffed by volunteers who regularly pay short visits (less than two hours) to someone who is frail or living alone. You can also purchase these services from home health agencies.

Senior Transportation Services

Transportation services help people get to and from medical appointments, shopping centers, and other places in the community. Some senior housing complexes and community groups offer transportation services. Many public transit agencies have services for people with disabilities. Some services are free. Others charge a fee.

Emergency Medical Alert Systems

Emergency response systems automatically respond to medical and other emergencies via electronic monitors. The user wears a necklace or bracelet with a button to push in an emergency. Pushing the button summons emergency help to the home. This type of service is especially useful for people who live alone or are at risk of falling. A monthly fee is charged.

LONG-TERM CARE PLANNING

You can never know for sure if you will need long-term care. Maybe you will never need it. But an unexpected accident, illness, or injury can change your needs, sometimes suddenly. The best time to think about long-term care is before you need it.

Planning for the possibility of long-term care gives you time to learn about services in your community and what they cost. It also allows you to make important decisions while you are still able.

People with Alzheimer disease (AD) or other cognitive impairments should begin planning for long-term care as soon as possible.

Making Decisions about Long-Term Care

Begin by thinking about what would happen if you became seriously ill or disabled. Talk with your family, friends, and lawyer about who would provide care if you needed help for a long time.

You might delay or prevent the need for long-term care by staying healthy and independent. Talk to your doctor about your medical and family history and lifestyle. He or she may suggest actions you can take to improve your health.

Healthy eating, regular physical activity, not smoking, and limited drinking of alcohol can help you stay healthy. So can an active social life, a safe home, and regular health care.

Making Housing Decisions: Aging in Place

In thinking about long-term care, it is important to consider where you will live as you age and how your place of residence can best support your needs if you can no longer fully care for yourself.

Most people prefer to stay in their own home for as long as possible.

Making Financial Decisions for Long-Term Care

Long-term care can be expensive. Americans spend billions of dollars a year on various services. How people pay for long-term care depends on their financial situation and the kinds of services they use. Often, they rely on a variety of payment sources, including:

- personal funds, including pensions, savings, and income from stocks
- government health insurance programs, such as Medicaid (Medicare does not cover long-term care but may cover some costs of short-term care in a nursing home after a hospital stay.)
- private financing options, such as long-term care insurance
- veterans benefits
- services through the Older Americans Act (OAA)[1]

---

[1] National Institute on Aging (NIA), "What Is Long-Term Care?" National Institutes of Health (NIH), May 1, 2017. Available online. URL: www.nia.nih.gov/health/what-long-term-care. Accessed August 23, 2023.

RESIDENTIAL FACILITIES, ASSISTED LIVING, AND NURSING HOMES

At some point, support from family, friends, and local programs may not be enough. People who require help full-time might move to a residential facility that provides many or all of the long-term care services they need.

Facility-based long-term care services include board and care homes, assisted living facilities, nursing homes, and continuing care retirement communities (CCRCs).

Some facilities have only housing and housekeeping, but many also provide personal care and medical services. Many facilities offer special programs for people with AD and other types of dementia.

What Are Board and Care Homes?

Board and care homes, also called "residential care facilities" or "group homes," are small private facilities, usually with 20 or fewer residents. Rooms may be private or shared. Residents receive personal care and meals and have staff available around the clock. Nursing and medical care usually are not provided on-site.

What Is Assisted Living?

Assisted living is for people who need help with daily care, but not as much help as a nursing home provides. Assisted living facilities range in size from as few as 25 residents to 120 or more. Typically, a few "levels of care" are offered, with residents paying more for higher levels of care.

Assisted living residents usually live in their own apartments or rooms and share common areas. They have access to many services, including up to three meals a day; assistance with personal care; help with medications, housekeeping, and laundry; 24-hour supervision, security, and on-site staff; and social and recreational activities. Exact arrangements vary from state to state.

What Are Nursing Homes?

Nursing homes, also called "skilled nursing facilities," provide a wide range of health and personal care services. Their services focus on medical care more than most assisted living facilities. These services typically include nursing care, 24-hour supervision, three meals a day, and assistance with everyday activities. Rehabilitation services, such as physical, occupational, and speech therapy, are also available.

Some people stay at a nursing home for a short time after being in the hospital. After they recover, they go home. However, most nursing home residents live there permanently because they have ongoing physical or mental conditions that require constant care and supervision.[2]

HOW TO CHOOSE A NURSING HOME

A nursing home, also known as a "skilled nursing facility," provides a wide range of health-care and personal care services.

If you need to go to a nursing home after a hospital stay, the hospital staff can help you find one that will provide the kind of care that is best for you. If you are looking for a nursing home, ask your doctor's office for recommendations. Once you know what choices you have, the following are a few good ideas:

- **Consider what you want**. What is important to you—nursing care, meals, physical therapy, a religious connection, hospice care, or special care units for dementia patients? Do you want a place close to family and friends, so they can easily visit?
- **Talk to friends and family**. Talk with friends, relatives, social workers, and religious groups to find out what places they suggest. Check with health-care providers about which nursing homes they feel provide good care.
- **Call different nursing homes**. Get in touch with each place on your list. Ask questions about how many people live there and what it costs. Find out about waiting lists.

---

[2] National Institute on Aging (NIA), "Residential Facilities, Assisted Living, and Nursing Homes," National Institutes of Health (NIH), May 1, 2017. Available online. URL: www.nia.nih.gov/health/residential-facilities-assisted-living-and-nursing-homes. Accessed August 23, 2023.

- **Visit the facility**. Make plans to meet with the director and the nursing director. For example, look for:
  - Medicare and Medicaid certification
  - handicap access
  - residents who look well cared for
  - warm interaction between staff and residents
- **Ask questions during your visit**. Do not be afraid to ask questions. For example, ask the staff to explain any strong odors. Bad smells might indicate a problem; good ones might hide a problem. You might want to find out how long the director and heads of nursing, food, and social services departments have worked at the nursing home. If key members of the staff change often, that could mean there is something wrong.
- **Visit the facility again**. Make a second visit without calling ahead. Try another day of the week or time of day, so you will meet other staff members and see different activities. Stop by at mealtime. Is the dining room attractive and clean? Does the food look tempting?
- **Carefully read your contract**. Once you select a nursing home, carefully read the contract. Question the director or assistant director about anything you do not understand. Ask a good friend or family member to read over the contract before you sign it.

The Centers for Medicare and Medicaid Services (CMS) requires each state to inspect any nursing home that gets money from the government. Homes that do not pass inspection are not certified. Ask to see the current inspection report and certification of any nursing home you are considering.[3]

What Are Continuing Care Retirement Communities?

Continuing care retirement communities, also called "life-care communities," offer different levels of service in one location.

---

[3] National Institute on Aging (NIA), "How to Choose a Nursing Home," National Institutes of Health (NIH), May 1, 2017. Available online. URL: www.nia.nih.gov/health/how-choose-nursing-home. Accessed August 23, 2023.

Many of them offer independent housing (houses or apartments), assisted living, and skilled nursing care all on one campus. Health-care services and recreation programs are also provided.

In a CCRC, where you live depends on the level of service you need. People who can no longer live independently move to the assisted living facility or sometimes receive home care in their independent living unit. If necessary, they can enter the CCRC's nursing home.

There are many sources of information about facility-based long-term care. A good place to start is the Eldercare Locator at 800-677-1116 or https://eldercare.acl.gov/Public/Index.aspx. You can also call your local area agency on aging (AAA), an aging and disability resource center (ADRC), the Department of Human Services or Aging, or a social service agency.[4]

WHAT ARE THE OTHER LONG-TERM CARE CHOICES?

You may have other long-term care options (besides nursing home care) available to you. Before you make any decisions about long-term care, talk to someone you trust to understand more about other long-term care services and support. You might want to talk to your family, your doctor or other health-care provider, a person-centered counselor, or a social worker for help deciding what kind of long-term care you need.

If you are in a hospital, in a nursing home, or working with a home health agency (HHA), you can get support to help you understand your options or help you arrange care. Talk to:

- a discharge planner
- a social worker
- an organization in a "No Wrong Door System," such as an ADRC, AAA, or center for independent living (CIL)

LONG-TERM CARE OPTIONS TO CONSIDER
Home- and Community-Based Services

A variety of home- and community-based services may be available to help with your personal care and activities.

---

[4] See footnote [2].

210

Medicaid may cover some services, including:

- home care (such as cooking, cleaning, or helping with other daily activities)
- home health services (such as physical therapy or skilled nursing care)
- transportation to medical care
- personal care
- respite care
- hospice
- case management

Medicaid programs vary from state to state. Medicaid may offer more services in your state.

These types of services may also be available through other programs, such as the AAA, Medicare, or hospice programs.

Community sources, including volunteer groups that help with things such as shopping or transportation, which may be free or low cost (or may ask for a voluntary donation), are another option. Examples of the services and programs that may be available in your community are:

- adult day services
- adult day health care (which offers nursing and therapy)
- care coordination and case management (including transition services to leave a nursing home)
- home care (such as cooking, cleaning, or helping with other daily activities)
- meal programs (such as Meals on Wheels)
- senior centers
- friendly visitor programs
- help with shopping and transportation
- help with legal questions, bill pay, and other financial matters

Accessory Dwelling Unit

An accessory dwelling unit (ADU; sometimes called an "in-law apartment," "accessory apartment," or a "second unit") is a second living space within a home or on a lot. It has a separate living and sleeping area, a place to cook, and a bathroom. If you or a loved one owns a single-family home, adding an ADU to an existing home may help you keep your independence.

Space such as an upper floor, basement, attic, or over a garage may be turned into an ADU. Family members may be interested in living in an ADU in your home, or you may want to move into an ADU at a family member's home.

Check with your local zoning office to be sure ADUs are allowed in your area and find out if there are any special rules. The cost of an ADU can vary widely, depending on many factors, such as the size of the project.

Subsidized Senior Housing

There are state and federal programs that help pay for housing for some seniors with low-to-moderate incomes. Some of these housing programs also offer help with meals and other activities, such as housekeeping, shopping, and doing the laundry. Residents usually live in their own apartments within an apartment building. Rent payments are usually based on a percentage of a person's income.

Continuing Care Retirement Communities

Some retirement communities offer different kinds of housing and levels of care. In the same community, there may be:

- individual homes or apartments (for residents who still live on their own)
- an assisted living facility (for people who need some help with daily care)
- a nursing home (for people who require higher levels of care)

Residents can move from one level to another based on their needs but usually stay within the CCRC. If you are considering a CCRC, be sure to check the quality of its nursing home at www.medicare.gov/care-compare/?providerType=NursingHome and the inspection report.

Group Living Arrangements

Residential care communities (sometimes called "adult foster/family homes" or "personal care homes") and assisted living communities are types of group living arrangements. In some states, residential care and assisted living communities mean the same thing. Both can help with some of the ADLs, such as bathing, dressing, using the bathroom, and meals. Whether they offer nursing services or help with medications varies by state.

In most cases, residents of these communities pay a regular monthly rent and additional fees depending on the type of personal care services they get.

Hospice and Respite Care

Hospice is a program of care and support for people who are terminally ill. Hospice helps people who are terminally ill live comfortably. The focus is on comfort, not on curing an illness.

Respite care is a very short inpatient stay given to hospice patients so that their usual caregiver can rest.

Program of All-Inclusive Care for the Elderly

The Program of All-Inclusive Care for the Elderly (PACE) is a Medicare and Medicaid program that helps people meet their health-care needs in the community instead of going to a nursing home or other care facility.

If you join the PACE, a team of health-care professionals will work with you to help coordinate your care.

HOW DOES THE PROGRAM OF ALL-INCLUSIVE CARE FOR THE ELDERLY WORK?

The PACE covers all Medicare- and Medicaid-covered care and services and anything else the health-care professionals in your PACE team decide you need to improve and maintain your health. This includes prescription drugs and any medically necessary care.

Here are some of the services the PACE may cover:

- adult day primary care (including doctor and recreational therapy nursing services)

- dentistry
- emergency services
- home care
- hospital care
- laboratory/x-ray services
- meals
- nursing home care
- nutritional counseling
- occupational therapy
- physical therapy
- preventive care
- social work counseling
- transportation to the PACE center for activities or medical appointments

WHO CAN JOIN A PROGRAM OF ALL-INCLUSIVE CARE FOR THE ELDERLY?

The PACE is only available in some states that offer the PACE under Medicaid.

You can join the PACE, even if you do not have Medicare or Medicaid, if you:

- are at least 55
- live in the service area of a PACE organization
- need a nursing home level of care (as certified by your state)
- are able to live safely in the community with help from the PACE

WHAT DOES THE PROGRAM OF ALL-INCLUSIVE CARE FOR THE ELDERLY COST?

If you have Medicaid, you would not pay a monthly premium for the long-term care portion of the PACE benefit.

If you do not qualify for Medicaid but you have Medicare, you will pay:

- a monthly premium to cover the long-term care portion of the PACE benefit
- a premium for Medicare Part D drugs

There is no deductible or co-payment for any drug, service, or care approved by your health-care team. If you do not have Medicare or Medicaid, you can pay for the PACE yourself.

HOW DO YOU APPLY FOR A PROGRAM OF ALL-INCLUSIVE CARE FOR THE ELDERLY?

To find out if you are eligible and if there is a PACE center near you, search for PACE plans in your area at www.medicare.gov/plan-compare/#/pace?year=2023&lang=en or call your Medicaid office.[5]

---

[5] "What Are My Other Long-Term Care Choices?" Centers for Medicare & Medicaid Services (CMS), August 17, 2012. Available online. URL: www.medicare.gov/what-medicare-covers/what-part-a-covers/what-are-my-other-long-term-care-choices. Accessed August 23, 2023.

Chapter 22 | **Palliative and Hospice Care**

Many Americans die in facilities, such as hospitals or nursing homes, receiving care that is not consistent with their wishes. It is important for older adults to plan ahead and let their caregivers, doctors, or family members know their end-of-life preferences in advance. For example, if an older person wants to die at home, receiving end-of-life care for pain and other symptoms, and makes this known to health-care providers and family, it is less likely he or she will die in a hospital receiving unwanted treatments.

If the person is no longer able to make health-care decisions for themselves, a caregiver or family member may have to make those decisions. Caregivers have several factors to consider when choosing end-of-life care, including the older person's desire to pursue life-extending treatments, how long he or she has left to live, and the preferred setting for care.

PALLIATIVE CARE
What Is Palliative Care?
Palliative care is specialized medical care for people living with a serious illness, such as cancer or heart failure. Patients in palliative care may receive medical care for their symptoms, or palliative care, along with treatment intended to cure their serious illness. Palliative care is meant to enhance a person's current care by focusing on quality of life (QOL) for them and their family.

Who Can Benefit from Palliative Care?
Palliative care is a resource for anyone living with a serious illness, such as heart failure, chronic obstructive pulmonary disease

(COPD), cancer, dementia, Parkinson disease (PD), and many others. Palliative care can be helpful at any stage of illness and is best provided soon after a person is diagnosed.

In addition to improving QOL and helping with symptoms, palliative care can help patients understand their choices for medical treatment. The organized services available through palliative care may be helpful to any older person having a lot of general discomfort and disability very late in life.

Who Makes Up the Palliative Care Team?

A palliative care team is made up of multiple different professionals who work with the patient, family, and the patient's other doctors to provide medical, social, emotional, and practical support. The team comprises palliative care specialist doctors and nurses and includes others, such as social workers, nutritionists, and chaplains. A person's team may vary based on their needs and level of care. To begin palliative care, a person's health-care provider may refer him or her to a palliative care specialist. If he or she does not suggest it, the person can ask a health-care provider for a referral.

Where Is Palliative Care Provided?

Palliative care can be provided in hospitals, nursing homes, outpatient palliative care clinics, or certain other specialized clinics or at home. Medicare, Medicaid, and insurance policies may cover palliative care. Veterans may be eligible for palliative care through the U.S. Department of Veterans Affairs (VA). Private health insurance might pay for some services. Health insurance providers can answer questions about what they will cover.

In palliative care, a person does not have to give up treatment that might cure a serious illness. Palliative care can be provided along with curative treatment and may begin at the time of diagnosis. Over time, if the doctor or the palliative care team believes ongoing treatment is no longer helping, there are two possibilities. Palliative care could transition to hospice care if the doctor believes the person is likely to die within six months. Or the palliative care team could continue to help with increasing emphasis on comfort care.

HOSPICE CARE
What Is Hospice Care?

Increasingly, people are choosing hospice care at the end of life. Hospice care focuses on the care, comfort, and QOL of a person with a serious illness who is approaching the end of life.

At some point, it may not be possible to cure a serious illness, or a patient may choose not to undergo certain treatments. Hospice is designed for this situation. The patient beginning hospice care understands that his or her illness is not responding to medical attempts to cure it or to slow the disease's progress.

Like palliative care, hospice provides comprehensive comfort care as well as support for the family, but in hospice, attempts to cure the person's illness are stopped. Hospice is provided for a person with a terminal illness whose doctor believes he or she has six months or less to live if the illness runs its natural course.

It is important for a patient to discuss hospice care options with their doctor. Sometimes, people do not begin hospice care soon enough to take full advantage of the help it offers. Perhaps they wait too long to begin hospice, and they are too close to death. Or some people are not eligible for hospice care soon enough to receive its full benefits. Starting hospice early may be able to provide months of meaningful care and quality time with loved ones.

Where Is Hospice Care Provided, and Who Provides It?

Hospice is an approach to care, so it is not tied to a specific place. It can be offered in two types of settings: at home or in a facility such as a nursing home, a hospital, or even a separate hospice center.

Hospice care brings together a team of people with special skills—among them are nurses, doctors, social workers, spiritual advisors, and trained volunteers. Everyone works together with the person who is dying, along with the caregiver and/or the family, to provide the medical, emotional, and spiritual support needed.

A member of the hospice team visits regularly, and someone is usually always available by phone—24 hours a day, seven days a week. Hospice may be covered by Medicare and other insurance companies.

It is important to remember that stopping treatment aimed at curing an illness does not mean discontinuing all treatment. A good example is an older person with cancer. If the doctor determines that the cancer is not responding to chemotherapy and the patient chooses to enter hospice care, then the chemotherapy will be stopped. Other medical care may continue as long as it is helpful. For example, if the person has high blood pressure (HBP), he or she will still get medicine for that.

Although hospice provides a lot of support, the day-to-day care of a person dying at home is provided by family and friends. The hospice team coaches family members on how to care for the dying person and even provides respite care when caregivers need a break. Respite care can be for as short as a few hours or for as long as several weeks.

ADVANCE CARE PLANNING AND END-OF-LIFE DECISIONS

When a person is diagnosed with a serious illness, they should prioritize early advance care planning conversations with their family and doctors. Studies have shown that patients who have participated in advance care planning are more likely to be satisfied with their care and have care that is aligned with their wishes.

What Are the Benefits of Hospice Care?

Families of people who received care through a hospice program are more satisfied with end-of-life care than those who did not have hospice services. Also, hospice recipients are more likely to have their pain controlled and less likely to undergo tests or be given medicines they do not need compared with people who do not use hospice care.

WHAT DOES THE HOSPICE SIX-MONTH REQUIREMENT MEAN?

In the United States, people enrolled in Medicare can receive hospice care if their health-care provider thinks they have less than six months to live should the disease take its usual course. Doctors have a hard time predicting how long an older, sick person will live. Health often declines slowly, and some people might need a lot of help with daily living for more than six months before they die.

The person should talk with their doctor if they think a hospice program might be helpful. If he or she agrees but thinks it is too soon for Medicare to cover the services, then the person can investigate how to pay for the services that are needed.

WHAT HAPPENS IF SOMEONE UNDER HOSPICE CARE LIVES LONGER THAN SIX MONTHS?

If the doctor continues to certify that that person is still close to dying, Medicare can continue to pay for hospice services. It is also possible to leave hospice care for a while and then later return if the health-care provider still believes that the patient has less than six months to live.[1]

MYTHS ABOUT PALLIATIVE AND HOSPICE CARE

Do you know the differences between palliative and hospice care? Although these two types of care are similar, they also differ in many ways (see Table 22.1).[2]

Table 22.1. Myths about Palliative and Hospice Care

Palliative Care		Hospice Care	
Specialized medical care for people living with a serious illness		Focusing on the care, comfort, and quality of life of a person with a serious illness who is approaching the end of life	
Myth: When I begin palliative care, I can no longer receive treatment for my disease.	**Fact:** Palliative care can be provided along with curative treatment.	**Myth:** In hospice care, I can't receive any treatments.	**Fact:** People may receive medications to help manage symptoms but not treatments to help cure their illness.
Myth: I can no longer see my primary doctor when I start palliative care.	**Fact:** Palliative care teams work with primary doctors.	**Myth:** Hospice care is only provided in a hospital or hospice facility.	**Fact:** It can be provided at home, in a hospital or nursing home, or in a separate hospice center.

[1] National Institute on Aging (NIA), "What Are Palliative Care and Hospice Care?" National Institutes of Health (NIH), May 14, 2021. Available online. URL: www.nia.nih.gov/health/what-are-palliative-care-and-hospice-care. Accessed July 27, 2023.
[2] National Institute on Aging (NIA), "Four Myths about Palliative and Hospice Care," National Institutes of Health (NIH), April 28, 2023. Available online. URL: www.nia.nih.gov/health/infographics/four-myths-about-palliative-and-hospice-care. Accessed July 27, 2023.

Chapter 23 | Telehealth and Virtual Support at the End of Life

When thinking about health care, most of us conjure up images of office visits or trips to the emergency room (ER). Whether it is for a routine checkup, lab tests, an outpatient procedure, or major surgery, the norm is for patients and caregivers to leave their homes (often sitting in traffic or rushing from work) to meet their doctor at a health-care facility of some kind. But things are changing.

Based on advances in information and communications technologies, medical professionals as well as other "health and care" providers can now offer increasingly robust, remote (from one location to another), and interactive (two-way) services to consumers, patients, and caregivers.

The terms used to describe these broadband-enabled interactions include "telehealth," "telemedicine," and "telecare." All three of these words are often—but not always—used interchangeably. They can also have different meanings depending on who you ask. And that is precisely why you should ask your doctor, your insurance provider, your nurse, or anyone who is part of your health and care universe.

- **Telemedicine.** It can be defined as using telecommunications technologies to support the delivery of all kinds of medical, diagnostic, and treatment-related services, usually by doctors. For example, this includes conducting diagnostic tests, closely monitoring a patient's progress after treatment or therapy, and facilitating access to specialists who are not located in the same place as the patient.

- **Telehealth**. It is similar to telemedicine but includes a wider variety of remote health-care services beyond the doctor-patient relationship. It often involves services provided by nurses, pharmacists, or social workers, for example, who help with patient health education, social support and medication adherence, and troubleshooting health issues for patients and their caregivers.
- **Telecare**. It generally refers to technology that allows consumers to stay safe and independent in their own homes. For example, telecare may include consumer-oriented health and fitness apps, sensors and tools that connect consumers with family members or other caregivers, exercise tracking tools, digital medication reminder systems, or early warning and detection technologies.[1]

WHAT DOES TELEHEALTH MEAN?

Telehealth lets your health-care provider care for you without an in-person office visit. Telehealth is done primarily online with Internet access on your computer, tablet, or smartphone.

There are several options for telehealth care:

- Talk to your health-care provider live over the phone or through video chat.
- Send and receive messages from your health-care provider using secure messaging, email, and secure file exchange.
- Use remote monitoring, so your health-care provider can check on you at home. For example, you might use a device to gather vital signs to help your health-care provider stay informed on your progress.

---

[1] "Telehealth, Telemedicine, and Telecare: What's What?" Federal Communications Commission (FCC), May 2, 2015. Available online. URL: www.fcc.gov/general/telehealth-telemedicine-and-telecare-whats-what. Accessed August 24, 2023.

There are many options to access telehealth if you do not have a stable Internet connection or a device connected to the Internet.

WHAT TYPES OF CARE CAN YOU GET USING TELEHEALTH?

You can get a variety of specialized care through telehealth. Telehealth is especially helpful in monitoring and improving ongoing health issues, such as medication changes or chronic health conditions. Your health-care provider will decide whether telehealth is right for your health needs.

Your health-care provider may also ask you to send information that will help improve your health:

- your weight, blood pressure, blood sugar, or vital information
- images of a wound, or eye, or skin condition
- a diary or document of your symptoms
- medical records that may be filed with another provider, such as x-rays

Health-care providers can send you information to manage your health at home:

- notifications or reminders to do rehabilitation exercises or take medication
- new suggestions for improving diet, mobility, or stress management
- detailed instructions on how to continue your care at home
- encouragement to stick with your treatment plan

BENEFITS OF TELEHEALTH

Virtual visits are growing in popularity. Though in-person office visits may be necessary in certain cases, there are many benefits of telehealth care:

- Limited physical contact reduces the risk of nosocomial infections.
- Virtual visits ensure you get health care wherever you are located—at home, at work, or even in your car.
- Virtual visits cut down on travel, time off from work, and the need for childcare.

- Virtual health-care tools can shorten the wait for an appointment.
- It increases access to specialists who are located far away from your hometown.

Telehealth is not a perfect fit for everyone or every medical condition. Make sure you discuss any disadvantages or risks with your health-care provider.[2]

---

[2] "What Is Telehealth?" U.S. Department of Health and Human Services (HHS), July 27, 2023. Available online. URL: https://telehealth.hhs.gov/patients/understanding-telehealth. Accessed August 24, 2023.

Part 5 | **End-of-Life Caregiving**

Chapter 24 |
Communication in End-of-Life Care

Chapter Contents

Section 24.1 | Communicating End-of-Life Wishes

MAKING DECISIONS FOR SOMEONE AT THE END OF LIFE

If someone close to you or someone you know is dying, you may wonder how you can comfort the person, prevent or ease suffering, and provide the best quality of life (QOL) possible in their remaining time. If the person can no longer communicate, you may be asked to make difficult decisions about their care and comfort. This can be overwhelming for family members, especially if they have not had a chance to discuss the person's wishes ahead of time or if multiple family members are involved and do not agree.

Some people have advance directives in place that outline the care they want if they are unable to speak for themselves. Or they may have communicated their wishes to family members verbally. Even if your loved one has provided written or verbal guidance, some decisions may not be clear, and you may be called upon to make decisions on their behalf.

DECISION-MAKING STRATEGIES

When making choices for someone else, you can consider different decision-making strategies to help determine the best approach for the person:

- **Substituted judgment.** For this approach, you put yourself in the place of the person who is dying and try to choose as they would. Some experts believe that decisions should be based on substituted judgment whenever possible.
- **Best interests.** For this, you determine what you, as their representative, think is best for the dying person. This is sometimes combined with substituted judgment.

If you are making decisions for someone at the end of life and are trying to use one of these approaches, it may be helpful to think about the following questions:

- Has the person ever talked about what they would want at the end of life?

- Has the person ever expressed an opinion about someone else's end-of-life treatment?
- What are their values?
- What gives meaning to their life?

QUESTIONS TO ASK THE HEALTH-CARE TEAM

To make a decision on someone's behalf, you will need as much information as possible from the health-care team. The decisions you are faced with and the questions you may ask can vary depending on whether the person is at home, in a hospital, or in a care facility.

The following are a few questions to consider asking:

- What might we expect to happen in the next few hours, days, or weeks if we continue our current course of treatment?
- Will treatment provide more quality time with family and friends?
- What if we do not want the treatment offered? What happens then?
- When should we begin hospice care? Can they receive this care at home or at the hospital?
- If we begin hospice, will the person be denied certain treatments?
- Which medicines will be given to help manage pain and other symptoms? What are the possible side effects?
- What will happen if our family member stops eating or drinking? Will a feeding tube be considered? What are the benefits and risks?
- If we try using a ventilator to help with breathing and decide to stop, how will that be done?

Understanding and making these decisions can be difficult. Consider having someone with you to take notes and help you remember details. Do not be afraid to ask the doctor or nurse to repeat or rephrase what they said if you are unclear about something they told you. Keep asking questions until you have all the information you need to make a decision.

ADVANCE CARE PLANNING: WHAT DOES YOUR LOVED ONE WANT?

Advance care planning involves sharing and discussing potential decisions about medical care if someone is unable to communicate their wishes. Having meaningful conversations with your loved ones about their preferences is the most important part of advance care planning. A loved one's requests can also be included in advance directives.

For example, a durable power of attorney for health care (DPOAHC) is an advance directive that identifies someone—called a "health-care proxy" (HCP) or a "health-care agent"—to make decisions for a person if they are unable to communicate their wishes themselves. The HCP can decide on care based on the person's values and what they believe the person would want.

Knowing about someone's wishes and having these documents in place can help alleviate the pressure family members and friends may feel if asked to make difficult medical decisions.[1]

Section 24.2 | Enhancing Communication in Cancer Care

Good communication with your family and the health-care team can create a trusting relationship that positively affects many parts of your cancer journey.

The following are the goals of good communication in cancer care:

- Build a trusting relationship with your health-care team.
- Learn from your health-care team about your cancer diagnosis.
- Discuss your options for treatment and care throughout your cancer journey.
- Improve your well-being and quality of life (QOL).

---

[1] National Institute on Aging (NIA), "End-of-Life Care—Providing Care and Comfort," National Institutes of Health (NIH), November 2022. Available online. URL: https://order.nia.nih.gov/sites/default/files/2023-01/end-of-life-older-adults.pdf. Accessed August 29, 2023.

You will face many decisions when you are diagnosed with cancer. Tell your health-care team about concerns you may have during treatment and if you have problems coping with the cancer diagnosis and journey.

Studies show that there are many positive results when people with cancer and their doctors communicate well during cancer care. Positive results include:

- more satisfaction with care
- more likely to follow through with treatment
- better QOL
- reduced anxiety and other symptoms
- more likely to take part in a clinical trial
- improved knowledge of the disease and prognosis
- preferred care, which is received at the end of life

Ask for a patient navigator if you need help communicating with your doctor. A patient navigator can guide you through the health-care system and help you communicate with your health-care team, so you get the information you need to make decisions about your care.

FAMILIES MAY EXPERIENCE COMMUNICATION CHALLENGES

Cancer can be an emotional experience. You may want to hide feelings of distress and sadness and act normal to protect your family and friends. This is also often true for friends and family. Talking about cancer-related issues may help reduce stress for you and your family. Family-focused psychotherapy may also benefit you and your family.

CULTURAL AND DEMOGRAPHIC FACTORS IN COMMUNICATION
People May Have a Preferred Way to Receive Information from Their Health-Care Team

You may ask for written instructions and phone calls, or you may prefer texts and emails. Let your health-care team know how you want to receive information about your cancer and cancer treatment.

Culture Can Also Affect Communication

Some cultures place a greater emphasis on communication with the family as a whole unit, while other cultures focus more on the patient's ability to make their own decisions. Tell your health-care team how much information you want to receive.

Your religious beliefs may be a source of strength and coping for you. Tell your health-care team about any spiritual and religious needs and concerns you want them to know about.

COMMUNICATION IN PEDIATRIC CANCER CARE
Parents Want to Know Their Child's Prognosis

When your child has cancer, you will likely have questions about how serious the cancer is and your child's chances of survival. The likely outcome or course of a disease is called "prognosis." Learning your child's prognosis may be upsetting, but knowing this information can help you and your loved ones make decisions. Your child's doctor is in the best position to talk with you about your child's prognosis if you want to know that information.

Children with Cancer Need Information That Is Right for Their Age

Studies show that children with cancer want to know about their illness and how it will be treated. The amount of information a child may want to know depends in part on their age. Most children worry about how their illness and treatment will affect their daily lives and the people around them. Studies also show that children have less doubt and fear when they are given age-appropriate information about their illness, even if it is bad news.

What Happens to Children When a Loved One is Diagnosed with Cancer?

When a parent has cancer, the child may have high levels of distress. Children may also experience anxiety and distress when they see a sibling going through cancer therapy or dying. Children do better when family members or the health-care team talks with them about what to expect and answers their questions.

ELECTRONIC COMMUNICATION IN CANCER CARE

Many health-care teams reach out to people with cancer using electronic methods. A method of communication that is used frequently in medicine is eHealth. eHealth refers to the "use of digital technology," such as home computers, mobile devices, and the Internet, to seek and communicate health information. eHealth helps:

- promote clear communication among patients, family members, and the health-care team
- enhance shared decision-making
- improve how patients communicate their concerns to the health-care team
- provide social support to patients
- provide clinical trial information[2]

---

[2] "Communication in Cancer Care (PDQ®)—Patient Version," National Cancer Institute (NCI), May 25, 2023. Available online. URL: www.cancer.gov/about-cancer/coping/adjusting-to-cancer/communication-pdq. Accessed August 29, 2023.

Chapter 25 | Long-Distance Caregiving

WHO IS A LONG-DISTANCE CAREGIVER?

Anyone anywhere can be a long-distance caregiver, no matter your gender, income, age, social status, or employment. If you are living an hour or more away from a person who needs your help, you are probably a long-distance caregiver. Anyone who is caring for an aging friend, relative, or parent from afar can be considered a long-distance caregiver.

WHAT CAN A CAREGIVER REALLY DO FROM AFAR?

Long-distance caregivers take on different roles. As a long-distance caregiver, you may:
- help with finances, money management, or bill-paying
- arrange for in-home care—hire professional caregivers or home health or nursing aides and help get needed durable medical equipment
- locate care in an assisted living facility or nursing home (also known as a "skilled nursing facility")
- provide emotional support and occasional respite care for a primary caregiver (the person who takes on most of the everyday caregiving responsibilities)
- serve as an information coordinator—research health problems or medicines, help navigate through a maze of new needs, and clarify insurance benefits and claims
- keep family and friends updated and informed
- create a plan and get the paperwork in order in case of an emergency

- evaluate the house and make sure it is safe for the older person's needs

Over time, as your family member's needs change, so will your role as a long-distance caregiver.

FIRST STEP FOR NEW LONG-DISTANCE CAREGIVERS

To get started, do the following:
- Ask the primary caregiver, if there is one, and the care recipient how you can be most helpful.
- Talk to friends who are caregivers to see if they have suggestions about ways to help.
- Find out more about local resources that might be useful.
- Develop a good understanding of the person's health issues and other needs.
- Visit as often as you can. (You might not only notice something that needs to be done and can be taken care of from a distance, but you can also relieve a primary caregiver for a short time.)

Many of us do not automatically have a lot of caregiver skills. Information about training opportunities is available. Some local chapters of the American Red Cross might offer courses, as do some nonprofit organizations focused on caregiving. Medicare and Medicaid will sometimes pay for this training.

WHAT DO CAREGIVERS NEED TO KNOW ABOUT THEIR FAMILY MEMBER'S HEALTH?

Learn as much as you can about your family member's condition and any treatment. This can help you understand what is going on, anticipate the course of an illness, prevent crises, and assist in health-care management. It can also make talking with the doctor easier.

Get written permission, as needed under the Health Insurance Portability and Accountability Act of 1996 (HIPAA) Privacy Rule, to receive medical and financial information. To the extent possible, the family member with permission should be the one to talk with all health-care providers. Try putting together a notebook, on paper or online, that includes all the vital information about medical care, social services, contact numbers, financial issues, and so on. Make copies for other caregivers and keep them up to date.

MAKING THE MOST OUT OF VISITS WITH AGING PARENTS OR RELATIVES

Talk to the care recipient ahead of time and find out what he or she would like to do during your visit. Also, check with the primary caregiver, if appropriate, to learn what he or she needs, such as handling some caregiving responsibilities while you are in town. This may help you set clear-cut and realistic goals for the visit. Decide on the priorities and leave other tasks to another visit.

Remember to actually spend time visiting with your family members. Try to make time to do things unrelated to being a caregiver, such as watching a movie, playing a game, or taking a drive. Finding time to do something simple and relaxing can help everyone—it can be fun and build family memories. And try to let outside distractions wait until you are home again.

HOW CAN YOU STAY CONNECTED WITH AN AGING PARENT OR RELATIVE FROM AFAR?

Try to find people who live near your loved one and can provide a realistic view of what is going on. This may be your other parent. A social worker may be able to provide updates and help with making decisions.

Do not underestimate the value of a phone and email contact list. It is a simple way to keep everyone updated on your parents' needs.

You may also want to give the person you care for a cell phone (and make sure he or she knows how to use it). Or, if your family member lives in a nursing home, consider having a private phone line installed in his or her room. Program telephone numbers of doctors, friends, family members, and yourself into the phone and perhaps provide a list of the speed-dial numbers to keep with the phone. Such simple strategies can be a lifeline. But try to be prepared should you find yourself inundated with calls from your parents.[1]

Long-distance caregiving presents unique challenges. If you find yourself in a long-distance caregiving role, here is a summary of things to keep in mind.

KNOW WHAT YOU NEED TO KNOW AS A LONG-DISTANCE CAREGIVER

Experienced caregivers recommend that you learn as much as you can about your family member or friend's illness, medicines, and resources that might be available. Make sure at least one family member has written permission to receive medical and financial information. To the extent possible, one family member should handle conversations with all health-care providers. Try putting all the vital information in one place—perhaps in a notebook or in a shared, secure online document. This includes all the important information about medical care, social services, contact numbers, financial issues, and so on. Make copies for other caregivers and keep the information up to date.

PLAN YOUR VISITS WITH AN AGING PARENT OR RELATIVE

When visiting your loved one, you may feel that there is just too much to do in the time that you have. You can get more done and feel less stressed by talking to your family member or friend ahead of time and finding out what he or she would like to do. Also, check with the primary caregiver, if appropriate, to learn what he or she needs, such as handling some caregiving responsibilities while you are in town. This may help you set clear-cut and realistic goals for the visit. For instance, does your mother need to get some new winter clothes or visit another family member? Could your father

---

[1] National Institute on Aging (NIA), "Getting Started with Long-Distance Caregiving," National Institutes of Health (NIH), May 2, 2017. Available online. URL: www.nia.nih.gov/health/getting-started-long-distance-caregiving. Accessed August 22, 2023.

use help in fixing things around the house? Would you like to talk to your mother's physician? Decide on the priorities and leave other tasks for another visit.

ACTIVITIES TO DO WHEN VISITING AN AGING PARENT OR RELATIVE

Try to make time to do things unrelated to being a caregiver. Maybe you could find a movie to watch with your relatives or plan a visit with old friends or other family members. Perhaps they would like to attend worship services. Offer to play a game of cards or a board game. Take a drive or go to the library together. Finding a little bit of time to do something simple and relaxing can help everyone, and it builds more family memories. And keep in mind that your friend or relative is the focus of your trip—try to let outside distractions wait until you are home again.

ORGANIZE PAPERWORK FOR AN AGING PARENT

Organizing paperwork is one way that a long-distance caregiver can be a big help. An important part of effective caregiving depends on keeping a great deal of information in order and up to date. Often, long-distance caregivers will need access to a parent or relative's personal, health, financial, and legal records.

Getting all this material together is a lot of work at first, and from afar, it can seem even more challenging. But, once you have gathered everything together, many other caregiving tasks will be easier. Maintaining current information about your parent's health and medical care, as well as finances, homeownership, and other legal issues, lets you get a handle on what is going on and allows you to respond more quickly if there is a crisis.

As you are getting started, try to focus on gathering the essentials first and fill in the blanks as you go along. Talk with the older person and the primary caregiver about any missing information or documentation and how you might help organize the records. It is also a good idea to make sure that all financial matters, including wills and life insurance policies, are in order. It will also help if someone has a durable power of attorney (the legal document naming one person to handle financial and property issues for another).

241

Your family member or friend may be reluctant to share personal information with you. Explain that you are not trying to invade their privacy or take over their personal lives—you are only trying to assemble what will be needed in the event of an emergency. Assure them that you will respect their privacy and then keep your promise. If they are still uncomfortable, ask if they would be willing to work with an attorney (some lawyers specialize in elder affairs) or perhaps with another trusted family member or friend.[2]

---

[2] National Institute on Aging (NIA), "Eight Tips for Long-Distance Caregiving," National Institutes of Health (NIH), May 16, 2017. Available online. URL: www.nia.nih.gov/health/eight-tips-long-distance-caregiving. Accessed August 22, 2023.

Chapter 26 | Self-Care for Caregivers

Chapter Contents

Section 26.1 | Shared Caregiving within Families

Caring for an older family member often requires teamwork. While one sibling might be local and take on most of the everyday caregiving responsibilities, a long-distance caregiver can also have an important role. As a long-distance caregiver, you can provide important respite to the primary caregiver and support to the aging family member.

TALK ABOUT CAREGIVING RESPONSIBILITIES

First, try to define the caregiving responsibilities. You could start by setting up a family meeting and, if it makes sense, include the care recipient in the discussion. This is best done when there is not an emergency. A calm conversation about what kind of care is wanted and needed now and what might be needed in the future can help avoid a lot of confusion.

Decide who will be responsible for which tasks. Many families find the best first step is to name a primary caregiver, even if one is not needed immediately. That way, the primary caregiver can step in if there is a crisis.

Agree in advance on how each of your efforts can complement one another so that you can be an effective team. Ideally, each of you will be able to take on tasks best suited to your skills or interests.

CONSIDER YOUR STRENGTHS WHEN SHARING CAREGIVING RESPONSIBILITIES

When thinking about who should be responsible for what, start with your strengths. Consider what you are particularly good at and how those skills might help in the current situation:

- Are you good at finding information, keeping people up to date on changing conditions, and offering cheer, whether on the phone or online?
- Are you good at supervising and leading others?
- Are you comfortable speaking with medical staff and interpreting what they say to others?

- Is your strongest suit doing the numbers—paying bills, keeping track of bank statements, and reviewing insurance policies and reimbursement reports?
- Are you the one in the family who can fix anything, while no one else knows the difference between pliers and a wrench?

CONSIDER YOUR LIMITS WHEN SHARING CAREGIVING RESPONSIBILITIES

When thinking about who should be responsible for what, consider your limits. Ask yourself the following questions:
- How often, both mentally and financially, can you afford to travel?
- Are you emotionally prepared to take on what may feel like a reversal of roles between you and your parents—taking care of your parent instead of your parents taking care of you? Can you continue to respect your parent's independence?
- Can you be both calm and assertive when communicating from a distance?
- How will your decision to take on caregiving responsibilities affect your work and home life?

Be realistic about how much you can do and what you are willing to do. Think about your schedule and how it might be adapted to give respite to a primary caregiver. For example, you might try to coordinate holiday and vacation times. Remember that over time, responsibilities may need to be revised to reflect changes in the situation, your care recipient's needs, and each family member's abilities and limitations.

HOW TO SUPPORT A LOCAL CAREGIVER FROM AFAR

A spouse or the sibling who lives closest to an aging parent often becomes the primary caregiver. Long-distance caregivers can help by providing emotional support and occasional respite to the primary caregiver. Ask the primary caregiver what you can do to help.

Staying in contact with your parents by phone or email might also take some pressure off your parents or siblings. Just listening may not sound like much help, but often it is.

Long-distance caregivers can also play a part in arranging for professional caregivers, hiring home health and nursing aides, or locating care in an assisted living facility or nursing home (also known as a "skilled nursing facility").

Long-distance caregivers may find they can be helpful by handling things online—for example, researching health problems or medicines, paying bills, or keeping family and friends updated. Some long-distance caregivers help a parent pay for care; others step in to manage finances.

HOW TO HELP A PARENT WHO IS THE PRIMARY CAREGIVER

A primary caregiver—especially a spouse—may be hesitant to ask for help or a break. Be sure to acknowledge how important the caregiver has been for the care recipient. Also, discuss the physical and emotional effects caregiving can have on people. Although caregiving can be satisfying, it can also be very hard work.

Offer to arrange for respite care. Respite care will give your parents a break from caregiving responsibilities. It can be arranged for an afternoon or for several days. Care can be provided in the family home through an adult day services program or at a skilled nursing facility.

The Access to Respite Care and Help (ARCH) National Respite Locator Service can help you find services in your parents' community. You might suggest contacting the Well Spouse Association. It offers support to the wives, husbands, and partners of chronically ill or disabled people and has a nationwide listing of local support groups.

Your parents may need more help from home-based care to continue to live in their own homes. Some people find it hard to have paid caregivers in the house, but most also say that the assistance is invaluable. If the primary caregiver is reluctant, point out that with an in-home aide, he or she may have more energy to devote to caregiving and some time for himself/herself. Suggest him/her to try it for a short time and then decide.

In time, the person receiving care may have to move to assisted living or a nursing home. If that happens, the primary caregiver will need your support. You can help select a facility. The primary caregiver may need help adjusting to the person's absence or to living alone at home. Just listening may not sound like much help, but often it is.[1]

Section 26.2 | Tips for Caregiver Self-Care

Being a caregiver to a patient is an important and challenging role. Caregivers are so often focused on the medical, physical, and emotional needs of their loved ones—they forget to care for themselves. But, caregivers, your health and wellness are important, too.

It is time to make caregiver self-care a priority. Doing so can help you as a caregiver manage your needs in a healthy way to avoid stress, burnout, sickness, and fatigue. It will also ensure you find a good balance between caring for your loved one and yourself.

Here are our self-care tips for caregivers of patients with a brain or spine tumor. We encourage you to follow the following tips to stay healthy:

- **Schedule self-care time**. Make time to focus on your needs each day or week. Make it a priority by scheduling a recurring one-hour appointment with yourself. Your self-care time should include an activity you enjoy or an event that provides comfort: exercise, go shopping, meditate, have coffee with a friend, or take a nap. The scheduled time will rejuvenate you and help you make your physical and mental health a priority. Your loved one needs you healthy, too.
  - For any of the activities that you incorporate into a consistent routine, make sure you stay in the

[1] National Institute on Aging (NIA), "How to Share Caregiving Responsibilities with Family Members," National Institutes of Health (NIH), May 9, 2017. Available online. URL: www.nia.nih.gov/health/how-share-caregiving-responsibilities-family-members. Accessed August 14, 2023.

moment and enjoy yourself. You can think about anything you need to get done after you have taken this time for yourself.

- **Write down your positive qualities**. Show yourself self-love by writing down the qualities that make you a great caregiver and a person. This can help build your self-esteem and help you stay motivated. The following is an activity to try:
  - Write the letters of the alphabet. Find one positive quality about yourself for each letter. Write it next to the letter. Keep this list handy and refer to it when you need a mental boost.
- **Make a self-care emergency plan**. Having a plan can help you when you feel overwhelmed. In these moments, it can be difficult to think of things to do for yourself. The plan keeps you ready with a list of things you can do to stay calm and in control of how you feel. You can also include things to avoid that might make you feel worse. And keep this plan in a place where you see it consistently. Your plan should include the following:
  - **A list of activities that help you relax**. Take a 30-minute walk or meditate for 10 minutes. Include activities that boost your mood and tips to remind you to stay calm and in the moment. And remember to breathe.
  - **A list of people to reach out to for help or support**. It can include a friend or loved one who can provide comfort or distraction or groups to attend to meet other caregivers.
  - **Positive messages to say to yourself**. This helps keep you motivated.

Caregivers, remember that your health and wellness are as important as your loved one. And your loved one wants and needs you healthy, too. So you should take care of yourself today and every day.[2]

---

[2] "3 Tips for Caregiver Self-Care," National Cancer Institute (NCI), February 8, 2019. Available online. URL: www.cancer.gov/rare-brain-spine-tumor/blog/2019/caregiver-tips. Accessed August 4, 2023.

TAKE CARE OF YOURSELF AS A CAREGIVER

Caregiving can be rewarding, but it is also challenging. Taking time for yourself can make you a better caregiver. You may have to do the following:

- Make time for a hobby you enjoy.
- Go to sleep a half hour earlier.
- Take a short walk outside.
- Try a yoga class.
- Meet a friend for lunch.
- Join a support group.

Give yourself credit for everything you are doing. Ask for help when you need it. Your caregiving makes a big difference in someone else's life.[3]

Section 26.3 | Coping with Caregiving Challenges

Caregiving can be a labor of love and sometimes a job of necessity. These often-unsung heroes provide hours of assistance to others, yet the stress and strain of caregiving can take a toll on their own health. Researchers funded by the National Institutes of Health (NIH) are working to understand the risks these caregivers face. And scientists are seeking better ways to protect caregivers' health.

Many of us will end up becoming a caregiver at some point in our lives. Chances are we will be helping out older family members who cannot fully care for themselves. Such caregiving can include everyday tasks, such as helping with meals, schedules, and bathing and dressing. It can also include managing medicines, doctor visits, health insurance, and money. Caregivers often give emotional support as well.

---

[3] National Institute on Aging (NIA), "Take Care of Yourself as a Caregiver," National Institutes of Health (NIH), November 9, 2016. Available online. URL: www.nia.nih.gov/health/infographics/take-care-yourself-caregiver. Accessed August 4, 2023.

People who provide unpaid care for an elderly, ill, or disabled family member or friend in the home are called "informal caregivers." Most are middle-aged. Roughly two-thirds are women. Nearly half of informal caregivers assist someone who is aged 75 or older. As the elderly population continues to grow nationwide, so will the need for informal caregivers.

Studies have shown that some people can thrive when caring for others. Caregiving may help strengthen connections to a loved one. Some find joy or fulfillment in looking after others. But, for many, the strain of caregiving can become overwhelming. Friends and family often take on the caregiving role without any training. They are expected to meet many complex demands without much help. Most caregivers hold down a full-time job in addition to the hours of unpaid help they give to someone else.

"With all of its rewards, there is a substantial cost to caregiving—financially, physically, and emotionally," says Dr. Richard J. Hodes, director of the National Institute on Aging (NIA) of NIH. "One important insight from our research is that because of the stress and time demands placed on caregivers, they are less likely to find time to address their own health problems."

Informal caregivers, for example, may be less likely to fill a needed prescription for themselves or get a screening test for breast cancer. "Caregivers also tend to report lower levels of physical activity, poorer nutrition, and poorer sleep or sleep disturbance," says Dr. Erin Kent, an NIH expert on cancer caregiving.

Studies have linked informal caregiving to a variety of long-term health problems. Caregivers are more likely to have heart disease, cancer, diabetes, arthritis, and excess weight. Caregivers are also at risk for depression or anxiety. And they are more likely to have problems with memory and paying attention.

"Caregivers may even suffer from physical health problems related to caregiving tasks, such as back or muscle injuries from lifting patients," Dr. Kent adds.

Caregivers may face different challenges and risks depending on the health of the person they are caring for. Taking care of loved ones with cancer or dementia can be especially demanding. Research suggests that these caregivers bear greater levels of physical and mental burdens than caregivers of the frail elderly or people with diabetes.

"Cancer caregivers often spend more hours per day providing more intensive care over a shorter period of time," Dr. Kent says. "The health of cancer patients can deteriorate quickly, which can cause heightened stress for caregivers. And, aggressive cancer treatments can leave patients greatly weakened. They may need extra care, and their medications may need to be monitored more often."

Cancer survivorship, too, can bring intense levels of uncertainty and anxiety. "A hallmark of cancer is that it may return months or even years later," Dr. Kent says. "Both cancer survivors and their caregivers may struggle to live with ongoing fear and stress of a cancer recurrence."

Dementia can also create unique challenges for caregivers. The health-care costs alone can take an enormous toll. A study found that out-of-pocket spending for families of dementia patients during the past five years of life averaged $61,522, which was 81 percent higher than for older people who died from other causes.

Research has found that caregivers for people with dementia have particularly high levels of potentially harmful stress hormones. Caregivers and care recipients often struggle with problems related to dementia, such as agitation, aggression, trouble sleeping, wandering, and confusion. These caregivers spend more days sick with an infectious disease, have a weaker immune response to the flu vaccine, and have slower wound healing.

One major successful and expanding effort to help ease caregiver stress is known as "Resources for Enhancing Alzheimer Caregiver Health" (REACH). Nearly a decade ago, researchers funded by the NIH showed that a supportive, educational program for dementia caregivers could greatly improve their quality of life (QOL) and reduce rates of clinical depression. As part of the program, trained staff connected with caregivers over six months by making several home visits, telephone calls, and structured telephone support sessions.

"REACH showed that what caregivers need is support. They need to know that there are people out there and resources available to help them," says Dr. John Haaga, who oversees the NIH's behavioral and social research related to aging.

The REACH program is now being more widely employed. It has been adapted for use in free community-based programs, such as in local area agencies on aging (AAA). It is also being used by the U.S. Department of Veterans Affairs (VA) and by the Indian Health Service (IHS) in collaboration with the Administration for Community Living (ACL).

"We know how to support families caring for an older adult. But that knowledge is not easily accessible to the families who need it," says Dr. Laura Gitlin, a coauthor of the REACH study and an expert on caregiving and aging at Johns Hopkins University. "Caregivers need to know it is not only acceptable but recommended that they find time to care for themselves. They should consider joining a caregiver's support group, taking breaks each day, and keeping up with their own hobbies and interests."[4]

---

[4] *NIH News in Health*, "Coping with Caregiving," National Institutes of Health (NIH), December 2015. Available online. URL: https://newsinhealth.nih.gov/2015/12/coping-caregiving. Accessed August 14, 2023.

Chapter 27 | **Preparing for the Inevitable**

What to do after someone dies depends on where the person died. If someone dies at home, there is no need to move the body right away. If the person was in hospice, a plan for what happens after death would likely already be in place. If the person was not in hospice, talk with the doctor, local medical examiner (coroner), local health department, or a funeral home representative about how to proceed. You might want to have someone make sure the body is lying flat before the joints become stiff. This rigor mortis begins sometime during the first few hours after death.

When a loved one passes, some people want to stay in the room with the body; others prefer to leave. Some families want time to sit quietly with the body, console each other, and maybe share memories. This is the time for any special religious, ethnic, or cultural customs that are performed soon after death.

If your loved one died in a facility, such as a hospital or nursing home, discuss any important customs or rituals with the staff early on, if possible. You could ask a member of your religious community or a spiritual counselor to come. If you have a list of people to notify, this is the time to call those who might want to come and see the body before it is moved.

COPING WITH LOSS

When your spouse or loved one dies, your entire world may change. You may feel a variety of different emotions, such as anger, guilt, or sadness. Remember that everyone grieves differently, and there is no sole right way to grieve. You may find that surrounding yourself with loved ones, joining a support group, or talking to a professional may help you cope with loss.

GET A LEGAL PRONOUNCEMENT OF DEATH

As soon as possible, the death must be officially pronounced by someone in authority, such as a doctor in a hospital or nursing facility or a hospice nurse. This person also fills out the forms certifying the cause, time, and place of death. These steps will make it possible for an official death certificate to be prepared. This legal form is necessary for many reasons, including life insurance and financial and property issues.

MAKE ARRANGEMENTS FOR AFTER DEATH

If the person was in hospice, a plan for what happens after death would already be in place. If death happens at home without hospice, try to talk with the doctor, local medical examiner (coroner), local health department, or a funeral home representative in advance about how to proceed. You can also consider a home funeral, which is legal in most states.

Arrangements should be made to pick up the body as soon as the family is ready and according to local laws. This can be done by a funeral home or by the family themselves in most states. The hospital or nursing facility, if that is where the death took place, may help with these arrangements. If at home, you will need to contact the funeral home directly, make arrangements yourself, or ask a friend or family member to do that for you.

The doctor may ask if you want an autopsy. This is a medical procedure conducted by a specially trained physician to learn more about what caused the death. For example, if the person who died was believed to have Alzheimer disease (AD), a brain autopsy will allow for a definitive diagnosis. If your religion or culture objects to autopsies, talk to the doctor. Some people planning a funeral with a viewing worry about having an autopsy, but the physical signs of an autopsy are usually hidden by clothing and other body preparation techniques.

WHAT TO DO WITHIN A FEW WEEKS OF DEATH

Over the next few weeks, you may want to notify a few places about your loved one's death. This may include the following:

- **Social Security Administration (SSA).** If the deceased was receiving Social Security benefits, you need to stop the checks.
- **Life insurance companies.** You will need a death certificate and policy numbers to make claims on any policies.
- **Credit agencies.** To prevent identity theft, you will want to send copies of the death certificate to three major firms: Equifax, Experian, and TransUnion.
- **Banks and financial institutions.** If your loved one left a list of accounts and passwords, it will be much easier to close or change accounts. You will need a copy of the death certificate if the person did not leave a list.

WHAT ABOUT ORGAN AND BRAIN DONATION?

At some time before death or right after it, the doctor may ask about donating organs such as the heart, lungs, pancreas, kidneys, cornea, liver, and skin. Organ donation allows healthy organs from someone who died to be transplanted into living people who need them. People of any age can be organ donors.

The person who is dying may have already said that he or she would like to be an organ donor. Some states list this information on the driver's license. If not, the decision has to be made quickly. There is no cost to the donor's family for this gift of life. If the person has requested a do-not-resuscitate (DNR) order but wants to donate organs, he or she might have to indicate that the desire to donate supersedes the DNR. That is because it might be necessary to use machines to keep the heart beating until the medical staff is ready to remove the donated organs.

Brain donation is a separate process, and registering as an organ donor does not mean you are choosing to donate your brain. If the person is registered as a brain donor, their point of contact will need to be notified within two hours after death.[1]

[1] National Institute on Aging (NIA), "What to Do after Someone Dies," National Institutes of Health (NIH), November 17, 2022. Available online. URL: www.nia.nih.gov/health/what-do-after-someone-dies. Accessed July 27, 2023.

Part 6 | Death and Children: A Guide for Parents and Caregivers

Chapter 28 | **Stillbirth, Miscarriage, and Infant Death**

Chapter Contents

Section 28.1 | Understanding Stillbirth

WHAT IS STILLBIRTH?

In the United States, stillbirth refers to the death of a fetus at or after the 20th week of pregnancy. The death of a fetus before the 20th week of pregnancy is usually called a "miscarriage" or "pregnancy loss."

Stillbirths can occur in the following instances:

- **In the womb, before labor begins.** This kind of stillbirth is also called an "antepartum stillbirth." In the United States, slightly more than one-half of all stillbirths occur before the start of labor. Researchers may further categorize stillbirths into early (20–27 weeks of pregnancy) and late (28–36 weeks of pregnancy).
- **During labor and delivery.** These deaths may be called "preterm stillbirths" (occurring before 37 weeks of pregnancy) or "term" or "intrapartum stillbirths" (occurring at 37 weeks of pregnancy or later). The causes of stillbirths during labor and delivery tend to be different from the causes of stillbirths before labor.

Some of the risk factors that can lead to stillbirth can also lead to a baby's death just after birth.

HOW COMMON IS STILLBIRTH?

Because of improvements in prenatal care, labor and delivery practices, and other factors, the rate of stillbirths in the United States has been dropping since the Centers for Disease Control and Prevention (CDC) began collecting data in 1950. However, rates have leveled off in recent years. Nonetheless, the rate of early stillbirth decreased by 3 percent in 2020 over 2019. The rate of late stillbirth was relatively unchanged from 2019.

Different countries and regions of the world have different stillbirth definitions, rates, and characteristics. The World Health Organization (WHO) defines stillbirth as fetal deaths at or after

28 weeks of pregnancy but before or during birth. Using this definition, the WHO estimates that there are more than 2 million stillbirths worldwide each year; about 40 percent of those occur before labor.

WHAT ARE THE RISK FACTORS FOR STILLBIRTH?

Stillbirth can happen in any pregnancy. Even after an autopsy and other tests, the cause of stillbirth may not be known.

Research shows that some factors increase the risk for stillbirth among U.S. women, while other factors may increase the risk among women worldwide. Here, we focus on U.S. risk factors. Many of these factors are not changeable, meaning there is nothing the pregnant woman, her family, or her health-care provider can do to prevent the stillbirth.

Despite some known risk factors, most U.S. stillbirths occur in pregnant people who do not have any risk factors.

Risks for Stillbirth in the United States

Studies have found several factors that increase the risk for stillbirths among pregnant people in the United States. However, these factors do not cause stillbirths; they only increase the chances that one will occur.

FEATURES OF THE PREGNANT PERSON OR THE PREGNANCY

- low socioeconomic status
- age 35 years or older
- tobacco, marijuana, or alcohol use during or just before pregnancy
- exposure to secondhand smoke during pregnancy
- illegal drug use before or during pregnancy
- Black/African-American race/ethnicity
- certain medical conditions or diseases, such as diabetes or high blood pressure (HBP) before pregnancy and some infections
- having overweight or obesity
- never having given birth before

- previous pregnancy loss, miscarriage, or stillbirth
- previous low birth weight or small infant for the stage of pregnancy, called "small for gestational age" (SGA)
- pregnancy with twins, triplets, or other multiples
- using assisted reproductive technology
- stressful life events, such as major financial, emotional, traumatic, or partner-related events, in the year before pregnancy
- environmental exposures, including pollution and high temperatures

FEATURES OF THE FETUS

For the fetus, one known risk factor for stillbirth is small size, sometimes called "SGA." SGA can result from growth restriction, a condition in which the fetus does not grow as quickly or as well as it should because of a problem with the pregnancy.

WHAT ARE POSSIBLE CAUSES OF STILLBIRTH?

Researchers have identified several possible causes of or contributors to stillbirth. However, in many stillbirths, the cause remains unknown even after extensive testing.

Beginning in 2003, the *Eunice Kennedy Shriver* National Institute of Child Health and Human Development (NICHD) supported the Stillbirth Collaborative Research Network (SCRN) to learn more about the possible causes of and contributors to stillbirth. This first-of-its-kind resource examined more than 500 stillbirths at 59 medical centers around the United States over five years. In almost one-quarter of these cases, the researchers could not determine a probable or even a possible cause of death. Also, many of the stillbirths had more than one likely cause.

Although analyses of data from the SCRN continue, the research identified the following possible causes of stillbirth in the United States, in order from most to least common:

- **Pregnancy and labor complications**. These include preterm labor, pregnancy with twins or triplets, and the separation of the placenta, which provides oxygen and nutrition to the fetus from the womb (also called "placental abruption"). These were more common causes of stillbirths before 24 weeks of pregnancy.

- **Problems with the placenta.** Placental problems, such as insufficient blood flow, were the leading causes of stillbirths in the womb, usually after 24 weeks of pregnancy.
- **Fetal genetic problems and birth defects.** In defects such as the neural tube defect anencephaly, most or all of the fetal brain and skull fail to develop.
- **Infection in the pregnant person, womb, placenta, or fetus.** Stillbirths from *Escherichia coli*, group B streptococcus, and enterococcus were most common. Infection-related stillbirths were more common before 24 weeks of pregnancy.
- **Problems with the umbilical cord.** Umbilical cord problems, such as when it gets knotted or squeezed, cutting off oxygen to the fetus, were more likely to cause term stillbirths and those during labor and delivery.
- **HBP disorders.** Disorders such as chronic HBP before pregnancy and preeclampsia were more common causes of late stillbirths and term stillbirths than early stillbirths.
- **Medical problems in the pregnant person.** Certain medical problems, such as diabetes, before pregnancy can also be causes of stillbirth.

RACIAL DISPARITIES IN STILLBIRTH

In the United States, stillbirths are more than twice as likely among Black women than among White women. However, the reasons for this disparity are not entirely clear.

The SCRN study found that the most common causes of stillbirth were different for Black women than for White women and for Hispanic women. For non-Hispanic Black women in the SCRN, stillbirths were more likely to be caused by infection or by complications of pregnancy and labor. Also, the timing of stillbirth in Black women was different than that of White and Hispanic women: Stillbirths were more likely during labor and delivery and early (before 24 weeks) in pregnancy for non-Hispanic Black women.

As mentioned previously, SCRN research found that the risk for stillbirth was higher among women who had experienced major financial, emotional, traumatic, or partner-related events in the year before delivery. Black women were more likely than women in general to have experienced at least three such stressful events in the past year, which could help explain some of the disparity. However, it is more likely that the higher number of stillbirths among non-Hispanic Black women results from a combination of risk factors and causes.

HOW IS STILLBIRTH DIAGNOSED?

Before delivery, the only way to diagnose a stillbirth is to determine if the fetus' heart is beating. Providers often use ultrasound, a type of imaging that projects harmless sound waves through the pregnant person's body to create an image, to look for the fetal heartbeat.

After labor and delivery, caregivers look for the following signs of life:

- breathing
- heartbeat
- pulsations in the umbilical cord
- voluntary movements

If one or more of these signs are not present, life-saving measures will be taken, such as neonatal resuscitation methods. If these measures are not successful, the situation may be diagnosed as a stillbirth.

Fetal Movement Monitoring

In some cases, health-care providers may recommend that pregnant people keep track of feelings of fetal movements or kicks. It is important to note, however, that the absence of feelings of fetal movement does not mean stillbirth has occurred in all cases.

In some first-time pregnancies, for example, movement is difficult to detect.

The Count the Kicks campaign aims to raise awareness about fetal movement and possible prevention of stillbirth. They offer an app, educational information, and data for providers about counting fetal kicks and movements.

HOW DO HEALTH-CARE PROVIDERS MANAGE STILLBIRTH?

Care after a stillbirth depends on when it occurs.

If a stillbirth occurs in the womb, then the fetus and the placenta need to be removed or delivered. If it occurs during labor or delivery, then the placenta will still need to be removed or delivered.

Health-care providers will then try to determine a cause for the stillbirth by examining the fetus, the placenta, and other tissues from the pregnancy and possibly by performing an autopsy.

At the same time, providers will offer support to help the family cope with their loss.

When or if the family wants to try for another pregnancy, providers can work with them to discuss any risk factors and possible ways to prevent another stillbirth.

Learn more about each aspect of managing a stillbirth.

Delivering the Fetus

If the stillbirth occurs in the womb, the next step is to deliver it and the placenta. This delivery does not always have to happen right away. Some parents might take time to cope or to make arrangements. Others might prefer to complete the process as soon as possible.

Health-care providers usually use one of the following methods to deliver the fetus and placenta:

- **Induction**. Providers give the pregnant person medicine to start labor. Then they rupture the pregnancy membranes and proceed with regular labor and delivery. This method is used more often later in pregnancy.
- **Dilation and evacuation**. In this procedure, providers first give the pregnant person medicine to help

the cervix open or dilate. Once the cervix is open, providers give medicine to numb the birth canal and uterus. Then they surgically remove the fetus, the placenta, and other pregnancy material by inserting instruments through the vagina and cervix into the womb. Dilation and evacuation is only an option in the second trimester.

Removing the placenta once the fetus is removed or delivered is an important part of all pregnancies. The placenta provides for the transfer of oxygen and nutrients through blood. If it is not removed or is only partially removed after the pregnancy has ended, the risk for life-threatening problems, such as hemorrhage or sepsis, is very high.

Examining the Fetus

Providers will try to figure out a cause for the stillbirth, if possible. According to the American College of Obstetricians and Gynecologists (ACOG), knowing a cause can provide some closure to families, and it can help identify risks that might affect future pregnancies.

Health-care providers might examine a stillbirth in one of the following ways:

- **Inspecting the exterior of the fetus, placenta, and other tissues.** This examination can reveal problems, such as a knot in the umbilical cord or a problem with the development of the placenta, that could have caused or contributed to the death. The exam may include weighing and measuring the fetus and placenta and getting recordings or photographs to put in the medical record or to show to a specialist.
- **Examining individual cells and genetic material.** With parents' permission, providers may take tissue and fluid samples and send them to a lab for analysis. These tests may identify problems with cells, chromosomal or genetic abnormalities, or infection as a possible cause of the stillbirth.

- **Performing an autopsy.** With parents' permission, providers may do an autopsy. An autopsy involves examining the fetus to look for problems with the brain, heart, or other organs.

If an autopsy is not performed, x-rays or other types of imaging may be done to show the inside of the body and help find the cause of death.

Coping with Grief

Experiencing a stillbirth can be devastating for a pregnant person and their family. Getting support from providers, counselors, friends, and family is important for the healing process. People handle loss differently, and there are many ways to support someone through a stillbirth.

Managing Risk Factors

Managing factors to reduce the risk of future stillbirth is challenging. In some cases, no known risk factors are present when a stillbirth occurs, or the risk factors are not changeable. In other cases, no cause may be identified, or the cause may have been spontaneous.

Families that have experienced a stillbirth should work with health-care providers to identify and address any changeable risk factors before trying for another pregnancy. The families may also want to consult genetic counselors and others who may be able to provide additional insights.[1]

[1] "Stillbirth," *Eunice Kennedy Shriver* National Institute of Child Health and Human Development (NICHD), August 25, 2023. Available online. URL: www.nichd.nih.gov/health/topics/stillbirth. Accessed September 19, 2023.

Section 28.2 | **Pregnancy Loss**

Pregnancy loss is the unexpected loss of a fetus before the 20th week of pregnancy. It is sometimes called "miscarriage," "early pregnancy loss," "midtrimester pregnancy loss," "fetal demise," or "spontaneous abortion."

Health-care providers use a different term—stillbirth—to describe the loss of a fetus after 20 weeks of pregnancy.

Pregnancy loss may occur so early that a woman may not know she is pregnant.

Researchers can only estimate the number of women who experience pregnancy loss because some losses occur before a woman's pregnancy is confirmed by a health-care provider or pregnancy test. But the American College of Obstetricians and Gynecologists (ACOG) estimates that early pregnancy loss is common, occurring in about 10 percent of confirmed pregnancies.

WHAT ARE THE SYMPTOMS OF PREGNANCY LOSS (BEFORE 20 WEEKS OF PREGNANCY)?

Symptoms of pregnancy loss may include the following:
- bleeding from the vagina
- pain or cramps in the lower stomach area (abdomen)
- low back pain
- fluid, tissue, or clot-like material coming out of the vagina

However, bleeding from the vagina during pregnancy does not always mean a miscarriage. Many pregnant women have spotting and cramping in early pregnancy but do not miscarry. Your health-care provider might call this pregnancy "threatened." In any case, pregnant women who have any of the symptoms of miscarriage should contact their health-care provider immediately.

Some women do not experience any symptoms of pregnancy loss.

Although this is rare in the United States, some women who have a miscarriage may get an infection in the uterus, which can be life-threatening. Women who have the following symptoms for more than 24 hours should call 911:

- a fever higher than 100.4 °F (38 °C) on more than two occasions
- severe pain in the lower abdomen
- bloody discharge from the vagina (which can include pus and be foul smelling)

Recent research has also found that morning sickness—nausea and vomiting during pregnancy—is linked to a lower risk of pregnancy loss. The *Eunice Kennedy Shriver* National Institute of Child Health and Human Development (NICHD) researchers are continuing to look for other factors that may indicate a lower risk of pregnancy loss.

WHAT ARE THE CAUSES AND RISKS OF PREGNANCY LOSS (BEFORE 20 WEEKS OF PREGNANCY)?

Pregnancy loss may occur for many reasons, and sometimes, the cause remains unknown even after additional tests are completed.

Possible Causes

Pregnancy loss often happens when a pregnancy does not develop normally.

In many cases, miscarriages result from a problem with the chromosomes in the fetus. The number of chromosomes the fetus has—too many or too few—can affect survival.

Other possible causes of pregnancy loss include the following:

- being exposed to toxins in the environment
- problems of the placenta, cervix, or uterus
- problems with the father's sperm

In many cases, though, health-care providers cannot identify a cause or causes of pregnancy loss.

Risk Factors

Problems with chromosomes happen more often in the fetuses of older parents, particularly among women who are older than 35.

For this reason, the risk for pregnancy loss increases as the parents age; it is much higher at age 45 than at age 35.

Women who have had previous miscarriages are also at a higher risk for pregnancy loss.

Health issues, such as chronic diseases, in the mother that can also increase the risk for pregnancy loss include the following:

- chronic diseases, such as high blood pressure (HBP), diabetes, thyroid disease, or polycystic ovary syndrome (PCOS)
- problems with the immune system, such as an autoimmune disorder
- infections (such as untreated gonorrhea or Zika)
- hormone problems
- extremes in weight, such as obesity or being too thin
- lifestyle factors, such as using drugs or alcohol, smoking, or consuming more than 200 milligrams of caffeine per day (equal to about one 12-ounce cup of coffee)

HOW DO HEALTH-CARE PROVIDERS DIAGNOSE AND TREAT PREGNANCY LOSS (BEFORE 20 WEEKS OF PREGNANCY)?

If a pregnant woman has any of the symptoms of pregnancy loss, such as abdominal cramps, back pain, light spotting, or bleeding, she should contact her health-care provider immediately. Remember that vaginal bleeding during pregnancy does not definitely mean a pregnancy loss is occurring.

Diagnosing Pregnancy Loss

Depending on how far along the pregnancy is, health-care providers may use different methods to determine whether a pregnancy loss has occurred:

- a blood test to check the level of human chorionic gonadotropin (hCG), the pregnancy hormone
- a pelvic exam to see whether the woman's cervix is dilated or thinned, which can be a sign of pregnancy loss

- an ultrasound test, which allows the provider to look at the pregnancy, uterus, and placenta

If a woman has had more than one miscarriage, she may want to have a health-care provider check her blood for chromosome problems, hormone problems, or immune system disorders that may be contributing to pregnancy loss.

Treating Pregnancy Loss

Treatments for pregnancy loss focus on ensuring that the nonviable pregnancy leaves the woman's body safely and completely. Women going through pregnancy loss are at risk for bleeding, pain, and infection, especially if some of the pregnancy tissue remains behind in the uterus.

The specific treatment used depends on how far along the pregnancy is, the woman's overall health, her age, and other factors.

In many cases, pregnancy loss before 20 weeks may not require any special treatment. The bleeding that occurs with pregnancy loss empties the uterus without any further problems.

Women who have heavy bleeding during pregnancy loss should contact a health-care provider immediately. For reference, heavy bleeding refers to soaking at least two maxi pads an hour for at least two hours in a row.

Some women may need a surgical procedure called a "dilation and curettage" (D&C) to remove any pregnancy tissue that is still in the uterus. A D&C is recommended if a woman is bleeding heavily or if an ultrasound shows pregnancy tissue is still in the uterus. D&C may also be used if a woman has any signs of infection, such as a fever, or if she has other health problems, such as cardiovascular disease (CVD) or a bleeding disorder.

Some women are treated with a medication called "misoprostol," which helps the tissue pass out of the uterus and controls the resulting bleeding. Research shows that misoprostol is safe and effective in most cases.

Women who lose a pregnancy may also need other treatments to control mild-to-moderate bleeding, prevent infection, relieve pain, and help with emotional support.

IS THERE A WAY TO PREVENT PREGNANCY LOSS (BEFORE 20 WEEKS OF PREGNANCY)?

There is currently no known way to prevent pregnancy loss before 20 weeks from occurring, nor is there a way to stop pregnancy loss once it has started.

There are ways to lower the risk of general pregnancy complications, but none of them definitely prevent pregnancy loss. Some ways to lower overall risk include the following:

- staying in good health before becoming pregnant and getting regular care during pregnancy
- diagnosing any health conditions, such as diabetes or thyroid disorders, and taking steps to manage or treat the condition before getting pregnant
- avoiding environmental hazards, such as exposure to radiation, pollution, or toxic chemicals
- avoiding alcohol and drugs, including high levels of caffeine in both partners
- protecting yourself from certain infections by not traveling to certain areas and by preventing mosquito bites

An NICHD study found that women who are at a higher risk for pregnancy loss because of two or more previous losses may increase their chances of carrying the pregnancy to term by taking a low-dose aspirin every day if they have high levels of inflammation.[2]

COPING WITH LOSS

After the loss, you might be stunned or shocked. You might be asking, "Why me?" You might feel guilty that you did or did not do something to cause your pregnancy to end. You might feel cheated and angry. Or you might feel extremely sad as you come to terms with the baby that will never be. These emotions are all normal reactions to loss. With time, you will be able to accept the loss and

---

[2] "Pregnancy Loss (Before 20 Weeks of Pregnancy)," *Eunice Kennedy Shriver* National Institute of Child Health and Human Development (NICHD), September 1, 2017. Available online. URL: www.nichd.nih.gov/health/topics/pregnancyloss. Accessed July 31, 2023.

move on. You will never forget your baby. But you will be able to put this chapter behind you and look forward to life ahead. To help get you through this difficult time, try some of these ideas:

- Turn to loved ones and friends for support. Share your feelings and ask for help when you need it.
- Talk to your partner about your loss. Keep in mind that men and women cope with loss in different ways.
- Take care of yourself. Eating healthy foods, keeping active, and getting enough sleep will help restore energy and well-being.
- Join a support group. A support group might help you feel less alone.
- Do something in remembrance of your baby.
- Seek help from a grief counselor, especially if your grief does not ease with time.

TRYING AGAIN

Give yourself plenty of time to heal emotionally. It could take a few months or even a year. Once you and your partner are emotionally ready to try again, confirm with your doctor that you are in good physical health and that your body is ready for pregnancy. Following a miscarriage, most healthy women do not need to wait before trying to conceive again. You might worry that pregnancy loss could happen again. But take heart in knowing that most women who have gone through pregnancy loss go on to have healthy babies.[3]

---

[3] Office on Women's Health (OWH), "Pregnancy Loss," U.S. Department of Health and Human Services (HHS), February 22, 2021. Available online. URL: www.womenshealth.gov/pregnancy/youre-pregnant-now-what/pregnancy-loss. Accessed July 31, 2023.

Section 28.3 | **Addressing Infant Death**

Infant mortality is the death of an infant before his or her first birthday. The infant mortality rate is the number of infant deaths for every 1,000 live births. In addition to giving us key information about maternal and infant health, the infant mortality rate is an important marker of the overall health of a society. In 2020, the infant mortality rate in the United States was 5.4 deaths per 1,000 live births.

CAUSES OF INFANT MORTALITY

Almost 20,000 infants died in the United States in 2020. The five leading causes of infant death in 2020 were:
- birth defects
- preterm birth and low birth weight
- sudden infant death syndrome (SIDS)
- injuries (e.g., suffocation)
- maternal pregnancy complications

INFANT MORTALITY RATES BY STATE

See Figure 28.1 for state-wise mortality rates in 2020.

Healthy People provides science-based, 10-year national objectives for improving the health of all Americans. One of the objectives of Healthy People is to reduce the rate of all infant deaths. In 2020, 16 states met the Healthy People 2030 target of 5.0 infant deaths per 1,000 live births. Geographically, infant mortality rates in 2020 were highest among states in the south.

INFANT MORTALITY RATES BY RACE AND ETHNICITY

See Figure 28.2 for mortality rates by race and ethnicity in 2019.

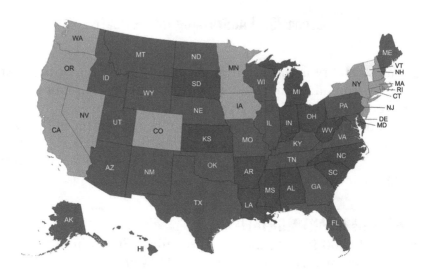

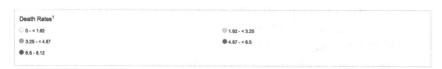

Figure 28.1. Infant Mortality Rates by State Map, 2020

Centers for Disease Control and Prevention (CDC)
*The number of infant deaths per 1,000 live births

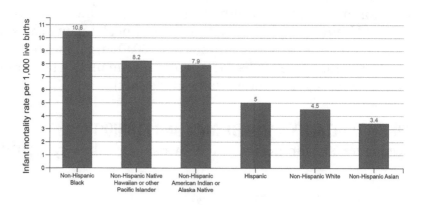

Figure 28.2. Infant Mortality Rates by Race and Ethnicity, 2019

Centers for Disease Control and Prevention (CDC)

In 2019, infant mortality rates by race and ethnicity were as follows:

- non-Hispanic Black: 10.6
- non-Hispanic Native Hawaiian or other Pacific Islander: 8.2
- non-Hispanic American Indian/Alaska Native: 7.9
- Hispanic: 5.0
- non-Hispanic White: 4.5
- non-Hispanic Asian: 3.4

Note: All records that indicate Hispanic ethnicity are classified as Hispanic regardless of race. For brevity, text references omit the term "single-race."[4]

ARE THERE WAYS TO REDUCE THE RISK OF INFANT MORTALITY?

Often, there are no definite ways to prevent many of the leading causes of infant mortality. However, there are ways to reduce a baby's risk. Researchers continue to study the best ways to prevent and treat the causes of infant mortality and affect the contributors to infant mortality. Consider the following ways to help reduce the risk.

Preventing Birth Defects

Birth defects are currently the leading cause of infant mortality in the United States. There are different kinds of birth defects, and they can happen in any pregnancy.

There are several things pregnant women can do to help reduce the risk of certain birth defects, such as getting enough folic acid before and during pregnancy to prevent neural tube defects.

Addressing Preterm Birth, Low Birth Weight, and Their Outcomes

There is currently no definitive way to prevent preterm birth, the second most common cause of infant mortality in the United

---

[4] "Infant Mortality," Centers for Disease Control and Prevention (CDC), June 22, 2022. Available online. URL: www.cdc.gov/reproductivehealth/maternalinfanthealth/infantmortality.htm. Accessed July 31, 2023.

States. However, researchers and health-care providers are working to address the issue on multiple fronts, including finding ways to stop preterm labor from progressing to a preterm delivery and identifying ways to improve health outcomes for infants who are born preterm. Preterm infants commonly have a low birth weight, but sometimes, full-term infants are also born underweight. Causes can include a mother's chronic health condition or poor nutrition. Adequate prenatal care is essential to ensure that full-term infants are born at a healthy weight.

There are some known risk factors for preterm birth—including having had a preterm birth with a previous pregnancy—and women with known risk factors may receive treatments to help reduce those risks. But, in most cases, the cause of preterm birth is not known, so there are not always effective treatments or actions that can prevent a preterm delivery.

Researchers and health-care providers are also working to understand the health challenges faced by infants born preterm or at a low birth weight as a way to develop treatments for these challenges. For instance, preterm infants are at high risk for serious breathing problems as a result of their underdeveloped lungs. Treatments such as ventilators and steroids can help stabilize breathing to allow the lungs to develop more fully. In addition, studies suggest that infants born at low birth weight are at increased risk of certain adult health problems, such as diabetes, high blood pressure, and heart disease.

GETTING PREPREGNANCY AND PRENATAL CARE

During pregnancy, the mother's health, environment, and experiences affect how her fetus develops and the course of the pregnancy. By taking good care of her own health before and during pregnancy, a mother can reduce her baby's risk of many of the leading causes of infant mortality in the United States, including birth defects, preterm birth, low birth weight, sudden infant death syndrome (SIDS), and certain pregnancy complications.

Women do not need to wait until they are pregnant to take steps to improve their health. Reaching a healthy weight, getting proper nutrition, managing chronic health conditions, and seeking help for substance use and abuse, for example, can help a woman achieve better health before she is pregnant. Her improved health, in turn, can help reduce infant mortality risks for any babies she has in the future.

Once she becomes pregnant, a mother should receive early and regular prenatal care. This type of care helps promote the best outcomes for mother and baby.

Creating a Safe Infant Sleep Environment

SIDS is defined as the sudden, unexplained death of an infant younger than one year of age that remains unexplained even after a thorough investigation. SIDS is the third-leading cause of infant mortality in the United States.

SIDS is one type of death within a broader category of causes of death called "sudden unexpected infant death" (SUID). The SUID category includes other sleep-related causes of infant death—such as accidental suffocation—as well as infections, vehicle collisions, and other causes.

As SIDS rates have been declining in the last few decades, rates of other sleep-related causes of infant death have been increasing. Accidental injury is the fifth-leading cause of infant mortality in the United States.

Although there is no definite way to prevent SIDS, there are ways to reduce the risk of SIDS and other sleep-related causes of infant death. For example, always placing a baby on his or her back to sleep and keeping the baby's sleep area free of soft objects, toys, crib bumpers, and loose bedding are important ways to reduce a baby's risk. The Safe to Sleep® campaign (formerly the Back to Sleep campaign) led by the *Eunice Kennedy Shriver* National Institute of Child Health and Human Development (NICHD) describes many ways that parents and caregivers can reduce the risk of SIDS and other sleep-related causes of infant death.

Using Newborn Screening to Detect Hidden Conditions

Newborn screening can detect certain conditions that are not noticeable at the time of birth but that can cause serious disability or even death if not treated quickly. Infants with these conditions may seem perfectly healthy and frequently come from families with no previous history of a condition.

To perform this screening, health-care providers take a few drops of blood from an infant's heel and apply them to special paper. The blood spots are then analyzed. If any conditions are detected, treatment can begin immediately.

Most states screen for at least 29 conditions, but some test for 50 or more conditions. Infants who are at increased or high risk for a condition because of their family history can undergo additional screening—beyond what states offer automatically—through a health-care specialist.

Since this public health program was initiated 50 years ago, it has saved countless lives by providing early detection and intervention and by improving the quality of life (QOL) for children and their families.[5]

[5] "Are There Ways to Reduce the Risk of Infant Mortality?" *Eunice Kennedy Shriver* National Institute of Child Health and Human Development (NICHD), October 29, 2021. Available online. URL: www.nichd.nih.gov/health/topics/infant-mortality/topicinfo/reduce-risk. Accessed July 31, 2023.

Chapter 29 | **Sudden Infant Death Syndrome**

Sudden infant death syndrome (SIDS) is the sudden, unexplained death of an infant younger than one year of age that remains unexplained after a complete investigation. This investigation can include an autopsy, a review of the death scene, and complete family and medical histories.

A diagnosis of SIDS is made by collecting information, conducting scientific or forensic tests, and talking with parents, other caregivers, and health-care providers. If, after this process is complete, there is still no identifiable cause of death, the infant's death might be labeled as SIDS.

WHAT FACTORS INCREASE THE RISK OF SUDDEN INFANT DEATH SYNDROME?

Currently, there is no known way to prevent SIDS, but there are ways to reduce the risk. Several factors present during pregnancy, at birth, and throughout the first year after birth can impact SIDS risk. Many of these factors can be controlled or changed to reduce the risk, but some cannot be controlled or changed.

One of the most effective actions that parents and caregivers can take to lower SIDS risk is to place their baby to sleep on his or her back for all sleep times.

Research shows the following:

- Back sleeping carries the lowest risk for SIDS and is recommended.
- Stomach sleeping carries the highest risk for SIDS— between 1.7 and 12.9 times the risk of back sleeping. It is not recommended.

- The side-lying position also increases the risk. It is unstable, and babies can easily roll to their stomach. It is not recommended.

Other known risk factors for SIDS include the following:
- **Preterm birth**. Infants born before 37 weeks in the womb are at higher risk for SIDS than infants born at full term.
- **Smoking**. Maternal smoking during pregnancy and smoking in the infant's environment increase the risk of SIDS.
- **Race/ethnic origin**. African-American and American-Indian/Alaska Native infants are at a higher risk for SIDS than are White, Hispanic-American, or Asian-/Pacific Islander-American infants.

WHAT CAUSES SUDDEN INFANT DEATH SYNDROME?

Health-care providers and researchers do not know the exact cause, but there are many theories.

More and more research evidence suggests that infants who die from SIDS are born with brain abnormalities or defects. These defects are typically found within a network of nerve cells that rely on a chemical called "serotonin" that allows one nerve cell to send a signal to another nerve cell. The cells are located in the part of the brain that probably controls breathing, heart rate, blood pressure, temperature, and waking from sleep.

However, scientists believe that brain defects alone may not be enough to cause a SIDS death. Evidence suggests that other events must also occur for an infant to die from SIDS. Researchers use the triple risk model to explain this concept. In this model, all three factors have to occur for an infant to die from SIDS. Having only one of these factors may not be enough to cause death from SIDS, but when all three combine, the chances of SIDS are high.

These factors are as follows:
- **At-risk infant**. An infant has an unknown problem—such as a genetic change or a brain defect—that puts

him or her at risk for SIDS. Health-care providers, parents, and caregivers do not know about these problems, so they do not know the infant is at risk.

- **Important time in an infant's development**. During the first six months after birth, infants go through many quick phases of growth that can change how well the body controls or regulates itself. Also, infant's bodies are learning how to respond to their environment.
- **Stressors in the environment**. All infants have stressors in their environments—sometimes called "external stressors" because they are outside the body. Being placed to sleep on the stomach, overheating during sleep, and exposure to cigarette smoke are all examples of external stressors. Infants who have no problems such as those explained previously can usually correct or overcome external stressors to survive and thrive. But an infant who has an unknown problem and whose body systems are immature and unstable might not be able to overcome these stressors.

According to the triple risk model, all three things have to be present for SIDS to occur.

Removing one of these factors—such as external stressors—may tip the balance in favor of the infant's survival. Because the first two situations cannot be seen or pinpointed, the most effective way to reduce the risk of SIDS is to remove or reduce environmental stressors. Strategies to remove these stressors form the basis of the Safe to Sleep® campaign messages.

HOW COULD YOU REDUCE BABY'S RISK OF SUDDEN INFANT DEATH SYNDROME?

The American Academy of Pediatrics (AAP) Task Force on SIDS reviews all the latest scientific and clinical evidence about SIDS and other sleep-related infant deaths and makes recommendations about the most effective ways to reduce baby's risk of SIDS and sleep-related deaths, such as suffocation.

It is important for all caregivers—parents, grandparents, aunts, uncles, babysitters, childcare providers, and everyone who might care for a baby—to learn about safe infant sleep to help reduce the baby's risk.[1]

Ways to Reduce Baby's Risk

Parents, caregivers, health-care providers, and others have made great progress in reducing sleep-related deaths in the United States. By placing babies on their backs to sleep for all sleep times, creating a safe sleep environment for baby, and following other evidence-based recommendations from the AAP Task Force on SIDS, everyone who cares for baby can help reduce baby's risk of SIDS and other sleep-related infant death, such as suffocation.

PLACE BABIES ON THEIR BACKS

Place babies on their backs to sleep for naps and at night.

- Place all babies—including those born preterm and those with reflux—on their backs to sleep until they are one year old.
- It is not safe to place babies on their sides or stomachs to sleep, not even for a nap. The safest sleep position is on the back.
- Babies who sleep on their backs are at lower risk for SIDS than babies who sleep on their stomachs or sides.
- If a baby usually sleeps on their back, putting them on the stomach or side to sleep, such as for a nap, increases the risk for SIDS by up to 45 times.
- Once babies can roll from back to stomach and from stomach to back on their own, you can leave them in the position they choose after starting to sleep on their back. If they can only roll one way on their own, you can reposition them to their back if they roll onto their stomach during sleep.

USE A FIRM/FLAT SLEEP SURFACE

Use a sleep surface for the baby that is firm (returns to its original shape quickly if pressed on), flat (such as a table, not a hammock), level (not at an angle or incline), and covered only with a fitted sheet.

- Both the sleep surface (such as a mattress) and the sleep space (such as a crib, bassinet, or portable play yard) should meet the safety standards of the Consumer Product Safety Commission (CPSC).
- Soft surfaces, such as couches, sofas, waterbeds, memory foam, air and pillow-top mattresses, quilts, thick blankets, and sheepskins, are not safe for babies to sleep on. Babies who sleep on soft surfaces may not be able to breathe due to entrapment or wedging, suffocation, or strangulation.
- Inclined or tilted sleep surfaces, with one end higher than the other, are not safe for babies to sleep on because the baby's body can slide down and their head can slump forward, which could block their airway and breathing.
- Do not use sitting devices, such as car seats and strollers, or carrying devices, such as carriers and slings, for a baby's regular sleep area or for naps. If a baby falls asleep in a sitting or carrying device, move them to their regular sleep space as soon as possible once you are out of the vehicle. The AAP offers travel safety tips, such as giving baby breaks from the sitting device every few hours.
- Avoid letting the baby sit slumped over, such as with their chin on their chest, because it could block their airway and breathing. Young babies and those unable to control their head and neck muscles risk suffocation and death from sitting this way.
- Keep comforters, quilts, pillows, and blankets out of the baby's sleep area.

FEED YOUR BABY BREAST MILK

Feed your baby human milk, as by breastfeeding. In most cases, pediatricians and other health-care providers recommend feeding only human milk, with nothing added, if possible, for at least the baby's first six months. Babies born preterm or with certain health conditions may need different care.

SHARE A ROOM WITH THE BABY

Share a room with the baby for at least the first six months. Give babies their own sleep space (crib, bassinet, or portable play yard) in your room, separate from your bed.

- Babies in their own sleep space are at lower risk for injury and death from SIDS and situations such as an adult or sibling accidentally rolling over them.
- Room sharing by putting the baby's sleep space near but not in your bed is safer than sharing your bed with the baby. It is also safer to share your room with the baby than to put the baby in their own room.
- Keeping the baby's sleep space close to your bed makes it easy to check on, feed, and comfort the baby without having to get all the way out of bed.
- If you are bringing a baby into your bed for feeding or comforting, before you start, remove or clear away all soft items and bedding from your side of the bed. This may help prevent suffocation in case you fall asleep. When finished, put the baby back in their own sleep space close to your bed.
- If you fall asleep while feeding or comforting a baby in your bed, put them back in a separate sleep area as soon as you wake up. Research shows that the longer an adult shares a bed with a baby, the higher the baby's risk for suffocation and other sleep-related death.
- Couches and armchairs are never safe places for babies to sleep. These surfaces are extremely dangerous when an adult falls asleep while feeding, comforting, or snuggling with a baby. Do not let babies sleep on these surfaces alone, with you, with someone else, or with pets.
- Sharing an adult bed, couch, or armchair with a baby can be risky, especially in some situations.

- Very high risk:
  - The sleep surface is soft, such as a waterbed, old adult mattress, couch, or armchair.
  - The adult is very tired, taking medication that makes them drowsy, or using substances such as alcohol, or their ability to respond is affected in some way.
  - The adult smokes cigarettes or uses tobacco products (even if they do not smoke in the bed).
- High risk:
  - The baby is younger than four months old (regardless of adult smoking or sleep surface).
  - The adult is a caregiver other than the baby's parent, such as a grandparent or sibling.
- Higher-than-normal risk:
  - The baby was born preterm (before 37 weeks) or at a low birth weight.
  - The sleep area includes unsafe items, such as pillows or blankets.

KEEP THINGS OUT OF THE SLEEP AREA

Keep things out of the baby's sleep area—no soft objects, toys, or other items.

- Remove everything from the baby's sleep area, except a fitted sheet covering the mattress.
- Things in the sleep area can pose dangers for the baby especially if they are:
  - soft or squishy (e.g., pillows, stuffed toys, crib bumpers)
  - under or over baby (e.g., comforters, quilts, blankets, positioners)
  - nonfitted, even if lightweight, small, or tucked in (e.g., loveys, cloths, nonfitted sheets, tucked-in blankets)
  - weighted (e.g., weighted blankets, weighted swaddles, weighted objects)

- Research links crib bumpers and bedding other than a fitted sheet covering the baby's mattress to serious injuries and deaths from SIDS, suffocation, entrapment, and strangulation.

OFFER A PACIFIER

Offer the baby a pacifier for naps and at night once they are feeding well.

- If feeding the baby human milk through direct breastfeeding, wait until breastfeeding is well established, based on your pediatrician's guidance, before trying a pacifier. Breastfeeding is "well-established" when the parent has enough milk to feed and satisfy the baby's hunger, parent and baby are comfortable during breastfeeding, and the baby is gaining enough weight to meet growth goals.
- If not breastfeeding, offer the baby a pacifier as soon as you like. Research shows that pacifiers are especially helpful for reducing SIDS risk in formula-fed babies.
- To reduce the risk of strangulation, choking, and suffocation, do not attach the pacifier to clothing, stuffed toys, blankets, or other items.
- Do not coat the pacifier with anything, such as a sweetened liquid or honey.
- If the pacifier falls out of the baby's mouth, you do not need to put it back in.
- It is OK if the baby does not want the pacifier; do not force the baby to take it.
- Finger- or thumb-sucking does not reduce SIDS risk.

STAY SMOKE- AND VAPE-FREE

Stay smoke- and vape-free during pregnancy and keep the baby's surroundings smoke- and vape-free.

- Smoking during pregnancy greatly increases a baby's risk of SIDS.

- Secondhand smoke in a baby's home, the car, or other spaces where the baby spends time also increases the risk of SIDS and other health problems.

STAY DRUG- AND ALCOHOL-FREE

Stay drug- and alcohol-free during pregnancy and make sure anyone caring for a baby is drug- and alcohol-free.

- Research shows that drug and alcohol use—during pregnancy and by infant caregivers—increases the risk of SIDS.
- Sharing an adult bed with a baby when using drugs or alcohol also increases the baby's risk of injury and death.

AVOID LETTING BABY GET TOO HOT

Avoid letting the baby get too hot and keep the baby's head and face uncovered during sleep.

- Baby can get hot or overheated if they are wearing too many layers of clothes and bedding for the room temperature (sometimes called "overbundling"). Overheated babies are at higher risk for SIDS and heat-related death.
- Dress the baby in clothes suitable for the temperature of the room.
- Wearing hats while indoors can make a baby too hot, so take off the baby's hat when inside.
- Watch for signs that the baby is too hot, such as sweating, flushing/red or hot skin, or the baby's chest feeling hot to the touch.
- Dress the baby in a wearable blanket or an extra layer of clothing to keep them warm without adding items to the sleep area.
- Do not leave the baby alone in a vehicle, no matter the temperature outside.

GET REGULAR MEDICAL CARE

Get regular medical care throughout pregnancy.

- Visiting a health-care provider as soon as you find out you are pregnant and then regularly until birth can help promote a healthy pregnancy.
- Research shows that in certain communities, regular prenatal care can also reduce the risk of SIDS.

FOLLOW YOUR HEALTH-CARE PROVIDER'S ADVICE

Follow your health-care provider's advice on vaccines, checkups, and other health issues for babies.

- Pediatricians and other medical providers have the most up-to-date information about safe sleep, growth and development, and other health topics for babies.
- Research shows that vaccinated babies are at lower risk for SIDS.
- Vaccines also protect people, including babies, from dangerous and deadly diseases.

AVOID PRODUCTS AND DEVICES THAT GO AGAINST SAFE SLEEP GUIDANCE

Avoid products and devices that go against safe sleep guidance, especially those that claim to prevent SIDS and other sleep-related infant deaths.

- Many wedges, positioners, or other products that claim to keep babies in one position or to reduce the risk of SIDS, suffocation, or reflux do not meet federal guidelines for sleep safety. These products, such as inclined sleepers, are linked to injury and death, especially when used in a baby's sleep area. You can help prevent injuries and death by not using these products and devices.
- No product can prevent SIDS.
- The CPSC has more information about safety standards for baby products at www.cpsc.gov.

AVOID USING HEART, BREATHING, MOTION, OR OTHER MONITORS

Avoid using heart, breathing, motion, or other monitors to reduce the risk of SIDS.

- These types of monitors are not effective at detecting or preventing SIDS.
- If you choose to use these devices for reasons other than detecting SIDS, make sure to follow safe sleep recommendations to reduce baby's risk of sleep-related death.
- If you have questions about using these devices for health problems or concerns other than SIDS, talk with your baby's health-care provider.

AVOID SWADDLING

Avoid swaddling once a baby starts to roll over (usually around three months of age) and keep in mind that swaddling does not reduce SIDS risk.

- Even though swaddling does not reduce the risk of SIDS, some babies are calmer and sleep better when they are swaddled.
- If you choose to swaddle your baby, make sure you follow the AAP safe sleep recommendations to reduce the baby's risk of sleep-related deaths.
- Once a baby starts to roll over on their own, swaddling increases the risk of suffocation and strangulation. Stop swaddling babies when they start rolling over, usually around three months of age.
- Using the back sleep position for swaddled babies is especially important. A swaddled baby may have trouble moving out of the stomach or side positions, which puts them at greater risk for SIDS and other sleep-related death than the back sleep position.

GIVE PLENTY OF TUMMY TIME

Give babies plenty of tummy time, that is, placing baby on their stomach, when they are awake and someone is watching them.[2]

---

[2] "Ways to Reduce Baby's Risk," *Eunice Kennedy Shriver* National Institute of Child Health and Human Development (NICHD), February 8, 2023. Available online. URL: https://safetosleep.nichd.nih.gov/reduce-risk/reduce. Accessed October 20, 2023.

Chapter 30 | **Talking to Children about Cancer**

When a child has cancer, every member of the family needs support. Parents often feel shocked and overwhelmed following their child's cancer diagnosis. Honest and calm conversations build trust as you talk with your child and his or her siblings. Taking care of yourself during this difficult time is important; it is not selfish. As you dig deep for strength, reach out to your child's treatment team and to people in your family and community for support.

HOW TO TALK TO CHILDREN ABOUT CANCER BY AGE

As you talk with your child, begin with the knowledge that you know your child best. Your child depends on you for helpful, accurate, and truthful information. Your child will learn a lot from your tone of voice and facial expressions, so stay calm when you talk with your child.

The following age-related suggestions may be helpful as you work with the health-care team so that your child knows what to expect during treatment, copes well with procedures, and feels supported:

- **If your child is less than 1 year old**. Comfort your baby by holding and gently touching them. Skin-to-skin contact is ideal. Bring familiar items from home, such as toys or a blanket. Talk or sing to your child, since the sound of your voice is soothing. Try to keep up feeding and bedtime routines as much as possible.
- **If your child is 1–2 years old**. Very young children understand things they can see and touch. Toddlers

like to play, so find safe ways to let your child play. Toddlers also like to start making choices, so let your child choose a sticker or a flavor of medicine when possible. Prepare your child ahead of time if something will hurt. Not doing so may cause your child to become fearful and anxious.

- **If your child is 3–5 years old.** To help your child understand their treatment better, ask the doctor if they can touch the models, machines, or supplies (tubes, bandages, or ports) ahead of time. If a procedure will hurt, prepare your child in advance. You can help distract your child by reading a story or giving them a stuffed animal to hold.
- **If your child is 6–12 years old.** School-aged children understand that medicines and treatments help them get better. They are able to cooperate with treatment but want to know what to expect. Children this age often have many questions, so be ready to answer them or to find the answers together. Relationships are important, so help your child stay in touch with friends and family.
- **If your child is a teenager.** Teens often focus on how cancer changes their lives—their friendships, their appearance, and their activities. They may be scared and angry about how cancer has isolated them from their friends. Look for ways to help your teen stay connected to friends. Give your teen some of the space and freedom they had before treatment and include them in treatment decisions.

TIPS FOR PARENTS OF A CHILD WITH CANCER

Talk with your child's health-care team to get your questions answered. You may also find the following suggestions helpful.

Who Should Tell Your Child?

Many parents receive their child's diagnosis from the doctor at the same time that their child learns of it. However, if you choose to be the one to tell your child, the doctor or nurse can help you decide what to say and how to answer their questions.

When Should Your Child Be Told?

Your child should be told as soon as possible. This will help build trust between you and your child. It does not mean that your child needs to hear everything all at once.

What Should You Tell Your Child?

The information you share with your child depends on their age and what they can understand. Children of all ages need clear, simple information that makes sense to them. As much as possible, help them know what to expect by using ideas and words that they understand. Tell your child how treatment will make them feel and when something will hurt. Explain that strong medicine and treatments have helped other children.

How Much Should You Tell Your Child?

Help your child understand the basic facts about the illness, the treatment, and what to expect. It may be hard for many children to process too many details or information given too far in advance. Start with small amounts of information that your child can understand. Children often use their imaginations to make up answers to unanswered questions and may fear the worst. Answering questions honestly and having ongoing conversations can help your child. Telling untruths can cause your child to distrust you or people on their health-care team.

How Might Your Child React?

Each child is different. Some worry. Others get upset or become quiet, afraid, or defiant. Some express their feelings in words; others express their feelings in actions. Some children regress to behaviors they had when they were younger. These are normal reactions to changes in life as they know it. Their schedule, the way they look and feel, and their friendships may all be changing.

Expect that some days will be rough, and others will be easier. Tell your child and find ways to show them that you will always be there for them.

What Could You Do to Help Your Child Cope?

Children take cues from their parents, so being calm and hopeful can help your child. Show your love. Think about how your child and family have handled difficult times in the past. Some children feel better after talking. Others prefer to draw, write, play games, or listen to music.

HOW TO EXPLAIN CANCER TO A CHILD AT DIAGNOSIS

Talk with your child's health-care team about how to answer questions your child may have. You may also find the following suggestions helpful.

What Is Cancer?

When talking about cancer with your child, start with simple words and concepts. Explain that cancer is not contagious—it is not an illness that children catch from someone or that they can give to someone else. Young children may understand that they have a lump (tumor) that is making them sick or that their blood is not working the way it should. Parents and older children may want to read about different types of childhood cancer.

Why Did You Get Cancer?

Some children think they did something bad or wrong to cause the cancer. Others wonder why they got sick. Tell your child that nothing they—or anyone else—did caused the cancer, and doctors are working to learn more about what causes cancer in children.

- **You may tell your child**. I do not know. Not even doctors know exactly why one child gets cancer and another does not. We do know that you did not do anything wrong, you did not catch it from someone, and it is not contagious.

Will You Get Better?

Being in the hospital or having many medical appointments can be scary for a child. Some children may know or have heard about a person who has died from cancer. Your child may wonder if they will get better.

- **You may tell your child.** Cancer is a serious illness, and your doctors and nurses are giving you treatments that have helped other children. We are going to do all we can to help you get better. Let us talk with your doctor and nurse to learn more about the type of cancer you have.

How Will You Feel during Treatment?

Your child may wonder how they may feel during treatment. Children with cancer often see others who have lost their hair or are very sick. Talk with the nurse or social worker to learn how your child's treatment may affect how your child looks and feels and about the side effects that they may have.

- **You may tell your child.** Even when two children have the same type of cancer, what happens to one child may not happen to the other. Your doctors and I will talk with you and explain what we know. We will all work together as a team to help you feel as comfortable as possible during treatment.

WAYS TO HELP CHILDREN WITH CANCER

Cancer treatment brings many changes to a child's life and outlook. You can help your child by letting him/her live as normal a life as possible. Talk with the health-care team to learn what to expect, as your child goes through treatment, so your child and family can prepare.

Helping Your Child Adjust to Physical Changes

Children can be sensitive about how they look and how others respond to them. Here are ways to help your child:

- **Prepare for physical changes.** If treatment causes your child's hair to fall out, let your child pick out a fun cap,

299

scarf, and/or wig ahead of time. Some treatments may cause changes in weight. Meeting with a registered dietitian can help your child get the nutrients their body needs to stay strong during treatment.

- **Side effects.** Your child's nurse will talk with you and your child about supportive care. This is a care that is given to manage the side effects and improve your child's quality of life (QOL).
- **Help your child know how to respond.** Sometimes, people will stare, mistake your child's gender, or ask personal questions. Talk with your child and come up with an approach that works. Your child may choose to respond or ignore comments.

HELPING YOUR CHILD CONNECT WITH FRIENDS

Your child's friendships are tested and may change during a serious illness, such as cancer. Sometimes, it may seem as though old friends are no longer "there for them." It may help if your child takes the first step and reaches out to friends. Children may also make new friends through this experience. Here are some steps you can take with your child:

- **Help your child stay in touch with friends.** You can encourage or help your child connect with friends through text messages, video chats, phone calls, and/or social media.
- **Get tips and advice.** A social worker or child life specialist can help your child think through what they would and would not like to share with friends. If possible and when your child is up to it, friends may be able to visit. Your child may also be able to participate in school and other activities based on the advice of their doctor.

HELPING YOUR CHILD COPE WITH DIFFICULT EMOTIONS

Although, over time, many children with cancer cope well, your child may feel anxious, sad, stressed, scared, or withdrawn at times.

Talk with your child about what they are feeling and help them find ways to cope. Your child can also meet with a child life specialist or psychologist about feelings that do not have easy solutions or seem to be getting worse over time. These tips may help your child cope with difficult emotions:

- **Find ways to distract and entertain your child.** Playing video games or watching movies can help your child to relax. You can also learn about other practices that can support your child during treatment, such as art therapy, biofeedback, guided imagery, hypnosis, laughter therapy, massage therapy, meditation, music therapy, and relaxation therapy, among others.
- **Stay calm but do not hide your feelings.** Your child can feel your emotions. If you often feel sad or anxious, talk with your doctor and child's health-care team, so you can manage these emotions. Yet keep in mind that if you often hide your feelings, your child may also hide their feelings from you.
- **Get help if you see emotional changes in your child.** While it is normal for your child to feel down or sad at times, if these feelings happen on most days over a long period of time, they may be signs that your child needs extra support. Meeting with your child's nurse, child life specialist, and/or psychologist can help your child learn how to manage stress, and they can assess your child for mental health conditions, such as anxiety disorder and depression.

HELPING YOUR CHILD ADJUST TO A NEW NORMAL

Your child may spend more time in the hospital and at home during treatment. Here are ways to help your child cope with periods of isolation and time away from friends.

- **Hospital stays.** Being in the hospital can be especially difficult for children. It is a different setting, with new people and routines, large machines, and sometimes painful procedures.

301

- **Bring in comfort items**. Let your child choose favorite things from home, such as photos, games, and music. These items can comfort children and help them relax.
- **Visit game rooms, playrooms, and teen rooms**. Many hospitals have places where patients can play, relax, and spend time with other patients. These rooms often have toys, games, crafts, music, and computers. Encourage your child to take part in social events and activities that are offered at the hospital.
- **Isolation at home**. While your child is receiving treatment, he/she may need to stay at home for extended periods of time due to the side effects of cancer treatment, such as fatigue, risk of infection, pain, and gastrointestinal complications, for example.
  - **Decorate your child's room**. Posters, pictures, and other decorations may brighten the room and help cheer up your child. Window markers are a fun way to decorate. Check to see if any items should be removed from your child's room since there are sometimes medical restrictions.
  - **Explore new activities**. If sports are off-limits, learn about other activities that can help your child stay active and have fun. Your child may also enjoy listening to music, reading, playing games, or writing. Some children with cancer discover new skills and interests they never knew they had.
- **Missing school**. While some children with cancer are able to attend school, many need to take a leave of absence for short or long periods of time. Here are ways to get the academic support your child needs during this time:
  - **Meet with your child's doctor**. It helps you learn more about how treatment may affect your child's energy level and ability to keep up with schoolwork. Ask the doctor to write a letter to your

child's teachers that describes your child's medical situation, limitations, and how much time your child is likely to miss.

- **Keep your child's teachers updated.** Tell your child's teachers and principal about your child's medical situation. Share the letter from your child's doctor. Learn what schoolwork your child will miss and about ways for your child to keep up, as they are able.
- **Learn about assistance from the hospital and your child's school.** Hospitals have education coordinators or nurses who can talk with you about academic resources and assistance for your child. You will also want to ask about an individualized education plan (IEP), also called a "504 plan," for your child.

HOW TO COPE AS PARENTS AND SIBLINGS OF CHILDREN WITH CANCER

These suggestions can help you care for yourself, your children, and your family. Parents often say that their child's diagnosis feels like a family diagnosis. Here is practical advice to help families cope and stay connected during this challenging time.

Work to Keep Relationships Strong

Relationships and partnerships are strained and under pressure when a child has cancer. However, marriages can also grow stronger during this time. Here is what parents said helped:

- **Keep lines of communication open.** Talk about how you each deal best with stress. Make time to connect, even when time is limited.
- **Remember that no two people cope the same way.** Couples often have different coping strategies. If your spouse or partner does not seem as distraught as you, it does not mean he or she is suffering any less than you are.
- **Make time.** Even a quick call, text message, or handwritten note can go a long way in making your spouse's or child's day a better one.

Get Support from Family, Friends, and People in Your Community

Research shows what you most likely already know—that help from others strengthens and encourages your child and family. Family and friends may want to assist but might not know what you need. It may help with the following:

- **Finding an easy way to update family and friends**. Consider posting updates and getting practical support through sites, such as Caring Bridge (www.caringbridge.org), My Cancer Circle (mycancercircle.lotsahelpinghands.com/caregiving/home), MyLifeLine (www.mylifeline.org), or Lotsa Helping Hands (https://lotsahelpinghands.com). Share only what you feel comfortable sharing.

- **Being specific about how people can support your family**. Keep a list handy of things that others can do for your family. For example, people can cook, clean, grocery shop, or drive siblings to their activities.

- **Joining a support group**. Some groups meet in person, whereas others meet online. Many parents benefit from the experiences and information shared by other parents.

- **Seeking professional help**. If you are not sleeping well or are depressed, talk with your primary care doctor or people on your child's health-care team. Ask them to recommend a mental health specialist, such as a psychiatrist, psychologist, counselor, or social worker.

Make Time to Renew Your Mind and Body

It can be tempting to put your own needs on hold and focus solely on your sick child. However, it is essential that you make time for yourself. Doing so can also give you the energy to care for your child. Here are some tips to help you get started:

- **Find ways to relax and lower stress**. Some parents try something new, such as a yoga or deep breathing class at the hospital. Others are refreshed by being outdoors, even for short periods. Whatever the method or place, find one that feels peaceful to you. You can use the techniques available at www.cancer.gov/about-cancer/coping/feelings/relaxation to relax.

- **Fill waiting time.** Pick a few activities that you enjoy and can do at the hospital, such as playing a game, reading, writing, or listening to music.
- **Stay physically active.** Plan to walk, jog, go to the gym, or follow a workout app. Exercising with a friend or family member can make it easier to keep up the routine. If it is hard to stay physically active at the hospital, try walking up and down the stairs or around the hospital or unit. Physical activity helps lower stress and can also help you sleep better at night.

Support Siblings When a Brother or Sister Has Cancer

As a parent, you want to be there for all your children, yet this can be challenging when a child is being treated for cancer. You may notice that siblings are having a difficult time yet struggling to address their needs.

Here are some more ways you can help siblings during this difficult time:

- **Listen to and connect with siblings.** Set aside some time every day, even if it is just a few minutes, to spend with your other children. Check in and ask how they are doing, even if you do not have an easy solution to every challenge they may be facing. It is important to connect with and listen to them.
- **Keep siblings informed and involved.** Talk with your children about their sibling's cancer and tell them what to expect during treatment. If possible, find ways to include them in hospital visits. If you are far from home, find ways to connect through video chat, text messages, and phone calls, for example.
- **Keep things as normal as you can.** Arrange to keep siblings involved in school-related events and activities that are important to them. Ask friends and neighbors for support. Most people want to help and will appreciate being asked.

HELPING YOUR CHILD DURING TREATMENT

The following suggestions can help you and your child establish strong and effective relationships with your child's health-care team:

- **Build strong partnerships**. Give respect to and expect to receive respect from the people on your child's health-care team. Open and honest communication will also make it easier for you to ask questions, discuss options, and feel confident that your child is in good hands.
- **Take advantage of the many specialists who can help your child**. Work with them to help your child learn about cancer and how it will be treated, prepare for tests, manage side effects, and cope.
- **If you get information online, make sure the source is credible**. It is important to get accurate information that you understand and can use to make decisions. Share what you find with the health-care team to confirm that it applies to your child.
- **Make sure you understand what your child's health-care team tells you**. Speak up when something is confusing or unclear, especially when decisions need to be made. Ask to see pictures or videos to help understand new medical information.
- **Keep your child's pediatrician updated**. Ask for updates to be sent to your child's regular pediatrician.[1]

---

[1] "Support for Families When a Child Has Cancer," National Cancer Institute (NCI), November 16, 2022. Available online. URL: www.cancer.gov/about-cancer/coping/caregiver-support/parents. Accessed July 31, 2023.

Chapter 31 | **Pediatric Palliative Care: Supporting Children at the End of Life**

When a child is seriously ill, each person in the family is affected differently. That is why, it is important that you, your child, and your family get the support and care you need during this difficult time. A special type of care called "palliative care" can help. Palliative care is a key part of care for children living with a serious illness. It is also an important source of support for their families.

WHAT IS PALLIATIVE CARE?
Palliative care can ease the symptoms, discomfort, and stress of a serious illness for your child and family. Palliative care can help with your child's illness and give support to your family. It can help with the following:
- easing your child's pain and other symptoms of illness
- providing emotional and social support that respects your family's cultural values
- helping your child's health-care providers work together and communicate with one another to support your goals
- starting open discussions with you, your child, and your health-care team about options for care

307

Palliative Care Provides Comfort for Your Child

Palliative care can help children and teenagers living with many serious illnesses, including genetic disorders, cancer, neurologic disorders, heart and lung conditions, and others. Palliative care is important for children at any age or stage of serious illness. It can begin as soon as you learn about your child's illness. Palliative care can help prevent symptoms and give relief from much more than physical pain. It can also enhance your child's quality of life (QOL).

Palliative Care Gives You and Your Family an Added Layer of Support

Serious illness in a child affects everyone in the family, including parents and siblings of all ages. Palliative care gives extra support for your whole family. It can ease the stress on all of your children, your spouse, and you during a hard time.

Palliative Care Surrounds Your Family with a Team of Experts Who Work Together to Support All of You

It is a partnership between your child, your family, and the health-care team. This team listens to your preferences and helps you think through the care options for your family. They will work with you and your child to make a care plan for your family. They can also help when your child moves from one care setting (e.g., the hospital) to another (e.g., outpatient care or care at home).

DOES ACCEPTING PALLIATIVE CARE MEAN YOUR FAMILY IS GIVING UP ON OTHER TREATMENTS?

No. The purpose of palliative care is to ease your child's pain and other symptoms and provide emotional and other support to your entire family. Palliative care can help children, newborns, young adults, and their families—at any stage of a serious illness. Palliative care works alongside other treatments your child may be receiving. In fact, your child can start getting palliative care as soon as you learn about your child's illness.

How Is Palliative Care Different from Hospice Care?

Your child does not need to be in hospice to get palliative care. Your child can get palliative care wherever they receive care: in the hospital, during clinic visits, or at home. Hospice care focuses on a person's final months of life, but palliative care is available to your child at any time during a serious illness. Some children receive palliative care for many years. Some hospice programs require that patients are no longer getting treatments to cure their illness, but palliative care is different—it can be given at the same time as other treatments for your child's illness.

PALLIATIVE CARE HELPS YOUR CHILD LIVE A MORE COMFORTABLE LIFE

Palliative care can provide direct support for your child by providing relief from distressing symptoms, including the following:

- pain
- shortness of breath
- fatigue
- depression
- anxiety
- nausea
- loss of appetite
- problems with sleep

Palliative care can help your child deal with the side effects of medicines and treatments. Perhaps, most importantly, palliative care can help enhance your child's QOL. For example, helping to cope with concerns about school and friends might be very valuable to your child.

Palliative care may also include direct support for families, such as assistance with:

- including siblings in conversations
- providing respite care for parents to be able to spend time with their other children
- locating community resources for services such as counseling and support groups

Palliative care is effective. Scientists have studied how palliative care can help children living with serious illnesses. Studies show that patients who get palliative care say that it helps with the following:

- pain and other distressing symptoms, such as nausea or shortness of breath
- communication between health-care providers and family members
- emotional support

Other studies show that palliative care includes the following:

- helping patients get the kind of care they want
- meeting the emotional, developmental, and spiritual needs of patients

PALLIATIVE CARE FOCUSES ON THE NEEDS OF YOUR CHILD AND FAMILY

How Do You Know If Your Child or Family Needs Palliative Care?

Children living with a serious illness often experience physical and emotional distress related to their disease. Emotional distress is also common among their parents, siblings, and other family members.

Ask your child's health-care provider about palliative care if your child or any member of your family (including you):

- suffers from pain or other symptoms due to serious illness
- experiences physical pain or emotional distress that is not under control
- needs help to understand your child's health condition
- needs support coordinating your child's care

THE PALLIATIVE CARE TEAM WORKS WITH YOU, YOUR CHILD, AND YOUR CARE TEAM

Together with your child's health-care providers, palliative care professionals will work with you and your child to make a care plan that is right for your child, your family, and you. The team will help you and your child include pain and other symptom management in every part of your child's care.

Palliative care experts spend as much time with you and your family as it takes to help you fully understand your child's condition, care options, and other needs. They also make sure your child experiences a smooth transition between the hospital and other services, such as getting care at home.

Your team will listen to your preferences and work with you and your child to plan care for all of your child's symptoms throughout the illness. This will include the care for your child's current needs and flexibility for future changes.

Your Child's Palliative Care Team Is Unique

Every palliative care team is different. Your child's palliative care team may include the following:

- doctors
- nurses
- social workers
- pharmacists
- chaplains
- counselors
- child life specialists
- nutritionists
- art and music therapists

How Can Your Family Get Palliative Care?

The palliative care process can begin when your child's health-care provider refers you to palliative care services. Or you or your child can ask your provider for a referral if you feel that palliative care would be helpful for your child, your family, or yourself.

If You Start Palliative Care, Can Your Child Still See the Same Primary Health-Care Provider?

Yes. Your child does not have to change to a new primary health-care provider when starting palliative care. The palliative care team and your child's health-care provider work together to help you and your child decide the best care plan for your child.

311

What If Your Child's Health-Care Provider Is Unsure about Referring Palliative Care?

Some parents fear that they might offend their child's current health-care providers by asking about palliative care, but this is unlikely. Most health-care providers appreciate the extra time and information the palliative care team provides their patients. Occasionally, a clinician may not refer a patient for palliative care services. If this happens, ask for an explanation. Let your child's health-care provider know why you think palliative care could help your family.

Who Pays for Palliative Care?

Many insurance plans cover palliative care. If you have questions or concerns about costs, you can ask your health-care team to put you in touch with a social worker, care manager, or financial advisor at your hospital or clinic to look at payment options.

Where Can Your Child Get Palliative Care?

Your palliative care team will help you know what services are available in your community. Your child and family may receive palliative care in a hospital, during clinic visits, or at home. You and your child will first likely meet with your palliative care team in the hospital or at a clinic. After the first visit, some visits may still occur in the clinic or hospital. However, many palliative care programs offer services at home and in the community. Home services can occur through telephone calls or home visits.

If palliative care starts in the hospital, your care team can help your child make a successful move to your home or other health-care setting.

A home may feel most comfortable and safe to you and your child. Depending on your child's condition and treatment, the palliative care team may be able to help you find a nursing agency or community care agency to support palliative care for your child at home.

How Can Your Child's Pain Be Managed?

The palliative care team can bring your child comfort in many ways. Treating pain often involves medication, but there are also other methods to address a child's discomfort. Your child may feel better with changes, such as low lighting, comfortable room temperatures, pleasant smells, guided relaxation, and deep breathing techniques. Your child may welcome additional activities, such as video chats, social media, soothing music, and massage and art therapy, that may help decrease pain and anxiety.

If your child has an illness that causes pain that is not relieved by drugs, such as acetaminophen (Tylenol®) or ibuprofen (Motrin® or Advil®), your child's palliative care team may recommend trying stronger medicines.

Pain relief can be offered in a hospital, at home, or in other health-care settings. Your palliative care team will partner with you and your child to learn what is causing discomfort and how best to handle it.[1]

---

[1] "Palliative Care for Children," National Institute of Nursing Research (NINR), July 2015. Available online. URL: www.ninr.nih.gov/sites/files/docs/NINR_508cBrochure_2015-7-7.pdf. Accessed August 14, 2023.

Chapter 32 | **Helping Children Cope with Death**

Chapter Contents

Section 32.1 | Grief and Developmental Stages

At one time, children were considered miniature adults, and their behaviors were expected to be modeled as such. Today, there is a greater awareness of developmental differences between childhood and other developmental stages in the human life cycle. Differences between the grieving process for children and the grieving process for adults are recognized. It is now believed that the real issue for grieving children is not whether they grieve but how they exhibit their grief and mourning.

The primary difference between bereaved adults and bereaved children is that intense emotional and behavioral expressions are not continuous in children. A child's grief may appear more intermittent and briefer than that of an adult; in fact, a child's grief usually lasts longer.

The work of mourning in childhood needs to be addressed repeatedly at different developmental and chronological milestones. Because bereavement is a process that continues over time, children will revisit the loss repeatedly, especially during significant life events (e.g., going to camp, graduating from school, marrying, and experiencing the births of their own children). Children must complete the grieving process, eventually achieving a resolution of grief.

Although the experience of loss is unique and highly individualized, several factors can influence a child's grief:
- age
- personality
- stage of development
- previous experiences with death
- previous relationship with the deceased
- environment
- cause of death
- patterns of interaction and communication within the family
- stability of family life after the loss

- how the child's needs for sustained care are met
- availability of opportunities to share and express feelings and memories
- parental styles of coping with stress
- availability of consistent relationships with other adults

Children do not react to loss like adults do and may not display their feelings as openly as adults do. In addition to verbal communication, grieving children may employ play, drama, art, schoolwork, and stories. Bereaved children may not withdraw into preoccupation with thoughts of the deceased person; rather, they often immerse themselves in activities (e.g., they may be sad one minute and then play outside with friends the next). Families often incorrectly interpret this behavior to mean that the child does not really understand or has already gotten over the death. Neither assumption may be true; the minds of the children protect them from thoughts and feelings that are too powerful for them to handle.

Grief reactions are intermittent because children cannot explore all of their thoughts and feelings as rationally as adults can. Additionally, children often have difficulty articulating their feelings about grief. A grieving child's behavior may speak louder than any words he or she could speak. Strong feelings of anger and fear of abandonment or death may be evident in the behaviors of grieving children. Children often play death games as a way of working out their feelings and anxieties in a relatively safe setting. These games are familiar to the children and provide safe opportunities to express their feelings.

GRIEF AND DEVELOPMENTAL STAGES
A child's understanding of death and the events surrounding it depends on the child's age and developmental stage (see Table 32.1).

Table 32.1. Grief and Developmental Stages

Age (Years)	Understanding of Death	Expressions of Grief
0–2	The child is not yet able to understand death.	Quietness, crankiness, decreased activity, poor sleep, and weight loss
	Separation from the mother causes changes.	
2–6	Death is like sleeping.	Asking many questions (How does she go to the bathroom? How does he eat?)
		Problems in eating, sleeping, and bladder and bowel control
		Fear of abandonment
		Tantrums
	The dead person continues to live and function in some ways.	Magical thinking (Did I think something or do something that caused the death, like when I said I hate you and I wish you would die?)
	Death is temporary, not final.	
	A dead person can come back to life.	
6–9	Death is thought of as a person or spirit (skeleton, ghost, or bogeyman).	Curious about death
		Asking specific questions
		Having exaggerated fears about school
	Death is final and frightening.	Having aggressive behaviors (especially boys)
		Concerning about imaginary illnesses
	Death happens to others; it will not happen to me.	Feeling abandoned

Table 32.1. Continued

Age (Years)	Understanding of Death	Expressions of Grief
≥9	Everyone will die.	Heightened emotions, guilt, anger, and shame
		Increased anxiety over own death
		Mood swings
	Death is final and cannot be changed.	Fear of rejection; not wanting to be different from peers
	Even I will die.	Changes in eating habits
		Sleeping problems
		Regressive behaviors (loss of interest in outside activities)
		Impulsive behaviors
		Feeling guilty about being alive (especially related to the death of a sibling or peer)

Infants

Although infants do not recognize death, feelings of loss and separation are a part of developing awareness of death. Children who have been separated from their mothers and deprived of nurturing can exhibit changes such as listlessness, quietness, unresponsiveness to a smile or a coo, physical changes (including weight loss), and a decrease in activity and lack of sleep.

Ages Two to Three Years

In this age range, children often confuse death with sleep and can experience anxiety. In the early phases of grief, bereaved children can exhibit loss of speech and generalized distress.

Ages Three to Six Years

In this age range, children view death as a kind of sleep; the person is alive but in some limited way. They do not fully separate death from life and may believe that the deceased continues to live (i.e., in the ground where he or she was buried), and they often ask questions about the activities of the deceased person (e.g., how is the deceased eating, going to the toilet, breathing, or playing?). Young children can acknowledge physical death but consider it a temporary or gradual event, reversible and not final (such as leaving and returning or a game of peekaboo). A child's concept of death may involve magical thinking, that is, the idea that his or her thoughts can cause actions. Children may feel that they must have done or thought something bad to cause a loved one to become ill or that a loved one's death occurred because of the child's personal thought or wish. In response to death, children younger than five years will often exhibit disturbances in eating, sleeping, and bladder or bowel control.

Ages Six to Nine Years

It is not unusual for children in this age range to become very curious about death, asking very concrete questions about what happens to one's body when it stops working. Death is personified as a separate person or spirit, a skeleton, ghost, angel of death, or bogeyman. Although death is perceived as final and frightening, it is not universal. Children in this age range begin to compromise, recognizing that death is final and real but mostly happens to older people (not to themselves). Grieving children can:

- develop school phobias, learning problems, and antisocial or aggressive behaviors
- exhibit hypochondriacal concerns
- withdraw from others

Conversely, children in this age range can become overly attentive and clingy. Boys may show an increase in aggressive and destructive behavior (e.g., acting out in school), expressing their feelings in this way rather than by openly displaying sadness. When a parent dies, children may feel abandoned by both their deceased parent and their surviving parent because the surviving parent is frequently preoccupied with his or her own grief and is less able to emotionally support the child.

Ages Nine Years and Older
By the time a child is nine years old, death is understood as inevitable and is no longer viewed as a punishment. By the time the child is 12 years old, death is viewed as final and universal.[1]

Section 32.2 | Guiding Children through Grief

ISSUES FOR GRIEVING CHILDREN
The following are the three prominent themes in the grief expressions of bereaved children:

- Did I cause the death to happen?
- Is it going to happen to me?
- Who is going to take care of me?

---

[1] "Grief, Bereavement, and Coping with Loss (PDQ®)—Health Professional Version," National Cancer Institute (NCI), October 18, 2022. Available online. URL: www.cancer.gov/about-cancer/advanced-cancer/caregivers/planning/bereavement-hp-pdq. Accessed August 7, 2023.

Did I Cause the Death to Happen?

Children often engage in magical thinking, believing they have magical powers. If a mother says in exasperation, "You'll be the death of me," and later dies, her child may wonder whether he or she actually caused the death. Likewise, when two siblings argue, it is not unusual for one to say (or think), "I wish you were dead." If that sibling were to die, the surviving sibling might think that his or her thoughts or statements actually caused the death.

Is It Going to Happen to Me?

The death of a sibling or other child may be especially difficult because it strikes so close to the child's own peer group. If the child also perceives that the death could have been prevented (by either a parent or doctor), the child may think that he or she could also die.

Who Is Going to Take Care of Me?

Because children depend on parents and other adults for their safety and welfare, a child who is grieving the death of an important person in his or her life might begin to wonder who will provide the care that he or she needs now that the person is gone.

INTERVENTIONS FOR GRIEVING CHILDREN

There are interventions that may help facilitate and support the grieving process in children.

Explanation of Death

Silence about death (which indicates that the subject is taboo) does not help children deal with loss. When death is discussed with a child, explanations should be kept as simple and direct as possible. Each child needs to be told the truth with as much detail as can be comprehended at his or her age and stage of development. Questions should be addressed honestly and directly. Children need to be reassured about their own security (they frequently worry that they will also die or that their surviving parent will go away). A child's questions should be answered, and the child's processing of the information should be confirmed.

Correct Language

Although initiating this conversation with children is difficult, any discussion about death must include proper words (e.g., cancer, died, or death). Euphemisms (e.g., "he passed away," "he is sleeping," or "we lost him") should never be used because they can confuse children and lead to misinterpretations.

Planning Rituals

After a death occurs, children can and should be included in the planning of and participation in mourning rituals. As with bereaved adults, these rituals help children memorialize loved ones. Although children should never be forced to attend or participate in mourning rituals, their participation should be encouraged. Children can be encouraged to participate in aspects of the funeral or memorial service with which they feel comfortable. If the child wants to attend the funeral (or wake or memorial service), it is important that a full explanation of what to expect is given in advance. This preparation should include the layout of the room, who might be present (e.g., friends and family members), what the child will see (e.g., a casket and people crying), and what will happen. Surviving parents may be too involved in their own grief to give their children the attention they need. Therefore, it is often helpful to identify a familiar adult friend or family member who will be assigned to care for a grieving child during a funeral.[2]

---

[2] See footnote [1].

Chapter 33 | Collaborative Pediatric Critical Care Research Network

Pediatric critical care, or the effective and efficient care of children with critical or unstable conditions, is an important and growing subspecialty in pediatrics. Much of the technology and many therapies in pediatric critical care have evolved without adequate study or have been adopted uncritically from adult, neonatal, or anesthetic practice. As a result, the risks and benefits of intensive care practice remain largely unknown. Research is needed to make the best decisions regarding effective critical care practices. Rigorous use of appropriate scientific methodology, deployed across a network structure, achieves the numbers of patients required to provide answers more rapidly than individual sites acting alone.

The *Eunice Kennedy Shriver* National Institute of Child Health and Human Development (NICHD) funds the Collaborative Pediatric Critical Care Research Network (CPCCRN) through its Pediatric Trauma and Critical Illness Branch (PTCIB). The network, first established in 2004 and initially funded through a five-year cooperative agreement mechanism, has been recompeted multiple times. The most recent recompetition, in 2021, used a PL1, or linked-center grant, which allows the network to increase substantially in size and scope.

The most recent CPCCRN iteration includes 13 core clinical sites, 12 ancillary sites (hospitals), and a data coordinating center (DCC). It seeks to accelerate pediatric critical care research, leading to the evaluation of promising new approaches to life support and critical decision-making in complex childhood illnesses and injuries.

With its changed format and size, the network is primed to conduct large-scale multicenter randomized controlled trials, such as the ongoing effort on personalized testing and targeted management of immune function in infants and children with sepsis-induced multiple organ dysfunction syndrome (MODS). Results from this and other CPCCRN studies have the potential to be paradigm-shifting in critical care management and care.

TOPIC AREAS

Since its start, the CPCCRN has conducted controlled observations and objective evaluations of pediatric critical care practices, including new management and technology methodologies, in children with complex critical illnesses and injuries as well as coping, bereavement, and grief-related topics.

Current priority areas for the network include the following (in alphabetical order):

- critical illness in children with complex, chronic health conditions
- intensive care unit (ICU) processes, including (but not limited to) cardiopulmonary resuscitation (CPR), mechanical ventilation, extracorporeal therapies, and so on
- life-threatening pediatric trauma
- MODS in children
- palliative care in pediatric critical illness
- pediatric acute respiratory distress syndrome (ARDS)
- pediatric sepsis[1]

[1] "Collaborative Pediatric Critical Care Research Network (CPCCRN)," *Eunice Kennedy Shriver* National Institute of Child Health and Human Development (NICHD), August 29, 2023. Available online. URL: www.nichd.nih.gov/research/supported/cpccrn. Accessed August 30, 2023.

Part 7 | Legal and Economic Considerations at the End of Life

Chapter 34 | **Preparing End-of-Life Documents: Wills, Trusts, and More**

No one ever plans to be sick or disabled. Yet planning for the future can make all the difference in an emergency and at the end of life. Being prepared and having important documents in a single place can give you peace of mind, help ensure your wishes are honored, and ease the burden on your loved ones.

CHECKLIST FOR GETTING YOUR AFFAIRS IN ORDER

The following list provides common steps to consider when getting your affairs in order:

- **Plan for your estate and finances**. Depending on your situation, you may choose to prepare different types of legal documents to outline how your estate and finances will be handled in the future. The following are the common documents for estate and finances:
  - **Will**. This document specifies how your estate—your property, money, and other assets—will be distributed and managed when you die. A will can also address care for children under the age of 18, adult dependents, and pets, as well as gifts and end-of-life arrangements, such as a funeral or memorial service and burial or cremation. If you do not have a will, your estate will be distributed according to the laws in your state.

- **Durable power of attorney for finances**. This document names someone who will make financial decisions for you when you are unable to.
- **Living trust**. This document names and instructs a person, called the "trustee," to hold and distribute property and funds on your behalf when you are no longer able to manage your affairs.
- **Plan for your future health care**. Many people choose to prepare advance directives, which are legal documents that provide instructions for medical care and only go into effect if you cannot communicate your own wishes due to disease or severe injury. The following are the most common advance directives for health care:
  - **Living will**. This advance directive tells doctors how you want to be treated if you cannot make your own decisions about emergency treatment. You can say which common medical treatments or care you would want, which ones you would want to avoid, and under which conditions each of your choices applies.
  - **Durable power of attorney for health care (DPOAHC)**. This advance directive names your health-care proxy (HCP), a person who can make health-care decisions for you if you are unable to communicate these yourself. Your proxy—also known as a "representative," "surrogate," or "agent"—should be familiar with your values and wishes. A proxy can be chosen in addition to or instead of a living will. Having a HCP helps you plan for situations that cannot be foreseen, such as a serious auto accident or stroke. These documents are part of advance care planning, which involves preparing for future decisions about your medical care and discussing your wishes with your loved ones.
- **Put your important papers and copies of legal documents in one place**. You can set up a file, put everything in a desk or dresser drawer, or list the information and location of papers in a notebook.

For added security, you might consider getting a fireproof and waterproof safe to store your documents. If your papers are in a bank safe-deposit box, keep copies in a file at home.

- **Tell someone you know and trust or a lawyer where to find your important papers.** You do not need to discuss your personal affairs, but someone you trust should know where to find your papers in case of an emergency. If you do not have a relative or friend you trust, ask a lawyer to help.

- **Talk to your loved ones and a doctor about advance care planning.** A doctor can help you understand future health decisions you may face and plan the kinds of care or treatment you may want. Discussing advance care planning with your doctor is free through Medicare during your annual wellness visit. Private health insurance may also cover these discussions. Share your decisions with your loved ones to help avoid any surprises or misunderstandings about your wishes.

- **Give permission in advance for a doctor or lawyer to talk with your caregiver as needed.** If you need help managing your care, you can give your caregiver permission to talk with your doctors, your lawyer, your insurance provider, a credit card company, or your bank. You may need to sign and return a form. Giving permission for your doctor or lawyer to talk with your caregiver is different from naming a HCP. A HCP can only make decisions if you are unable to communicate them yourself.

- **Review your plans regularly.** It is important to review your plans at least once each year and when any major life event occurs, such as a divorce, move, or major change in your health.

WHICH DOCUMENTS DO YOU NEED TO HAVE IN PLACE?

When you are getting your affairs in order, it is important to prepare and organize important records and files all in one place.

Typically, you will want to include personal, financial, and health information. Remember, this is a starting place. You may have other information to add. For example, if you have a pet, you will want to include the name and address of your veterinarian.

Personal information
- full legal name
- Social Security number (SSN)
- legal residence
- date and place of birth
- names and addresses of spouse and children
- location of birth and death certificates and certificates of marriage, divorce, citizenship, and adoption
- employers and dates of employment
- education and military records
- names and phone numbers of religious contacts
- memberships in groups and awards received
- names and phone numbers of close friends, relatives, doctors, lawyers, and financial advisors

Financial Information
- sources of income and assets (pension from your employer, individual retirement account (IRA), 401(k)s, interest, etc.)
- Social Security information
- insurance information (life, long-term care, home, and car) with policy numbers and agents' names and phone numbers
- names of your banks and account numbers (checking, savings, and credit union)
- investment income (stocks, bonds, and property) and stockbrokers' names and phone numbers
- copy of most recent income tax return
- location of the most up-to-date will with an original signature
- liabilities, including property tax—what is owed, to whom, and when payments are due

- mortgages and debts—how and when they are paid
- location of the original deed of trust for the home
- car title and registration
- credit and debit card names and numbers
- location of the safe-deposit box and key

Health Information

- current prescriptions (be sure to update this regularly)
- living will
- DPOAHC
- copies of any medical orders or forms you have (e.g., a do-not-resuscitate (DNR) order)
- health insurance information with policy and phone numbers

WHO CAN HELP WITH GETTING YOUR AFFAIRS IN ORDER?

You may want to talk with a lawyer about setting up a general power of attorney, durable power of attorney, joint account, or trust. Be sure to ask about the lawyer's fees before you make an appointment.

You do not have to involve a lawyer in creating your advance directives for health care. Most states provide the forms for free, and you can complete them yourself.

You should be able to find a directory of local lawyers on the Internet or contact your local library, your local bar association for lawyers, or the Eldercare Locator (https://eldercare.acl.gov/Public/Index.aspx). Your local bar association can also help you find what free legal aid options your state has to offer. An informed family member may be able to help you manage some of these issues.

WHAT OTHER DECISIONS CAN YOU PREPARE FOR IN ADVANCE?

Getting your affairs in order can also mean making decisions about organ donation and funeral arrangements or what you want to happen to your body after you die. Deciding and sharing your decisions can help your loved ones during a stressful time and best ensure your wishes are understood and respected.

- **Organ donation and brain donation**. When someone dies, their healthy organs and tissues may be donated to help someone else. You can register to be an organ donor when you renew your driver's license or state identification documents (IDs) at your local Department of Motor Vehicles. You can also register online. Some people also choose to donate their brains to advance scientific research. It may be possible to donate organs for transplant as well as the brain for scientific research.

- **Funeral arrangements**. You can decide ahead of time what kind of funeral or memorial service you would like and where it will be held. You can also decide whether you would like to be buried or cremated and whether you want your body's ashes kept by your loved ones or scattered in a favorite place. Be sure and specify certain religious, spiritual, or cultural traditions that you would like to have during your visitation, funeral, or memorial service. You can make arrangements directly with a funeral home or crematory. If you choose not to be embalmed or cremated, most states allow families to take care of transportation, preparation of the body, and other needed arrangements. Put your preferences in writing and give copies to your loved ones and, if you have one, your lawyer.[1]

---

[1] National Institute on Aging (NIA), "Getting Your Affairs in Order Checklist: Documents to Prepare for the Future," National Institutes of Health (NIH), February 1, 2023. Available online. URL: www.nia.nih.gov/health/getting-your-affairs-order-checklist-documents-prepare-future. Accessed August 31, 2023.

Chapter 35 | Patients' Rights in End-of-Life Care

Chapter Contents

Section 35.1 | Informed Consent and Its Importance

WHAT IS INFORMED CONSENT?

Informed consent is a process through which you learn details about the trial before deciding whether to take part. This process includes learning about the trial's purpose and possible risks and benefits. It is a critical part of ensuring patient safety in research.

During the informed consent process, the research team, which is made up of doctors and nurses, first explains the trial to you. The team explains the trial's:

- purpose
- procedures
- risks and benefits

They will also discuss your rights, including your right to:
- make a decision about participating
- leave the study at any time

Before agreeing to take part in a trial, you have the right to:
- learn about all your treatment options
- learn all that is involved in the trial, including all details about treatment, tests, and possible risks and benefits
- discuss the trial with the principal investigator and other members of the research team
- both hear and read the information in a language you can understand

After discussing the study with you, the research team will give you an informed consent form to read. The form includes written details about the information that was discussed with you and describes the privacy of your medical records. If you agree to take part in the study, you sign the form. But, even after you sign the consent form, you can leave the study at any time.[1]

[1] "Informed Consent," National Cancer Institute (NCI), February 11, 2020. Available online. URL: www.cancer.gov/about-cancer/treatment/clinical-trials/patient-safety/informed-consent. Accessed August 28, 2023.

BASIC ELEMENTS OF INFORMED CONSENT
Description of Clinical Investigation

"A statement that the study involves research, an explanation of the purposes of the research and the expected duration of the subject's participation, a description of the procedures to be followed, and identification of any procedures that are experimental."

A clear statement that the clinical investigation involves research is important to make prospective subjects aware that although preliminary data (bench, animal, pilot studies, and literature) may exist, the purpose of the subject's participation is primarily to contribute to research (e.g., to evaluate the safety and effectiveness of the test article or to evaluate a different dose or route of administration of an approved drug) rather than to their own medical treatment.

The U.S. Food and Drug Administration (FDA) recommends that when discussing the required elements of informed consent with prospective subjects, there should first be a discussion of the care a patient would likely receive if not part of the research, if relevant, and then the potential subject should be provided with information about the research. This sequence allows prospective subjects to understand how the research differs from the care they might otherwise receive. The description of the clinical investigation should identify tests or procedures required by the protocol that would not be part of their care outside the research, for example, drawing blood samples for a pharmacokinetic study. Procedures related solely to research must be explained. In some cases, tests or procedures that would be considered part of usual clinical care will not be performed on study participants; when applicable, this should be discussed as part of the informed consent process.

The description of the clinical investigation must describe the test article. The description should include relevant information on what is known about both the test article and the control. For example, the description should indicate whether the test article is approved or cleared for marketing and describe the use(s) for which it has been approved or cleared. The description should also provide relevant information about any control used in the study, for example, whether the control is approved or cleared by the FDA for marketing, is considered a medically recognized standard of care, or is a placebo (including an explanation of what a placebo is). The information provided about the test article and control should include appropriate and reliable information about the potential benefits and risks of each to the extent such information is available.

The consent process should outline what the subject's participation will involve in order to comply with the protocol, for example, the number of clinic visits, maintenance of diaries, and medical or dietary restrictions (including the need to avoid specific medications or activities, such as participation in other clinical investigations). If describing every procedure would make the consent form too lengthy or detailed, the FDA recommends providing the general procedures in the consent form with an addendum describing the details of the study procedures to be performed at each visit. It may be helpful to provide a chart outlining what happens at each study visit to simplify the consent form and assist the prospective subject in understanding what participation in the clinical investigation will involve. The FDA believes that removing procedural details from the consent form will reduce its length, enhance its readability, and allow the consent document to focus on content related to the risks and anticipated benefits, if any.

The informed consent process must clearly describe the expected duration of the subject's participation in the clinical investigation, which includes their active participation as well as long-term follow-up, if appropriate. Prospective subjects must be informed of the procedures that will occur during such follow-up.

Risks and Discomforts

The informed consent process must describe the reasonably foreseeable risks or discomforts to the subject. This includes risks or discomforts of tests, interventions, and procedures required by the protocol (including protocol-specified standard medical procedures, exams, and tests) with a particular focus on those that carry a significant risk of morbidity or mortality. Possible risks or discomforts due to changes to a subject's medical care (e.g., by changing the subject's stable medication regimen or by stopping the subject's current treatment and randomizing them to either the investigational drug or placebo) should also be addressed. Where relevant, participants should also be made aware of the possibility of unintended disclosures of private information and be provided with an explanation of measures to protect a subject's privacy and data and limitations to those measures. The explanation of potential risks of the test article and control, if any, and an assessment of the likelihood of these risks occurring should be based on reliable and accurate information presented in the protocol, investigator's brochure, labeling, and/or previous research reports. Reasonably foreseeable discomforts to the subject must also be described. For example, the consent form should disclose that the subject may be uncomfortable having to stay in one position or experience claustrophobia-like symptoms during a magnetic resonance imaging (MRI).

Any reasonably foreseeable risks or discomforts to the subject need to be described in the informed consent form; however, it is not necessary to describe all possible risks, especially if doing so could make the form overwhelming for subjects to read. Information on risks that are more likely to occur and those that are serious should be described so that prospective subjects can understand the nature of the risk. The discussion may include information on whether a risk is reversible and the probability of the risk based on existing data. Information on what may be done to mitigate serious risks and risks and discomforts more likely to occur should also be considered for inclusion.

The description should not understate the probability and magnitude of the reasonably foreseeable risks and discomforts. If applicable, the consent document should include a description of the reasonably foreseeable risks to the subject but also the potential for risk to "others" (e.g., radiation therapy where close proximity to subjects postprocedure may create some risk to others). In situations where there may be a risk to others, efforts to mitigate the potential risk (e.g., using separate bathrooms) may be included in the consent document or provided in a separate document and given to the subject during the consent discussion.

Benefits

Potential benefits should be explained in terms of any direct impact on the prospective subject, in addition to the anticipated societal benefit of the research. The description of potential benefits to the subject from the use of the test article (and control, if appropriate) should include appropriate details and should be clear, balanced, and based on reliable information to the extent such information is available. This element requires a description of the potential benefits not only to the subject (e.g., "this product is intended to decrease XXX; however, we cannot guarantee that you will receive any benefit from it or from being in the study") but also to "others" (e.g., "your participation in this research may not benefit you, but information learned from this study may benefit patients with your disease or condition in the future").

Overly optimistic representations of the benefits of the test article being studied in the clinical investigation may be misleading and may violate the FDA regulations that prohibit the promotion of investigational drugs and devices. Where the purpose of the study is to determine the safety and/or effectiveness of the test article, there is usually significant uncertainty regarding whether and to what extent the test article provides a benefit.

If payments, including reimbursement for research-related expenses incurred by subjects due to participation, are provided, the consent process should not identify them as benefits.

Alternative Procedures or Treatments

To enable an informed decision about taking part in a clinical investigation, consent forms must disclose appropriate alternatives to entering the clinical investigation, if any, that might be advantageous to the subject. Prospective subjects must be informed of the appropriate alternatives available to them, including a description of the care they would be likely to receive if they choose not to participate in the research. This includes alternatives such as approved therapies for the patient's disease or condition, other forms of therapy (e.g., surgical) or diagnosis, and supportive care with no disease-directed therapy when appropriate. This disclosure must

341

include a description of the current medically recognized standard of care, particularly in studies of medical products intended to treat or diagnose serious diseases or conditions. The current medically recognized standard of care may include uses or treatment regimens for a legally marketed drug or device that are not included in the product's approved or cleared uses. When describing in the consent form an unapproved use or treatment regimen of an approved or cleared drug or device that the sponsor markets and such use or treatment regimen is a part of the medically recognized standard of care, the consent form can provide factual information concerning the unapproved use or treatment regimen of the drug or device.

When disclosing appropriate alternative procedures or courses of treatment, the FDA recommends that a description of any reasonably foreseeable risks or discomforts and potential benefits associated with these alternatives should be disclosed during the informed consent process although not necessarily included in the written informed consent document. Where such descriptions or disclosures can contain quantified comparative estimates of the reasonably foreseeable risks or discomforts and potential benefits (e.g., from the clinical literature) between the alternatives, they should do so. The agency does not believe that providing such quantified comparative estimates for every case would be realistic or appropriate. Where such well-defined estimates are not possible, the agency believes that a description of the risks and benefits should be sufficient.

It may be appropriate to refer the subject to their primary care provider or another health-care professional who can more fully discuss the alternatives, for example, when alternatives include various combinations of treatments, such as radiation, surgery, and chemotherapy for some cancers. Such discussions with an appropriate health-care professional should be completed prior to the subject signing and dating the consent form.

While an individual subject may be eligible for more than one clinical investigation, that determination and the decision as to which trial would be most appropriate for a particular subject would need to be made on a case-by-case basis. A discussion of other trials for which the subject may be eligible would generally be more appropriate to address as part of the informed consent discussion rather than the informed consent document. The subject may also wish to seek input from a primary care or other health-care provider on this issue.

As applicable, the informed consent process should advise that participation in one clinical investigation may preclude an individual's eligibility to participate in other clinical investigations. When there are multiple clinical investigations for evaluating the treatment of a particular disease for which a subject may be eligible, the sequence in which a subject may participate in the clinical investigations may be important and should be discussed with the prospective subject. For example, participation in a study of a drug for a specific therapeutic category may be an exclusion criterion for another study. The prospective subject may wish to discuss the study with their primary care provider, if appropriate.

Confidentiality

The consent process must describe the extent to which confidentiality of records identifying subjects will be maintained and should identify all entities, for example, the study sponsor, the research team, regulatory agencies, and/or ethics committee members, who may gain access to the records relating to the clinical investigation. The consent process must also note the possibility that the FDA may inspect records and should not state or imply that the FDA needs permission from the subject for access to the records. Under the Health Insurance Portability and Accountability Act (HIPAA) Privacy Rule, the FDA does not need permission to inspect records containing protected health information. The FDA may inspect study records to assess investigator compliance with the study protocol and the validity of the data reported by the sponsor.

Under the Federal Food, Drug, and Cosmetic Act (FD&C Act), the FDA may inspect and copy records relating to a clinical investigation. The FDA generally will not copy records that include the subject's name unless it is necessary to do so for the reasons described in 21 CFR 312.68 and 812.145, such as when there is reason to question whether the records represent the actual cases studied or results obtained. When the FDA requires subject names or other information that could connect the individual subject with

343

the personal health information contained in the record, the FDA will generally treat such information as confidential, but on rare occasions, the FDA may be required to disclose this information to third parties, for example, if required by a court of law. Therefore, the consent process should not promise or imply absolute confidentiality with regard to records that may be inspected by the FDA.

Compensation and Medical Treatment in the Event of Injury

For clinical investigations involving more than minimal risk, the informed consent process must describe any compensation and medical treatments available to subjects if injury occurs. Because available compensation and medical treatments may vary depending on the medical circumstances of the individual subject or the policies of the institution, the consent process should include an explanation to subjects of where they may obtain further information. An example of an adequate statement is, "the sponsor has made plans to pay for medical costs related to research-related injuries," followed by an explanation of how to obtain further information. If no compensation is available, the consent process should include a statement such as:

> "Because of hospital policy, the hospital is not able to pay for your medical care if you are injured as a result of being in this study. If you are injured as a result of being in this study, you or your insurance will be responsible for paying your medical expenses. However, you do not give up any of your legal rights by being in this study, and you may choose to pursue legal action if you are injured by being in the study."

Contacts

The consent document (or oral presentation, if a short form is used) must provide information on how to contact an appropriate individual for questions about the clinical investigation and the subjects' rights and whom to contact in the event that a research-related injury to the subject occurs. This information should include contact names (or offices), email addresses, and telephone numbers. The FDA recommends that the individual or office named for questions about subjects' rights not be part of the investigational team because subjects may be hesitant to report specific concerns or identify possible problems to someone who is part of the investigational team. In addition, the consent process should include information on whom to contact and what to do in the event of an emergency, including 24-hour contact information, if appropriate.

If contact information changes during the clinical investigation, then the new contact information must be provided to the subject. This may be done through a variety of ways; for example, a card providing the relevant contact information for the clinical investigation may be given to the subject during a visit or mailed to the subject in an envelope to protect the subject's privacy.

Voluntary Participation

This element requires that subjects be informed that they may decline to take part in the clinical investigation or may stop participation at any time without penalty or loss of benefits to which subjects are entitled. The language that limits the subject's right to decline to participate or withdraw from the clinical investigation must not be used. If special procedures should be followed for the subject to withdraw from the clinical investigation, the consent process must outline and explain the procedures. Also, note that subjects may not withdraw data that were collected about them prior to their withdrawal.[2]

IMPORTANCE OF INFORMED CONSENT

As new medical products are being developed, no one knows for sure how well they will work or what risks they will find. Clinical trials are used to answer the following questions:

- Are new medical products safe enough to outweigh the risks related to the underlying condition?

---

[2] "Informed Consent—Guidance for IRBs, Clinical Investigators, and Sponsors," U.S. Food and Drug Administration (FDA), August 2023. Available online. URL: www.fda.gov/media/88915/download. Accessed August 28, 2023.

- How should the product be used (e.g., the best dose, frequency, or any special precautions necessary to avoid problems)?
- How effective is the medical product at relieving symptoms or treating or curing a condition?

The main purpose of clinical trials is to "study" new medical products in people. It is important for people who are considering participation in a clinical trial to understand their role as a "subject of research" and not as a patient.

While research subjects may get personal treatment benefits from participating in a clinical trial, they must understand that they:

- may not benefit from the clinical trial
- may be exposed to unknown risks
- are entering into a study that may be very different from the standard medical practices that they currently know

To make an informed decision about whether to participate or not in a clinical trial, people need to be informed about:

- what will be done to them
- how the protocol (plan of research) works
- what risks or discomforts they may experience
- participation, which is a voluntary decision on their part

This information is provided to potential participants through the informed consent process. Informed consent means that the purpose of the research is explained to them, including what their role would be and how the trial will work.

A central part of the informed consent process is the informed consent document. The FDA does not dictate the specific language required for the informed consent document but does require certain basic elements of consent to be included.

Before enrolling in a clinical trial, the following information must be given to each potential research subject:

- a statement explaining that the study involves research
- an explanation of the purposes of the research

- the expected length of time for participation
- a description of all the procedures that will be completed during enrollment in the clinical trial
- information about all experimental procedures that will be completed during the clinical trial
- a description of any predictable risks
- any possible discomforts (e.g., injections, frequency of blood tests, etc.) that could occur as a result of the research
- any possible benefits that may be expected from the research
- information about any alternative procedures or treatment (if any) that might benefit the research subject
- a statement describing:
  - the confidentiality of information collected during the clinical trial
  - how records that identify the subject will be kept
  - the possibility that the FDA may inspect the records
- for research involving more than minimal risk information, including:
  - an explanation as to whether any compensation or medical treatments are available if an injury occurs
  - what they consist of
  - where more information may be found
  - questions about the research
  - research subjects' rights
  - injury related to the clinical trial
- a statement stating research subject participation is voluntary
- a statement stating research subjects have the right to refuse treatment without losing any benefits to which they are entitled
- a statement stating research subjects may choose to stop participation in the clinical trial at any time without losing the benefits to which they are entitled

- contact information to be provided for answers to questions about the research
- an explanation of whom to contact with questions about subjects' rights

When appropriate, one or more of the following elements of information must also be provided in the informed consent document:

- a statement that the research treatment or procedure may involve unexpected risks (to the subject and/or unborn baby, if the subject is or may become pregnant)
- any reasons why the research subject participation may be ended by the clinical trial investigator (e.g., failing to follow the requirements of the trial or changes in lab values that fall outside the clinical trial limits)
- added costs to the research subject that may result from participating in the trial
- the consequence of leaving a trial before it is completed (e.g., if the research and procedures require a slow and organized end of participation)
- a statement that important findings discovered during the clinical trial will be provided to the research subject
- the approximate number of research subjects that will be enrolled in the study

A potential research subject must have an opportunity to:
- read the consent document
- ask questions about anything they do not understand

Usually, if one is considering participating in a clinical trial, he or she may take the consent document home to discuss with family, friend, or advocate.

An investigator should only get consent from a potential research subject if:

- enough time was given to the research subject to consider whether or not to participate
- the investigator has not persuaded or influenced the potential research subject

348

The information must be in a language that is understandable to the research subject.

Informed consent may not include language that:

- the research subject is made to ignore or appear to ignore any of the research subject's legal rights
- releases or appears to release the investigator, the sponsor, the institution, or its agents from their liability for negligence

Participating in clinical trials is voluntary. You have the right not to participate or to end your participation in the clinical trial at any time.[3]

Section 35.2 | Protecting Health Information Privacy Rights

Most of us feel that our health information is private and should be protected. That is why there is a federal law that sets rules for health-care providers and health insurance companies about who can look at and receive our health information. This law called the "Health Insurance Portability and Accountability Act of 1996" (HIPAA) gives you rights over your health information, including the right to get a copy of your information, make sure it is correct, and know who has seen it.

GET IT

You can ask to see or get a copy of your medical record and other health information. If you want a copy, you may have to put your request in writing and pay for the cost of copying and mailing. In most cases, your copies must be given to you within 30 days.

---

[3] "Informed Consent for Clinical Trials," U.S. Food and Drug Administration (FDA), January 4, 2018. Available online. URL: www.fda.gov/patients/clinical-trials-what-patients-need-know/informed-consent-clinical-trials. Accessed August 28, 2023.

CHECK IT

You can ask to change any wrong information in your file or add information to your file if you think something is missing or incomplete. For example, if you and your hospital agree that your file has the wrong result for a test, the hospital must change it. Even if the hospital believes the test result is correct, you still have the right to have your disagreement noted in your file. In most cases, the file should be updated within 60 days.

KNOW WHO HAS SEEN IT

By law, your health information can be used and shared for specific reasons not directly related to your care, such as making sure doctors give good care, making sure nursing homes are clean and safe, reporting when the flu is in your area, or reporting as required by state or federal law. In many of these cases, you can find out who has seen your health information. You can do the following:

- **Learn how your health information is used and shared by your doctor or health insurer**. Generally, your health information cannot be used for purposes not directly related to your care without your permission. For example, your doctor cannot give it to your employer or share it for things such as marketing and advertising without your written authorization. You probably received a notice telling you how your health information may be used on your first visit to a new health-care provider or when you got new health insurance, but you can ask for another copy anytime.

- **Let your providers or health insurance companies know if there is information you do not want to share**. You can ask that your health information not be shared with certain people, groups, or companies. If you go to a clinic, for example, you can ask the doctor not to share your medical records with other doctors or nurses at the clinic. You can ask for other kinds of restrictions, but they do not always have to agree to do what you ask, particularly if it could affect your care. Finally, you can also ask your health-care provider or pharmacy not to tell your health insurance company about the care you receive or drugs you take if you pay for the care or drugs in full and the provider or pharmacy does not need to get paid by your insurance company.

- **Ask to be reached somewhere other than home.** You can make reasonable requests to be contacted at different places or in a different way. For example, you can ask to have a nurse call you at your office instead of your home or to send mail to you in an envelope instead of on a postcard.

If you think your rights are being denied or your health information is not being protected, you have the right to file a complaint with your provider, health insurer, or the U.S. Department of Health and Human Services (HHS).[4]

---

[4] "Your Health Information Privacy Rights," U.S. Department of Health and Human Services (HHS), March 14, 2013. Available online. URL: www.hhs.gov/sites/default/files/ocr/privacy/hipaa/understanding/consumers/consumer_rights.pdf. Accessed August 28, 2023.

Chapter 36 | **Advance Directives and Their Significance**

During an emergency or at the end of life, you may face questions about your loved one's medical treatment and not be able to answer them. You may assume your loved ones know what you would want, but that is not always true. In one study, people guessed nearly one out of three end-of-life decisions for their loved one incorrectly.

Research shows that you are more likely to get the care you want if you have conversations about your future medical treatment and put a plan in place. It may also help your loved ones grieve more easily and feel less burden, guilt, and depression.

WHAT IS ADVANCE CARE PLANNING?

Advance care planning involves discussing and preparing for future decisions about your medical care if you become seriously ill or unable to communicate your wishes. Having meaningful conversations with your loved ones is the most important part of advance care planning. Many people also choose to put their preferences in writing by completing legal documents called "advance directives."

WHAT ARE ADVANCE DIRECTIVES?

Advance directives are legal documents that provide instructions for medical care and only go into effect if you cannot communicate your own wishes.

The following are the two most common advance directives for health care:

- **Living will**. This is a legal document that tells doctors how you want to be treated if you cannot make your own decisions about emergency treatment. In a living will, you can say which common medical treatments or care you would want, which ones you would want to avoid, and under which conditions each of your choices applies.
- **Durable power of attorney for health care (DPOAHC)**. This is a legal document that names your health-care proxy, (HCP) a person who can make health-care decisions for you if you are unable to communicate these yourself. Your proxy, also known as a "representative," "surrogate," or "agent," should be familiar with your values and wishes. A proxy can be chosen in addition to or instead of a living will. Having a HCP helps you plan for situations that cannot be foreseen, such as a serious car accident or stroke.

Think of your advance directives as living documents that you review at least once each year and update if a major life event occurs, such as retirement, moving out of state, or a significant change in your health.

WHO NEEDS AN ADVANCE CARE PLAN?

Advance care planning is not just for people who are very old or ill. At any age, a medical crisis could leave you unable to communicate your own health-care decisions. Planning now for your future health care can help ensure you get the medical care you want and that someone you trust will be there to make decisions for you.

WHAT HAPPENS IF YOU DO NOT HAVE AN ADVANCE DIRECTIVE?

If you do not have an advance directive and you are unable to make decisions on your own, the laws of the state where you live will determine who may make medical decisions on your behalf. This is typically your spouse, your parents if they are available, or your children if they are adults. If you are unmarried and have not named your partner as your proxy, it is possible they could be excluded from decision-making. If you have no family members, some states allow a close friend who is familiar with your values to help. Or they may assign a physician to represent your best interests. To find out the laws in your state, contact your state legal aid office or state bar association.

WILL AN ADVANCE DIRECTIVE GUARANTEE YOUR WISHES ARE FOLLOWED?

An advance directive is legally recognized but not legally binding. This means that your health-care provider and proxy will do their best to respect your advance directives, but there may be circumstances in which they cannot follow your wishes exactly. For example, you may be in a complex medical situation where it is unclear what you would want. This is another key reason why having conversations about your preferences is so important. Talking with your loved ones ahead of time may help them better navigate unanticipated issues.

There is the possibility that a health-care provider refuses to follow your advance directives. This might happen if the decision goes against:

- the health-care provider's conscience
- the health-care institution's policy
- the accepted health-care standards

In these situations, the health-care provider must inform your HCP immediately and consider transferring your care to another provider.

OTHER ADVANCE CARE PLANNING FORMS AND ORDERS

You might want to prepare documents to express your wishes about a single medical issue or something else not already covered in your advance directives, such as an emergency. For these types of situations, you can talk with a doctor about establishing the following orders:

- **Do-not-resuscitate (DNR) order.** A DNR becomes part of your medical chart to inform medical staff in a hospital or nursing facility that you do not want cardiopulmonary resuscitation (CPR) or other life-support measures to be attempted if your heartbeat and breathing stop. Sometimes, this document is referred to as a "do-not-attempt-resuscitation (DNAR) order" or an "allow natural death (AND) order." Even though a living will might state that CPR is not wanted, it is helpful to have a DNR order as part of your medical file if you go to a hospital. Posting a DNR next to your hospital bed might avoid confusion in an emergency. Without a DNR order, medical staff will attempt every effort to restore your breathing and the normal rhythm of your heart.

- **Do-not-intubate (DNI) order.** A similar document, a DNI informs medical staff in a hospital or nursing facility that you do not want to be on a ventilator.

- **Do-not-hospitalize (DNH) order.** A DNH indicates to long-term care providers, such as nursing home staff, that you prefer not to be sent to a hospital for treatment at the end of life.

- **Out-of-hospital DNR order.** An out-of-hospital DNR alerts emergency medical personnel to your wishes regarding measures to restore your heartbeat or breathing if you are not in a hospital.

- **Physician orders for life-sustaining treatment (POLST) and medical orders for life-sustaining treatment (MOLST) forms.** These forms provide guidance about your medical care that health-care professionals can act on immediately in an emergency. They serve as a medical order in addition to your advance directive. Typically, you create a POLST or MOLST when you are near the end of life or critically ill and understand the specific decisions that might need to be made on your behalf. These forms may also be called "portable medical orders" or "physician orders for scope of treatment" (POST). Check with your state department of health to find out if these forms are available where you live.

You may also want to document your wishes about organ and tissue donation and brain donation. As well, learning about care options such as palliative care and hospice care can help you plan ahead.

HOW CAN YOU GET STARTED WITH ADVANCE CARE PLANNING?

To get started with advance care planning, consider the following steps:

- **Reflect on your values and wishes**. This can help you think through what matters most at the end of life and guide your decisions about future care and medical treatment.
- **Talk with your doctor about advance directives**. Advance care planning is covered by Medicare as part of your annual wellness visit. If you have private health insurance, check with your insurance provider. Talking to a health-care provider can help you learn about your current health and the kinds of decisions that are likely to come up. For example, you might ask about the decisions you may face if your high blood pressure (HBP) leads to a stroke.
- **Choose someone you trust to make medical decisions for you**. Whether it is a family member, a loved one, or your lawyer, it is important to choose someone you trust as your HCP. Once you have decided, discuss your values and preferences with them. If you are not ready to discuss specific treatments or care decisions yet, try talking about your general preferences. You can also try other ways to share your wishes, such as writing a letter or watching a video on the topic together.
- **Complete your advance directive forms**. To make your care and treatment decisions official, you can

complete a living will. Similarly, once you decide on your HCP, you can make it official by completing a DPOAHC.

- **Share your forms with your HCP, doctors, and loved ones.** After you have completed your advance directives, make copies and store them in a safe place. Give copies to your HCP, health-care providers, and lawyer. Some states have registries that can store your advance directive for quick access by health-care providers and your proxy.
- **Keep the conversation going.** Continue to talk about your wishes and update your forms at least once each year or after major life changes. If you update your forms, file and keep your previous versions. Note the date the older copy was replaced by a new one. If you use a registry, make sure the latest version is on record.

Everyone approaches the process differently. Remember to be flexible and take it one step at a time. Start small. For example, try simply talking with your loved ones about what you appreciate and enjoy most about life. Your values, treatment preferences, and even the people you involve in your plan may change over time. The most important part is to start the conversation.

HOW TO FIND ADVANCE DIRECTIVE FORMS

You can establish your advance directives for little or no cost. Many states have their own forms that you can access and complete for free. The following are some ways you might find free advance directive forms in your state:

- Contact your State Attorney General's Office.
- Contact your local Area Agency on Aging (AAA; https://eldercare.acl.gov/Public/About/Aging_ Network/AAA.aspx). You can find your area agency phone number by visiting the Eldercare Locator (https://eldercare.acl.gov/Public/Index.aspx) or by calling 800-677-1116.

- Download your state's form online from one of these national organizations: the American Association of Retired Persons (AARP; www.aarp.org/caregiving/financial-legal/free-printable-advance-directives/), the American Bar Association (ABA; www.americanbar.org/groups/law_aging/resources/health_care_decision_making/Stateforms/), or the National Hospice and Palliative Care Organization (NHPCO; www.caringinfo.org/planning/advance-directives/).
- If you are a veteran, contact your local Veterans Affairs (VA) office (www.va.gov/contact-us/#contact-your-local-va-facility). The VA offers an advance directive specifically for veterans.

Some people spend a lot of time in more than one state. If that is your situation, consider preparing advance directives using the form for each state and keep a copy in each place, too.

There are also organizations that enable you to create, download, and print your forms online, but they may charge fees. Before you pay, remember there are several ways to get your forms for free. The following are some free online resources:

- **PREPARE for Your Care**. This is an interactive online program that was funded in part by the National Institute on Aging (NIA; https://prepareforyourcare.org). It is available in English and Spanish.
- **The Conversation Project**. A series of online conversation guides and advance care documents available in English, Spanish, and Chinese. The Conversation Project is a public engagement initiative led by the Institute for Healthcare Improvement (IHI; https://theconversationproject.org).

If you use forms from a website, check to make sure they are legally recognized in your state. You should also make sure the website is secure and will protect your personal information. Read the website's privacy policy and check that the website link begins with "https" (make sure it has an "s") and that it has a small lock icon next to its web address.

Some people also choose to carry a card (e.g., from the American Hospital Association (AHA)) in their wallet, indicating they have an advance directive and where it is kept.[1]

[1] National Institute on Aging (NIA), "Advance Care Planning: Advance Directives for Health Care," National Institutes of Health (NIH), October 31, 2022. Available online. URL: www.nia.nih.gov/health/advance-care-planning-advance-directives-health-care. Accessed August 7, 2023.

Chapter 37 | **Financial Assistance for Long-Term Care**

Many older adults and caregivers worry about the cost of medical care and other help they may need. These expenses can use up a significant part of monthly income, even for families who thought they had saved enough.

How people pay for long-term care—whether delivered at home or in a hospital, assisted living facility, or nursing home—depends on their financial situation and the kinds of services they use. Some people believe that their current health or disability insurance will pay for their long-term care needs, but most of these insurance policies include limited, if any, long-term care benefits. Often, people must rely on a variety of payment sources, including personal funds, government programs, and private financing options.

PERSONAL FUNDS (OUT-OF-POCKET EXPENSES)

At first, many older adults pay for care in part with their own money. They may use personal savings, a pension or other retirement fund, income from stocks and bonds, or proceeds from the sale of a home.

Much home-based care is paid for using personal out-of-pocket funds. Initially, family and friends may provide personal care and other services, such as transportation, for free. But, as a person's needs increase, paid services may be needed.

Many older adults also pay out of pocket to participate in adult day service programs, receive meals, and get other community-based services provided by local governments and nonprofit groups. These services help them remain in their homes.

Professional care given in assisted living facilities and continuing care retirement communities is almost always paid for out of pocket though, in some states, Medicaid may cover some costs for people who meet financial and health requirements.

GOVERNMENT PROGRAMS

Older adults may be eligible for some government health-care benefits. Caregivers can help by learning more about possible sources of financial help and assisting older adults in applying for aid as appropriate.

Several federal and state programs provide help with health-care-related costs. Over time, the benefits and eligibility requirements of these programs can change, and some benefits differ from state to state.

Medicare

This federal government health insurance program helps pay some medical costs for people aged 65 and older and for people under the age of 65 with certain disabilities and serious health conditions. Covered services include hospital stays, doctor visits, some home health care, hospice care, and preventive services such as vaccinations. The program does not cover assisted living or long-term care. Medicare components include Part A (Hospital Insurance), Part B (Medical Insurance), and Part D (Drug Coverage). Medicare Advantage is another option for obtaining Part A and Part B coverage. Call Medicare at 800-633-4227 or visit Medicare.gov (www.medicare.gov) for more information.

Medicaid

Medicaid is a combined federal and state program for low-income people. This program covers the costs of medical care and some types of long-term care for people who have limited income and meet other eligibility requirements. Eligibility and covered services vary from state to state.

To learn more about Medicaid, visit Medicaid.gov (www.medicaid.gov), call 877-267-2323 (TTY: 866-226-1819), or contact your state health department.

Program of All-Inclusive Care for the Elderly

Some states offer the Program of All-Inclusive Care for the Elderly (PACE), a combined Medicare and Medicaid program that provides care and services to people who otherwise would need care in a nursing home. PACE covers medical, social service, and long-term care costs. It may pay for some or all of the long-term care needs of a person with Alzheimer disease (AD; www.nia.nih.gov/health/alzheimers). PACE enables most people who qualify to continue living at home instead of moving to a long-term care facility. Participants receive coordinated care from a team of health-care professionals.

You will need to find out if the person who needs care qualifies for PACE and if there is a PACE program near you. There may be a monthly charge. PACE is available only in certain states and locations within those states.

To find out more, contact Medicare at 800-633-4227 or visit Medicare's PACE website (www.medicare.gov/health-drug-plans/health-plans/your-coverage-options/other-medicare-health-plans/PACE). You can also search for local programs by state or ZIP code using PACEFinder (www.npaonline.org/find-a-pace-program), an online service of the National PACE Association (NPA).

State Health Insurance Assistance Program

The State Health Insurance Assistance Program (SHIP) is a national program offered in each state that provides one-on-one counseling and assistance with Medicaid, Medicare, and Medicare supplemental insurance (Medigap). SHIP can help you navigate eligibility, coverage, appeals, and out-of-pocket costs and answer questions about your family's unique situation and needs.

To find contact information for SHIP in your state, visit the SHIP website (www.shiphelp.org) or call 877-839-2675.

Department of Veterans Affairs

The U.S. Department of Veterans Affairs (VA) provides coverage for long-term care at a facility or at home for some veterans. If your family member or relative is eligible for veterans' benefits, check with the VA or get in touch with the VA medical center nearest you. There could be a waiting list for VA nursing homes.

To learn more about VA health-care benefits, call 877-222-8387 or visit the Veterans Health Administration (VHA) website (www. va.gov/health) or the Veterans Affairs Caregiver Support website (www.caregiver.va.gov). You can also find more information in Geriatrics and Extended Care: Paying for Long-Term Care (www. va.gov/GERIATRICS/pages/Paying_for_Long_Term_Care.asp).

Social Security Administration Programs

The Social Security Disability Insurance (SSDI; www.ssa.gov/benefits/disability) and the Supplemental Security Income (SSI; www. ssa.gov/ssi) programs provide financial assistance to people with disabilities.

The SSDI is for people under the age of 65 who are disabled, according to the Social Security Administration's definition. To qualify, you must be able to show that:

- you worked in a job covered by Social Security
- you are unable to work because of your medical condition
- your medical condition will last at least a year or is expected to result in death

Processing an SSDI application can take three to five months. However, Social Security has "compassionate allowances" to help people with certain serious medical conditions, such as early-onset AD and other forms of dementia, get disability benefits more quickly.

The SSI is another program that provides monthly payments to adults aged 65 and older who have a disability. To qualify, your income and resources must be under certain limits.

To find out more about these programs, call 800-772-1213 (TTY: 800-325-0778) or visit the Social Security Administration website (www.ssa.gov).

National Council on Aging

The National Council on Aging (NCOA), a private group, has a free service called "BenefitsCheckUp." This service can help you find federal and state benefit programs for older adults. After providing some general information about the person who needs care, you can see a list of possible benefit programs to explore. These programs can help pay for prescription drugs, heating bills, housing, meal programs, and legal services. You do not have to give a name, address, or Social Security number (SSN) to use this service.

Benefits.gov

For more information about federal, state, and local government benefits, visit the Benefits.gov website (www.benefits.gov) or call 800-FED-INFO (800-333-4636).

PRIVATE FINANCING OPTIONS FOR LONG-TERM CARE

In addition to personal funds and government programs, there are several private payment options for long-term care, including long-term care insurance, reverse mortgages, certain life insurance policies, annuities, and trusts. Which option is best for a person depends on many factors, including the person's age, health status, personal finances, and likelihood of needing care.

Long-Term Care Insurance

This type of insurance covers services and support for people needing long-term care, including help with the activities of daily living (ADL), as well as palliative and hospice care. Policies cover a wide range of benefits in a variety of settings, including the person's home, an assisted living facility, or a nursing home. The exact coverage depends on the type of policy and the services it includes. You can purchase nursing-home-only coverage or a comprehensive policy that includes both home care and facility care.

Many companies sell long-term care insurance. Costs and benefits vary, so it is a good idea to shop around and compare policies. The cost of a policy is based on the type and amount of services, how old you are when you buy the policy, and any optional benefits you choose. Some employers are starting to offer group long-term care insurance programs as a benefit. It may be easier to qualify for long-term care insurance through an employer-sponsored program, and group rates may be cheaper than the cost of an individual policy.

Buying long-term care insurance can be a good choice for younger, relatively healthy people at low risk of needing long-term care in the next 25 years. Costs go up for people who are older, have health problems, or want more benefits. Someone who is in poor health or already receiving end-of-life care services may not qualify for long-term care insurance.

Reverse Mortgages for Seniors

A reverse mortgage is a special type of home loan that lets a homeowner convert part of the ownership value in their home into cash without having to sell the home. Unlike a traditional home loan, no repayment is required until the borrower sells the home, no longer uses it as a main residence, or dies.

There are no income or medical requirements to get a reverse mortgage, but you must be aged 62 or older. The loan amount is tax-free and can be used for any expense, including long-term care. However, if you have an existing mortgage or other debt against your home, you must use the funds to pay off those debts first.

If you are thinking about a reverse mortgage, talk to an expert. A reverse mortgage can be complicated, and other borrowing options may be available. These might include a home equity loan or refinancing an existing mortgage to lower the monthly payments. Like a reverse mortgage, these options can free up cash for covering long-term care expenses. Additional information about reverse mortgages and other borrowing options is available from the Consumer Financial Protection Bureau. Visit the Consumer Financial Protection Bureau website (www.consumerfinance.gov) or call 855-411-2372.

Life Insurance Policies for Long-Term Care

Some life insurance policies can help pay for long-term care. Some policies offer a combination product that includes both life insurance and long-term care insurance.

Policies with an "accelerated death benefit" provide tax-free cash advances while you are still alive. The advance is subtracted from the amount your beneficiaries (the people who get the insurance proceeds) will receive when you die.

You can get an accelerated death benefit if you live permanently in a nursing home, need long-term care for an extended time, are terminally ill, or have a life-threatening diagnosis such as acquired immunodeficiency syndrome (AIDS). Check your life insurance policy to see exactly what it covers.

You may be able to raise cash by selling your life insurance policy for its current value. This option, known as a "life settlement," is usually available only to women aged 74 and older and men aged 70 and older. The proceeds are taxable and can be used for any reason, including paying for long-term care.

A similar arrangement, called a "viatical settlement," allows a terminally ill person to sell their life insurance policy to an insurance company for a percentage of the death benefit on the policy. This option is typically used by people who are expected to live two years or less. A viatical settlement provides immediate cash and is tax-free, but it can be hard to get. Companies decline more than half of the people who apply.

Keep in mind that if a person chooses to take life insurance benefits early or to sell their policy, there will be little or no money left from the policy to pass on to heirs.

Using Annuities to Pay for Long-Term Care

You may choose to enter into an annuity contract with an insurance company to help pay for long-term care services. In exchange for a single payment or a series of payments, the insurance company will send you an annuity, which is a series of regular payments over a specified period. These payments, however, may not be enough to cover all of a person's expenses. Annuities can have complicated effects on a person's taxes, so speak with a tax professional before buying one.

Trusts

A trust is a legal arrangement that allows a person to transfer assets, such as cash, property, or insurance benefits, to another person, called the "trustee." Once the trust is established, the trustee manages and controls the assets for the person or another beneficiary. You may choose to use a trust to provide flexible control of assets for an older adult or a person with a disability, which could include yourself or your spouse.

CAN FAMILY CAREGIVERS GET PAID TO TAKE CARE OF A FAMILY MEMBER?

Family caregivers make a lot of sacrifices to care for older, sick, or disabled relatives. Some even quit their jobs to care for the person full-time. There are many costs involved in caregiving, for example, covering travel expenses, paying bills, and buying household essentials. These costs can add up to create a significant financial burden for caregivers.

Many states offer some form of payment for family caregivers. But the laws, eligibility, and funding for this support vary by state. The most common source of assistance is Medicaid, which offers several state-based programs to people who are eligible based on income or disability. These programs include home and community-based services, adult foster care, and Medicaid personal care services.

Veterans and people living with certain diseases may also be eligible for financial assistance through federal and state agencies or private organizations. For more information, visit the Eldercare Locator website (www.eldercare.acl.gov/Public/Index.aspx) or call 800-677-1116.

Long-term care insurance usually provides coverage for care at home. However, policies differ regarding who can deliver that care. In some cases, only a professional service will be paid for long-term care. In other cases, the policy will pay for a family member to provide care. Contact your long-term care insurer to find out the details of your policy.[1]

---

[1] National Institute on Aging (NIA), "Paying for Long-Term Care," National Institutes of Health (NIH), November 2, 2022. Available online. URL: www.nia.nih.gov/health/paying-long-term-care. Accessed August 7, 2023.

Chapter 38 | **Insurance for Comprehensive End-of-Life Care**

Chapter Contents

Section 38.1 | Hospice Care Insurance

WHERE IS HOSPICE CARE RECEIVED?

Hospice care is usually provided in your home. If you live in a facility, such as a nursing home, Medicaid considers the facility to be your home. There are also other locations, such as assisted living facilities, rehabilitation centers, or hospitals, where hospice services can be covered. Check with your State Medicaid Agency (SMA) for other facilities that may be considered your home under the Medicaid hospice benefit. In June 2013, Medicare and Medicaid set rules about coordination between hospice and long-term care facilities. The following are the reasons for the change in the rules:

- to improve the quality of care you receive
- to improve communication between nursing homes and hospice providers

Communication among your various health-care providers is important. Communication is also necessary, so you, your providers, and your family members can stay informed. If you live in a nursing home or other facility and you are not sure about something, you should ask questions.

WHAT DOES THE MEDICAID HOSPICE PROGRAM COVER?

Hospice services are covered as part of your Medicaid benefits. Services are provided by a team to meet your needs. The hospice team may include you, your family, and others who can help meet your physical, psychosocial, spiritual, and emotional needs. Your needs are written in a plan of care (POC), also called a "plan."

The following benefits are examples of hospice services you may receive:

- physician services provided by the hospice agency
- nursing care
- medical equipment
- medical supplies
- drugs for symptom control and pain relief
- hospice aide and homemaker services

371

- physical therapy
- occupational therapy
- speech-language pathology services
- social worker services
- dietary counseling
- short-term inpatient care for pain control, symptom management, and respite care

Hospice benefits may also include anything needed to manage your terminal illness and related conditions that are normally covered by Medicaid. The following hospice services must be provided directly by hospice employees:

- nursing care
- physician services
- medical social services
- counseling

Other hospice services may be provided, such as visits by a physician who specializes in your illness. Hospice benefits may be different in each state. Check with your SMA about hospice benefits in the area.

ARE YOU RECEIVING QUALITY CARE?

If you are receiving hospice services, you have a right to quality care. Some examples of quality care are as follows:

- Care is focused on you and your family.
- Information is provided to you and your family, so you can make decisions.
- Staff members respect decisions made by you and your family.
- Care addresses your total needs.
- You are not denied access to care because of your race, gender, religion, or sexual orientation.
- Staff members are trained in how to care for you and your family.
- Care is coordinated between your medical team and the hospice agency.

If you feel you are not getting quality care, you should tell the hospice provider who helped you enroll in hospice. You can also call the following agencies:

- Adult Protective Services (APS) agency
- SMA
- Office of Ombudsman for Long-Term Care (OOLTC) if you live in a nursing home

WHAT CAN YOU DO TO HELP?

You play an important role in protecting the quality of care you receive and the Medicaid program. By knowing the Medicaid rules, you can ask the right questions about the services you are receiving. You should also report things that do not seem right. The following are some things you can do to help:

- Talk to your physician to see if you are eligible for hospice care. Your physician must certify that you have a reduced life expectancy resulting from your condition(s).
- Check with your SMA about what services may be covered under hospice.
- Remember, the choice to get the hospice benefit is up to you. If you are too ill, a representative can complete and sign the forms. No one should pressure you to enroll. Never sign a blank form without asking questions.
- Ask the hospice agency about the type of care you receive.
- Ask the hospice agency or SMA about what services you will receive and which services will no longer be covered after you elect hospice.
- Ask questions about bills you receive or services you are getting.
- Be careful to whom you give the details of your Medicaid, Medicare, or Social Security number (SSN).

WHERE SHOULD YOU REPORT CONCERNS RELATED TO HOSPICE CARE?

Report any acts of physical abuse or suspected fraud to your state Medicaid Fraud Control Unit (MFCU) or SMA. If you are receiving hospice care or are being pressured to enroll in hospice care but believe hospice care may not be appropriate for you, report it. If hospice services were billed but were not provided to you, report it. Information on contacting your SMA or MFCU is available at www.cms.gov/medicare-medicaid-coordination/fraud-prevention/ fraudabuseforconsumers/report_fraud_and_suspected_fraud.html on the Centers for Medicare & Medicaid Services (CMS) website, or contact the U.S. Department of Health and Human Services, Office of Inspector General (HHS-OIG). You can also call the toll-free number 800-HHS-TIPS (800-447-8477).

You play an important role in protecting the quality of care you receive and the Medicaid program. Discussing end-of-life care and choosing services that will help make you comfortable may be difficult and confusing. It is best to learn about hospice care and understand what Medicaid covers in the early stages of an illness. This helps make the decision to choose hospice easier if you become terminally ill.

You should talk to your physician to see if you are eligible for hospice care. Ask questions and stay informed. Report mistakes to your SMA. By knowing the answers to the questions, you can help protect yourself (and the Medicaid program) from fraud and abuse.[1]

Section 38.2 | Long-Term Care Insurance

WHAT IS LONG-TERM CARE INSURANCE?

Unlike traditional health insurance, long-term care insurance is designed to cover long-term services and support, including personal and custodial care, in a variety of settings such as your home, a community organization, or other facility.

Long-term care insurance policies reimburse policyholders a daily amount (up to a preselected limit) for services to assist them

---

[1] "Hospice Toolkit—An Overview of the Medicaid Hospice Benefit," Centers for Medicare & Medicaid Services (CMS), February 2016. Available online. URL: www.cms.gov/Medicare-Medicaid-Coordination/Fraud-Prevention/ Medicaid-Integrity-Education/Downloads/hospice-overviewbooklet.pdf. Accessed August 28, 2023.

with activities of daily living (ADLs), such as bathing, dressing, or eating. You can select a range of care options and benefits that allow you to get the services you need where you need them.

The cost of your long-term care policy is based on the following:

- how old you are when you buy the policy
- the maximum amount that a policy will pay per day
- the maximum number of days (years) that a policy will pay
- the maximum amount per day times the number of days that determines the lifetime maximum amount that the policy will pay
- any optional benefits you choose, such as benefits that increase with inflation

If you are in poor health or already receiving long-term care services, you may not qualify for long-term care insurance as most individual policies require medical underwriting. In some cases, you may be able to buy a limited amount of coverage or coverage at a higher "nonstandard" rate. Some group policies do not require underwriting.

What Does Long-Term Care Insurance Cover?

Most policies sold today are comprehensive. They typically allow you to use your daily benefit in a variety of settings, including:

- your home
- adult day service centers
- hospice care
- respite care
- assisted living facilities (also called "residential care facilities" or "alternate care facilities")
- Alzheimer special care facilities
- nursing homes

In the home setting, comprehensive policies generally cover the following services:

- skilled nursing care
- occupational, speech, physical, and rehabilitation therapy

- help with personal care, such as bathing and dressing

Receiving Long-Term Care Insurance Benefits

In order to receive benefits from your long-term care insurance policy, you meet the following two criteria:

- **Benefit triggers**. These are the criteria that an insurance company will use to determine if you are eligible for long-term benefits. Most companies use a specific assessment form that will be filled out by a nurse/social worker team.
  - Usually, these are defined in terms of ADLs or cognitive impairments.
  - Most policies pay benefits when you need help with two or more of six ADLs or when you have a cognitive impairment.
  - Once you have been assessed, your care manager from the insurance company will approve a plan of care (POC) that outlines the benefits for which you are eligible.
- **Elimination period**. This is the amount of time that must pass after a benefit trigger occurs but before you start receiving payment for services.
  - An elimination period is like the deductible you have on car insurance, except it is measured in time rather than by dollar amount.
  - Most policies allow you to choose an elimination period of 30, 60, or 90 days at the time you purchased your policy.
  - During this period, you must cover the cost of any services you receive.
  - Some policies specify that in order to satisfy an elimination period, you must receive paid care or pay for services during that time.

Once your benefits begin:

- most policies pay your costs up to a preset daily limit until the lifetime maximum is reached

- other policies pay a preset cash amount for each day that you meet the benefit trigger, whether you receive paid long-term care services on those days or not
- these "cash disability" policies offer more flexibility but are potentially more expensive

Where to Look for Long-Term Care Insurance
INSURANCE SPECIALIST

Most people buy long-term care insurance directly from an insurance agent, a financial planner, or a broker. The following are some important points to be noted:

- States regulate which companies can sell long-term care insurance.
- States regulate the products that companies can sell.
- There are more than 100 companies offering long-term care insurance nationally, but 15–20 insurers sell most policies.
- The best way to find out which insurance companies offer long-term care coverage in your state is to contact the Department of Insurance of your state.

STATE PARTNERSHIP PROGRAMS

Residents of some states may be able to find long-term care coverage through a State Partnership Program that links special partnership-qualified (PQ) long-term policies provided by private insurance companies with Medicaid. The uses of PQ policies to find long-term care coverage are as follows:

- Help people purchase shorter-term, more complete long-term care insurance.
- Include inflation protection, so the dollar amount of benefits you receive can be higher than the amount of insurance coverage you purchased.
- Help all of you apply for Medicaid under modified eligibility rules if you continue to need long-term care and your policy maximum is reached.

- Include a special "asset disregard" feature that allows you to keep assets such as personal savings above the usual $2,000 Medicaid limit.

Since PQ policies must include inflation protection, the amount of the benefits you receive can be higher than the amount of insurance protection you purchased. For example, if you have a PQ long-term care insurance policy and receive $100,000 in benefits from it, you can apply for Medicaid and, if eligible, retain $100,000 worth of assets over and above the state's Medicaid asset threshold. In most states, the asset limit is $2,000 for a single person. Asset limits for married couples are often higher.

States must certify that partnership policies meet the specific requirements for their partnership program, including that those who sell partnership policies are trained and understand how these policies relate to public and private coverage options. To find out more about your state's program, including which insurance agents are selling partnership policies, or to find out if your state offers a partnership program, contact the Department of Insurance of your state.

EMPLOYER

Many private and public employers, including the federal government and a growing number of state governments, offer group long-term care programs as a voluntary benefit:

- Employers do not typically contribute to the premium cost (as they do with health insurance), but they often negotiate a favorable group rate.
- If you are currently employed, it may be easier to qualify for long-term care insurance through your employer than it is to purchase a policy on your own.
- You should check with your benefit or pension office to see if your employer offers long-term care insurance.

The U.S. Office of Personnel Management (OPM) has additional information about the Federal Long Term Care Insurance Program (FLTCIP) for employees of the federal government.

Long-Term Care Insurance Costs

If you have a long-term care insurance policy, the buyer pays a preset premium. The policy then pays for the services you need when you need them (up to its coverage limits). On occasion, if the assumptions used to price the policy prove wrong, the insurance company can increase your premiums beyond the preset amount. Typically, you are not expected to pay premiums while you receive long-term care.

The cost of a long-term care policy varies greatly based on the following:

- your age at the time of purchase
- the policy type
- the coverage you select[2]

---

[2] "What Is Long-Term Care Insurance?" Administration for Community Living (ACL), February 18, 2020. Available online. URL: https://acl.gov/ltc/costs-and-who-pays/what-is-long-term-care-insurance. Accessed August 7, 2023.

Chapter 39 | **Navigating Social Security Benefits**

Social Security is here to support you when you lose a family member. Contacting them when you lose a loved one is very important. This ensures that they are able to provide information regarding benefits you may be entitled to.

You may be able to receive Social Security benefits if your loved one worked long enough in jobs insured under Social Security to qualify for benefits.

WHAT TO DO

The following are a few things you need to do:
- You should give the Social Security number (SSN) of the deceased to the funeral director because they usually report the person's death to the U.S. Social Security Administration (SSA).
- Contact them as soon as you can to make sure your family gets all the benefits they are entitled to.

WHO CAN GET SOCIAL SECURITY SURVIVORS BENEFITS?

- Social Security can pay a one-time lump-sum death payment (LSDP) of $255 to the surviving spouse under one of the following conditions:
  - If they were living with the deceased, they can receive this payment.
  - If they were living apart from the deceased and eligible for certain Social Security benefits on the deceased's record, they can receive this payment.

- If there is no surviving spouse, a child who is eligible for benefits on the deceased's record in the month of death can receive this payment.
- Certain family members may be eligible to receive monthly benefits, including the following:
  - **Surviving spouse**. A surviving spouse who is aged 60 or older (aged 50 or older if they have a disability) or any age and caring for the deceased's child who is under the age of 16 or who has a disability and is receiving Social Security benefits may be eligible to receive monthly benefits.
  - **Unmarried child of the deceased**. An unmarried child of the deceased who is under the age of 18 (or up to age 19 if they are a full-time student in an elementary or secondary school) or aged 18 or older with a disability that began before age 22 may be eligible to receive monthly benefits.
  - **Stepchild, grandchild, step-grandchild, or adopted child**. They may be eligible to receive monthly benefits under certain circumstances.
  - **Parents**. Parents aged 62 or older who were dependent on the deceased for at least half of their support may be eligible to receive monthly benefits.
  - **Surviving divorced spouse**. A surviving divorced spouse may be eligible to receive monthly benefits under certain circumstances.[1]

WHO IS ELIGIBLE FOR SOCIAL SECURITY LUMP-SUM DEATH PAYMENT?

To be eligible for this payment, the surviving spouse must be living in the same household with the worker when he or she died. If they were living apart, the surviving spouse could still receive the lump sum if, during the month the worker died, the spouse met one of the following requirements:

- He/she was already receiving benefits on the worker's record.

[1] "How Social Security Can Help You When a Family Member Dies," U.S. Social Security Administration (SSA), January 2023. Available online. URL: www.ssa.gov/pubs/EN-05-10008.pdf. Accessed August 10, 2023.

- He/she became eligible for benefits upon the worker's death.

If there is no eligible surviving spouse, the lump sum can be paid to the worker's child (or children) if, during the month the worker died, the child met one of the following requirements:
- He/she was already receiving benefits on the worker's record.
- He/she became eligible for benefits upon the worker's death.[2]

WHAT IS A BURIAL FUND?

A burial fund is money set aside to pay for burial expenses. For example, this money can be in a bank account, other financial instruments, or a prepaid burial arrangement.

Some states allow individuals to prepay for their burial by contracting with a funeral home and paying in advance for their funeral. You should discuss this with your local Social Security office.

DOES A BURIAL FUND COUNT AS A RESOURCE FOR SUPPLEMENTAL SECURITY INCOME?

Generally, you and your spouse can set aside up to $1,500 each to pay for burial expenses. In most cases, this money will not count as a resource for Supplemental Security Income (SSI).

If you (or your spouse) own life insurance policies or have other burial arrangements in addition to your $1,500 burial funds, some of the money in the burial fund may count toward the resource limit of $2,000 for an individual or $3,000 for a couple.

DOES INTEREST EARNED ON YOUR (AND YOUR SPOUSE'S) BURIAL FUND COUNT AS A RESOURCE OR INCOME FOR SUPPLEMENTAL SECURITY INCOME?

No. Interest earned on your (and your spouse's) burial fund that you leave in the fund does not count as a resource or income for SSI and does not affect your SSI benefit.

---

[2] Benefits.gov, "Social Security Lump Sum Death Payment," USA.gov, October 10, 2018. Available online. URL: www.benefits.gov/benefit/4392. Accessed August 10, 2023.

HOW CAN YOU SET UP A BURIAL FUND?

Any account you set up must clearly show that the money is set aside to pay burial expenses. You can do this by:

- titling the account as a burial fund
- signing a statement saying:
  - how much has been set aside for burial expenses
  - for whose burial the money is set aside
  - how the money has been set aside
  - the date you first considered the money set aside for burial expenses

WHAT HAPPENS WHEN YOU SPEND MONEY FROM A BURIAL FUND?

If you spend any money from a burial fund on items unrelated to burial expenses, there may be a penalty.[3]

---

[3] "Spotlight on Burial Funds," U.S. Social Security Administration (SSA), July 5, 2007. Available online. URL: www.ssa.gov/ssi/spotlights/spot-burial-funds.htm. Accessed August 10, 2023.

Chapter 40 | Duties and Responsibilities of Personal Representatives

PERSONAL REPRESENTATIVES

Generally, a health-care provider or health plan covered by the Health Insurance Portability and Accountability Act (HIPAA) must allow your personal representative to inspect and receive a copy of protected health information about you that they maintain.

Naming a Personal Representative

Your personal representative can be named in several ways. A state law may affect this process.

If a person can make health-care decisions for you using a health-care power of attorney, the person is your personal representative.

Children

The personal representative of a minor child is usually the child's parent or legal guardian. State laws may affect guardianship.

In cases where a custody decree exists, the personal representative is the parent(s) who can make health-care decisions for the child under the custody decree.

Deceased Persons

When an individual dies, the personal representative of the deceased is the executor or administrator of the deceased individual's estate or the person who is legally authorized by a court or by state law to act on behalf of the deceased individual or his or her estate.

Exceptions

A provider or plan may choose not to treat a person as your personal representative if the provider or plan reasonably believes that the person might endanger you in situations of domestic violence, abuse, or neglect.[1]

RECOGNIZING THE INDIVIDUAL'S PERSONAL REPRESENTATIVE

Table 40.1 displays who must be recognized as the personal representative for a category of individuals.

Table 40.1. The Personal Representative for a Category of Individuals

Individual	Personal Representative
An adult or an emancipated minor	A person with legal authority to make health-care decisions on behalf of the individual **Examples:** Health-care power of attorney, court-appointed legal guardian, and general power of attorney or durable power of attorney that includes the power to make health-care decisions **Exceptions:** See the Abuse, Neglect, and Endangerment Situations section
An unemancipated minor	A parent, guardian, or other person acting in loco parentis with legal authority to make health-care decisions on behalf of the minor child **Exceptions:** See the Parents and Unemancipated Minors and Abuse, Neglect, and Endangerment Situations sections
Deceased	A person with legal authority to act on behalf of the decedent or the estate (not restricted to persons with authority to make health-care decisions) **Examples:** Executor or administrator of the estate and next of kin or other family member (if relevant law provides authority)

---

[1] "Personal Representatives," U.S. Department of Health and Human Services (HHS), November 2, 2020. Available online. URL: www.hhs.gov/hipaa/for-individuals/personal-representatives/index.html. Accessed September 1, 2023.

Parents and Unemancipated Minors

In most cases under the, a parent, guardian, or other person acting in loco parentis (collectively, "parent") is the personal representative of the minor child and can exercise the minor's rights with respect to protected health information because the parent usually has the authority to make health-care decisions about his or her minor child.

However, the specifies three circumstances in which the parent is not the "personal representative" with respect to certain health information about his or her minor child. These exceptions generally track the ability of certain minors to obtain specified health care without parental consent under state or other laws or standards of professional practice. In these situations, the parent does not control the minor's health-care decisions and, thus under the Rule, does not control the protected health information related to that care. The three exceptional circumstances when a parent is not the minor's personal representative are as follows:

- when a state or other law does not require the consent of a parent or other person before a minor can obtain a particular health-care service and the minor consents to the health-care service:
  - Example: A state law provides an adolescent with the right to obtain mental health treatment without the consent of his or her parent and the adolescent consents to such treatment without the parent's consent.
- when someone other than the parent is authorized by law to consent to the provision of a particular health service to a minor and provides such consent.
  - Example: A court may grant authority to make health-care decisions for the minor to an adult other than the parent or to the minor, or the court may make the decision(s) itself.
- when a parent agrees to a confidential relationship between the minor and a health-care provider:
  - Example: A physician asks the parent of a 16-year-old if the physician can talk with the child confidentially about a medical condition and the parent agrees.

387

Regardless, however, of whether a parent is the personal representative of a minor child, the Privacy Rule defers to state or other applicable laws that expressly address the ability of the parent to obtain health information about the minor child. In doing so, the Privacy Rule permits a covered entity to disclose to a parent, or provide the parent with access to, a minor child's protected health information when and to the extent it is permitted or required by state or other laws (including relevant case law). Likewise, the Privacy Rule prohibits a covered entity from disclosing a minor child's protected health information to a parent, or providing a parent with access to such information, when and to the extent it is prohibited under state or other laws (including relevant case law).

In cases in which a state or other applicable law is silent concerning parental access to the minor's protected health information, and a parent is not the personal representative of a minor child based on one of the exceptional circumstances described previously, a covered entity has discretion to provide or deny a parent access under 45 CFR 164.524 to the minor's health information, if doing so is consistent with state or other applicable laws, and provided the decision is made by a licensed health-care professional in the exercise of professional judgment.

Abuse, Neglect, and Endangerment Situations

When a physician or other covered entity reasonably believes that an individual, including an unemancipated minor, has been or may be subjected to domestic violence, abuse, or neglect by the personal representative or that treating a person as an individual's personal representative could endanger the individual, the covered entity may choose not to treat that person as the individual's personal representative if, in the exercise of professional judgment, doing so would not be in the best interests of the individual. For example, if a physician reasonably believes that providing the personal representative of an incompetent elderly individual with access to the individual's health information would endanger that individual, the Privacy Rule permits the physician to decline to provide such access.[2]

---

[2] "Personal Representatives," U.S. Department of Health and Human Services (HHS), September 19, 2013. Available online. URL: www.hhs.gov/hipaa/for-professionals/privacy/guidance/personal-representatives/index. html. Accessed September 1, 2023.

RESPONSIBILITIES OF AN ESTATE ADMINISTRATOR

When a person dies, a probate proceeding may be opened. Depending on state law, probate will generally open 30–90 days after the date of death. One of the probate court's first actions is to appoint an estate administrator.

An estate administrator is the appointed legal representative of the deceased. The legal representative may be a surviving spouse, other family members, an executor named in the will, or an attorney.

In general, the estate administrator:

- collects all the assets of the deceased
- pays creditors
- distributes the remaining assets to heirs or other beneficiaries

Probate Court

Your first responsibility as an estate administrator is to provide the probate court with an accounting of the assets and debts of the deceased.

You will need to:

- have all assets appraised to determine their value
- verify all debts
- contact the Internal Revenue Service (IRS) to file a proof of claim

The probate court will issue Letters of Testamentary or a similar document and authorize you, the estate administrator, to act on behalf of the deceased. You will need Letters of Testamentary to handle their tax and other matters.

Filing and Tax Returns

The tax return for the deceased and their estate are separate. To meet filing requirements, you may need to file different types of tax returns.

Some or all the information you need to file income tax returns for the deceased and their estate may be in their personal records. If you need other items, we can help provide copies of:

- income documents (e.g., Forms W-2 or 1099)
- filed tax returns
- tax transcripts

Income Tax Returns of the Deceased

File income tax returns for the deceased on Form 1040, U.S. Individual Tax Return, or Form 1040-SR, U.S. Tax Return for Seniors. You are required to file a return for the year of death and for any preceding years for which a return was not filed if their income for those years was above the filing requirement.

Income Tax Returns of the Estate

File income tax returns for the estate on Form 1041. You will need to get a tax identification number for the estate called an "employer identification number" (EIN). An estate is required to file an income tax return if the assets of the estate generate more than $600 in annual income. For example, if the deceased had interest, dividend, or rental income when alive, then after death, that income becomes income of the estate that you need to include on an estate income tax return.

If the estate operates a business after the owner's death, you are required to secure a new EIN for the business, report wages or income under the new EIN, and pay any taxes due.

Estate Tax Returns

File an estate tax return on Form 706, United States Estate (and Generation-Skipping Transfer) Tax Return. Estate tax is a tax on the transfer of assets from the deceased to their heirs and beneficiaries. In general, estate tax only applies to large estates.[3]

---

[3] "Responsibilities of an Estate Administrator," Internal Revenue Service (IRS), August 31, 2023. Available online. URL: www.irs.gov/individuals/responsibilities-of-an-estate-administrator. Accessed September 1, 2023.

Chapter 41 | Family and Medical Leave Act

WHAT IS THE FAMILY AND MEDICAL LEAVE ACT?

The Family and Medical Leave Act (FMLA) provides eligible employees of covered employers with job-protected leave for qualifying family and medical reasons and requires continuation of their group health benefits under the same conditions as if they had not taken leave. FMLA leave may be unpaid or used at the same time as employer-provided paid leave. Employees must be restored to the same or virtually identical position when they return to work after FMLA leave.

Eligible Employees

Employees are eligible if they work for a covered employer for at least 12 months, have at least 1,250 hours of service with the employer during the 12 months before their FMLA leave starts, and work at a location where the employer has at least 50 employees within 75 miles.

Covered Employers

Covered employers under the FMLA include:
- private-sector employers who employ 50 or more employees in 20 or more workweeks in either the current calendar year or the previous calendar year
- public agencies (including federal, state, and local government employers, regardless of the number of employees)

- local educational agencies (including public school boards, public elementary and secondary schools, and private elementary and secondary schools, regardless of the number of employees)

The FMLA protects leave for:
- the birth of a child or placement of a child with the employee for adoption or foster care
- the care for a child, spouse, or parent who has a serious health condition
- a serious health condition that makes the employee unable to work
- reasons related to a family member's service in the military, including the following:
  - **Qualifying exigency leave**. This leave is applicable for certain reasons related to a family member's foreign deployment.
  - **Military caregiver leave**. This leave is applicable when a family member is a current service member or recent veteran with a serious injury or illness.

USING FAMILY AND MEDICAL LEAVE ACT LEAVE
Eligible employees may take:
- up to 12 workweeks of leave in a 12-month period for any FMLA leave reason except military caregiver leave
- up to 26 workweeks of military caregiver leave during a single 12-month period

Intermittent or Reduced Schedule Leave
Employees have the right to take FMLA leave all at once or in separate blocks of time when medically necessary or by reducing the time they work each day or week. Intermittent or reduced schedule leave is also available for military family leave reasons. However, employees may use FMLA leave intermittently or on a reduced leave schedule for bonding with a newborn or newly placed child only if they and their employer agree.

Paid Leave

The FMLA is job-protected, unpaid leave. Employees may use employer-provided paid leave at the same time that they take FMLA leave if the reason they are using FMLA leave is covered by the employer's paid leave policy. An employer may also require an employee to use their paid leave during FMLA leave.

Requesting Family and Medical Leave Act Leave

Employees do not have to specifically ask for FMLA leave but do need to provide enough information, so the employer is aware the leave may be covered by the FMLA. Employees must provide notice to their employer as soon as possible and practical that they will need to use FMLA leave. For example, if an employee knows that they have a procedure for a serious medical condition scheduled in three weeks, the employee needs to provide notice to the employer as soon as the procedure is scheduled. Employers may ask for information from the heath-care provider before approving FMLA leave and must allow 15 calendar days to provide the information. In some circumstances, such as when the employee's health-care provider is not able to complete the certification information timely, employees must be allowed additional time.

FAMILY AND MEDICAL LEAVE ACT LEAVE BENEFITS AND PROTECTIONS
Job Protection

Employees who use FMLA leave have the right to go back to work at their same job or to an equivalent job that has the same pay, benefits, and other terms and conditions of employment at the end of their FMLA leave. Violations of an employee's FMLA rights may include changing the number of shifts assigned to the employee, moving the employee to a location outside their normal commuting area, or denying the employee a bonus for which they qualified before their FMLA leave.

An employer cannot threaten, discriminate against, punish, suspend, or fire an employee because they requested or used FMLA leave. Violations of an employee's FMLA rights may include actions such as writing up the employee for missing work when using FMLA leave, denying a promotion because the employee has used FMLA leave, or assessing negative attendance points for FMLA leave use.

Group Health Plan Benefits

Employers are required to continue group health insurance coverage for an employee on FMLA leave under the same terms and conditions as if the employee had not taken leave. For example, if family member coverage is provided to an employee, it must be maintained during the employee's FMLA leave.

SPECIAL FAMILY AND MEDICAL LEAVE ACT RULES FOR SOME WORKERS

- **Teachers**. Special rules apply to employees of elementary schools, secondary schools, and school boards. Generally, these rules apply when an employee needs intermittent leave or leave near the end of a school term.
- **Airline flight crew employees**. These employees have special hours of service eligibility requirements.

FAMILY AND MEDICAL LEAVE ACT ELIGIBILITY FOR SERVICE MEMBERS UNDER THE USERRA

Returning service members are entitled to receive all rights and benefits of employment that they would have obtained if they had been continuously employed. Any period of absence from work due to the service covered by the Uniformed Services Employment and Reemployment Rights Act (USERRA) counts toward an employee's months and hours of service requirements for FMLA leave eligibility.

ADDITIONAL PROTECTIONS
State Laws

Some states have their own family and medical leave laws. Nothing in the FMLA prevents employees from receiving protections under other laws. Workers have the right to benefit from all the laws that apply.

Protection from Retaliation

The FMLA is a federal worker protection law. Employers are prohibited from interfering with, restraining, or denying the exercise of (or the attempt to exercise) any FMLA right. Any violations of the FMLA or the FMLA regulations constitute interfering with, restraining, or denying the exercise of rights provided by the FMLA.

Enforcement

The Wage and Hour Division (WHD) is responsible for administering and enforcing the FMLA for most employees. If you believe that your rights under the FMLA have been violated, you may file a complaint with the WHD or file a private lawsuit against your employer in court. State employees may be subject to certain limitations in pursuit of direct lawsuits regarding leave for their own serious health conditions. Most federal and certain congressional employees are also covered by the law but are subject to the jurisdiction of the U.S. Office of Personnel Management or Congress (OPM).[1]

---

[1] "The Family and Medical Leave Act," U.S. Department of Labor (DOL), February 2023. Available online. URL: www.dol.gov/agencies/whd/fact-sheets/28-fmla. Accessed August 10, 2023.

Chapter 42 | Digital Memorials

Many traditional practices have moved to online or virtual platforms in this era. Books and photographs are available online. Classroom sessions and official meetings are conducted via virtual meeting platforms. A new inclusion to this is preserving and honoring the memories of loved ones online through messages, videos, photos, and so on. Mourning online on the deceased person's social media pages has become common. Their page can be converted to an online memorial. The online and offline electronic information that remains after the death of a person is known as a "digital legacy."

WHAT ARE DIGITAL ASSETS?

Digital assets include emails, social networks, cryptocurrency, Internet banking, streaming services, drives, cloud services, work platforms, and so on, which are available on mobile phones, laptops, and other similar devices.

When a person dies, their physical belongings are typically passed on to their heirs or close family members. However, their digital assets are left behind, many of which cannot be accessed without a password. It is best to deactivate the social accounts of loved ones or convert them into memorial pages.

DIGITAL COMMEMORATION

Paying tribute to people who have lost their lives can be done online through various means. A few types of digital commemoration are as follows:

- blogs that honor loved ones
- tribute pages on social media sites
- virtual funeral ceremonies
- solar-powered digital video screens on tombstones display information, photos, and videos about the deceased
- quick response (QR) codes engraved on tombstones to access the deceased's memorial page

HOW TO BUILD A DIGITAL MEMORIAL

Creating a digital memorial is as simple as opening a new account on social media with fundamental details to be filled in. Various tools or platforms are available to build these memorials. Follow these steps to build a memorial website to collect memories:

- **Identify a tool**. First, choose a platform to create the memorial page. A tool makes it easy to set up the page by following the step-by-step instructions. Various free and paid tools are available online.
- **Register**. You must then register by signing up for an account with a username and password you will use to access the tool. Some tools require you to create a domain name.
- **Log in**. Once registration is complete, you need to log in and fill in the basic details of the deceased. This information will include their full name, date of birth, and date of death.
- **Choose a template**. Many tools offer a variety of format options. Choose an appropriate template from those available.
- **Personalize the page**. You may upload a picture of the deceased and choose the final look of the overall page. Personalize the page with photos, messages, videos, and so on.

- **Change privacy settings.** Before you finish, change the privacy settings of the memorial website to determine the audience you wish to view it. This may include only people invited to the page, or it may be viewable to the general public.
- **Share the page link.** Finally, send invitations to family and friends to access the page and pay tribute to the loved one.
- **Keep the page alive.** Encourage family and friends to contribute to the page by sharing media and messages to keep the memories of your loved one alive.

BENEFITS OF DIGITAL MEMORIALS

Digital memorials offer numerous benefits, each contributing to a more meaningful and lasting way to commemorate the lives of loved ones. The following are the benefits of digital memorials:

- **Reach distant communities.** Digital memorials provide those who cannot physically attend wakes and funeral services due to distance, health, or financial reasons a means to participate in memorializing the deceased.
- **Moral support.** Many online friends and contacts may offer their condolences and support to the family of the deceased or share their own experiences with loss. Close friends and family may find solace in knowing they are not alone in their grief.
- **Cope with loss.** Sharing fond memories, writing tributes, and reminiscing about beautiful moments of the deceased's life and shared memories can help individuals cope with grief and cherish good times.
- **Honor through charity.** Memorial platforms may also offer opportunities to raise funds for good causes in the name of the deceased. These may include planting trees in the deceased's name, donating to the deceased's favored charity, contributing a scholarship in the deceased's name, and other activities.
- **Data protection.** Photos and videos that may otherwise get lost or deleted can be saved in the cloud. This keeps all the data safe and accessible from anywhere, anytime.

- **Inexpensive**. Memorial tools are often free or included in the cost of funeral arrangements. You only need to collect and upload data.

SORTING OUT DIGITAL LEGACY DURING END-OF-LIFE CARE

It is wise for those under palliative care or performing estate and end-of-life planning to share their passwords and digital assets with someone they trust to ensure that their wishes are carried out and their personal data are protected after their death. This can help ease the burden on loved ones and ensure their legacy is preserved according to their wishes.

References

Arthur, Paul. "Memory and Commemoration in the Digital Present," ResearchGate, January 2014. Available online. URL: www.researchgate.net/publication/343418142_ Memory_and_Commemoration_in_the_Digital_Present. Accessed August 24, 2023.

"Digital Legacy," Digital Guide IONOS, June 27, 2023. Available online. URL: www.ionos.com/digitalguide/websites/digital-law/digital-legacy. Accessed August 22, 2023.

"How to Build a Memorial Website," Farewelling, July 7, 2020. Available online. URL: www.myfarewelling.com/ article/how-to-build-a-memorial-website. Accessed August 24, 2023.

Norris, James, et al. "Digital Asset and Digital End of Life Framework," The Digital Legacy Association, May 2018. Available online. URL: https://digitallegacyassociation. org/wp-content/uploads/2017/07/Digital-Assets-and-Digital-Legacy-Framework-April-2018-1.pdf. Accessed August 22, 2023.

"What Is a Digital Tombstone?" Ever Loved, December 7, 2021. Available online. URL: https://everloved.com/ articles/memorial-products/what-digital-tombstone. Accessed August 24, 2023.

Part 8 | Funerals and Grief

Chapter 43 | **Funeral Services**

When a loved one dies, grieving family members and friends often are confronted with dozens of decisions about the funeral—all of which must be made quickly and often under great emotional duress. What kind of funeral should it be? What funeral provider should you use? Should you bury or cremate the body or donate it to science? What are you legally required to buy? What about the availability of environmentally friendly or "green" burials? What other arrangements should you plan? And, practically, how much is it all going to cost?

FUNERAL PLANNING TIPS

Many funeral providers offer various "packages" of goods and services for different kinds of funerals. When you arrange for a funeral, you have the right to buy goods and services separately. That is, you do not have to accept a package that may include items you do not want. Here are some tips to help you shop for funeral services:

- **Shop around in advance.** Compare prices from at least two funeral homes. Remember that you can supply your own casket or urn.
- **Ask for a price list.** The law requires funeral homes to give you written price lists for products and services.
- **Resist pressure.** Avoid buying goods and services that you do not really want or need.
- **Avoid emotional overspending.** It is not necessary to have the fanciest casket or the most elaborate funeral to properly honor a loved one.

- **Recognize your rights**. Laws regarding funerals and burials vary from state to state. It is a smart move to know which goods or services the law requires you to purchase and which are optional.
- **Apply the same smart shopping techniques you use for other major purchases**. You can cut costs by limiting the viewing to one day or one hour before the funeral and by dressing your loved one in a favorite outfit instead of costly burial clothing.
- **Shop in advance**. It allows you to comparison shop without time constraints, creates an opportunity for family discussion, and lifts some of the burden from your family.[1]

TYPES OF FUNERALS

Every family is different, and not everyone wants the same type of funeral. Funeral practices are influenced by religious and cultural traditions, costs, and personal preferences. These factors help determine whether the funeral will be elaborate or simple, public or private, religious or secular, and where it will be held. They also influence whether the body will be present at the funeral if there will be a viewing or visitation and, if so, whether the casket will be open or closed and whether the remains will be buried or cremated.

"Traditional" Full-Service Funeral

This type of funeral, often referred to by funeral providers as a "traditional" funeral, usually includes a viewing or visitation and formal funeral service, use of a hearse to transport the body to the funeral site and cemetery, and burial, entombment, or cremation of the remains.

It is generally the most expensive type of funeral. In addition to the funeral home's basic services fee, costs often include embalming and dressing the body, rental of the funeral home for the viewing or service, and use of vehicles to transport the family if they do not

---

[1] "Shopping for Funeral Services," Federal Trade Commission (FTC), July 2012. Available online. URL: https://consumer.ftc.gov/articles/shopping-funeral-services. Accessed July 31, 2023.

use their own. The costs of a casket, cemetery plot or crypt, and other funeral goods and services must also be factored in.

Direct Burial

The body is buried shortly after death, usually in a simple container. No viewing or visitation is involved, so no embalming is necessary. A memorial service may be held at the graveside or later. Direct burial usually costs less than the "traditional" full-service funeral. Costs include the funeral home's basic services fee, as well as transportation and care of the body, the purchase of a casket or burial container, and a cemetery plot or crypt. If the family chooses to be at the cemetery for the burial, the funeral home often charges an additional fee for a graveside service.

Direct Cremation

The body is cremated shortly after death without embalming. The cremated remains are placed in an urn or other container. No viewing or visitation is involved. The remains can be kept in the home, buried or placed in a crypt or niche in a cemetery, or buried or scattered in a favorite spot. Direct cremation usually costs less than the "traditional" full-service funeral. Costs include the funeral home's basic services fee, as well as transportation and care of the body. A crematory fee may be included, or if the funeral home does not own the crematory, the fee may be added on. There will also be a charge for an urn or other container. The cost of a cemetery plot or crypt is included only if the remains are buried or entombed.

Funeral providers who offer direct cremations must also offer to provide an alternative container that can be used in place of a casket.[2]

---

[2] "Types of Funerals," Federal Trade Commission (FTC), July 2012. Available online. URL: https://consumer.ftc.gov/articles/types-funerals. Accessed July 31, 2023.

Chapter 44 | **Planning a Meaningful Funeral**

CHOOSING A FUNERAL PROVIDER

Many people do not realize that in most states, they are not legally required to use a funeral home to plan and conduct a funeral. However, because they have little experience with the many details and legal requirements involved and may be emotionally distraught when it is time to make the plans, they find the services of a professional funeral home to be a comfort.

People often select a funeral home or cemetery because it is close to home, has served the family in the past, or has been recommended by someone they trust. But limiting the search to just one funeral home may risk paying more than necessary for the funeral or narrowing their choice of goods and services.

COMPARISON SHOPPING FOR A FUNERAL HOME/PROVIDER

Comparison shopping does not have to be difficult, especially if it is done before the need for a funeral arises. Thinking ahead can help you make informed and thoughtful decisions about funeral arrangements. It allows you to choose the specific items you want and need and to compare the prices several funeral providers charge.

If you visit a funeral home in person, the funeral provider is required by law to give you a general price list (GPL) itemizing the cost of the items and services the home offers. If the GPL does not include specific prices of caskets or outer burial containers, the law requires the funeral director to show you the price lists for those items before showing you the items.

Sometimes, it is more convenient and less stressful to "price shop" funeral homes by telephone. The Funeral Rule requires funeral directors to provide price information on the phone to any caller who asks for it. In addition, many funeral homes are happy to mail you their price lists although that is not required by law.

When comparing prices, be sure to consider the total cost of all the items together, in addition to the costs of single items. Every funeral home should have price lists that include all the items essential for the different types of arrangements it offers. Many funeral homes offer package funerals that may cost less than buying individual items or services. Offering package funerals is permitted by law as long as an itemized price list is also provided. But you cannot accurately compare total costs unless you use the price lists.

In addition, there is a trend toward consolidation in the funeral home industry, and many neighborhood funeral homes may appear to be locally owned when, in fact, they are owned by a national corporation. If this issue is important to you, you may want to ask if the funeral home is independent and locally owned.[1]

PLANNING YOUR OWN FUNERAL

To help relieve their families, an increasing number of people are planning their own funerals, designating their funeral preferences, and sometimes paying for them in advance. They see funeral planning as an extension of will and estate planning.

Funeral Planning Tips

Thinking ahead can help you make informed and thoughtful decisions about funeral arrangements. It allows you to choose the specific items you want and need and compare the prices offered by several funeral providers. It also spares your survivors the stress

---

[1] "Choosing a Funeral Provider," Federal Trade Commission (FTC), July 2012. Available online. URL: https://consumer.ftc.gov/articles/choosing-funeral-provider. Accessed August 28, 2023.

of making these decisions under the pressure of time and strong emotions. You can make arrangements directly with a funeral establishment.

An important consideration when planning a funeral preneed is where the remains will be buried, entombed, or scattered. In the short time between the death and burial of a loved one, many family members find themselves rushing to buy a cemetery plot or grave—often without careful thought or a personal visit to the site. That is why it is in the family's best interest to buy cemetery plots before you need them.

You may wish to make decisions about your arrangements in advance but not pay for them in advance. Keep in mind that over time, prices may go up and businesses may close or change ownership. However, in some areas with increased competition, prices may go down over time. It is a good idea to review and revise your decisions every few years and to make sure your family is aware of your wishes.

Put your preferences in writing, give copies to family members and your attorney, and keep a copy in a handy place. Do not designate your preferences in your will because a will often is not found or read until after the funeral. And avoid putting the only copy of your preferences in a safe deposit box. That is because your family may have to make arrangements on a weekend or holiday before the box can be opened.

Prepaying

Millions of Americans have entered into contracts to arrange their funerals and prepay some or all of the expenses involved. Laws of individual states govern the prepayment of funeral goods and services, and various states have laws to help ensure that these advance payments are available to pay for funeral products and services when they are needed. However, protections vary widely from state to state, and some state laws offer little or no effective protection. Some state laws require the funeral home or cemetery to place a percentage of the prepayment in a state-regulated trust or to purchase a life insurance policy with death benefits assigned to the funeral home or cemetery.

If you are thinking about prepaying for funeral goods and services, it is important to consider the following issues before putting down any money:

- What are you paying for? Are you buying only merchandise, such as a casket and vault, or are you purchasing funeral services as well?
- What happens to the money you have prepaid? States have different requirements for handling funds paid for prearranged funeral services.
- What happens to the interest income on money that is prepaid and put into a trust account?
- Are you protected if the firm you dealt with goes out of business?
- Can you cancel the contract and get a full refund if you change your mind?
- What happens if you move to a different area or die while away from home? Some prepaid funeral plans can be transferred but often at an added cost.

Be sure to tell your family about the plans you have made; let them know where the documents are filed. If your family is not aware that you have made plans, your wishes may not be carried out. If family members do not know that you have prepaid the funeral costs, they could end up paying for the same arrangements. You may wish to consult an attorney on the best way to ensure that your wishes are followed.[2]

---

[2] "Planning Your Own Funeral," Federal Trade Commission (FTC), July 2012. Available online. URL: https://consumer.ftc.gov/articles/planning-your-own-funeral. Accessed August 28, 2023.

Chapter 45 | **Honoring Military Funerals**

HOW DO YOU SCHEDULE A BURIAL FOR A VETERAN OR OTHER FAMILY MEMBER?

If You Have a Preneed Decision Letter That Confirms Eligibility

To start, you or the funeral director can call the National Cemetery Scheduling Office (NCSO) at 800-535-1117 (TTY: 711) to request a burial. They are there Monday through Friday, from 8:00 a.m. to 7:30 p.m. ET, and Saturday, from 9:00 a.m. to 5:30 p.m. ET.

Keep in mind that the preneed decision letter does not identify a specific cemetery or gravesite since it is not possible to reserve these in advance. In some cases, they may review your eligibility again at your time of death, as laws and circumstances may have changed since your preneed application.

You do not need to do anything else except prepare yourself and your family for the funeral.

If You Do Not Have a Preneed Decision Letter

To start, you may want to choose a funeral director to help you plan the burial. Then either you or the funeral director will need to take the following three steps to schedule the burial.

STEP 1: GATHER THE INFORMATION AND DOCUMENTS YOU WILL NEED TO IDENTIFY THE DECEASED WHEN YOU CALL THE NATIONAL CEMETERY SCHEDULING OFFICE

You will need the DD214 or other discharge documents of the veteran or service member whose military service will be used to determine eligibility for burial in a Veterans Affairs (VA) national

411

cemetery. Their discharge from service needs have to be under conditions other than dishonorable.

They may also need other documents to verify a relationship to a veteran or the status of a dependent. These may include a death certificate, letters from your doctor, a divorce decree, a statement from the Social Security Administration (SSA), or other documents to support your claim.

- Find out which discharge documents they accept along with your application (www.cem.va.gov/CEM/hmm/discharge_documents.asp).
- Find out how to request the veteran's DD214 (www.va.gov/records/get-military-service-records/#how-do-i-request-someone-elses).
- Use the helpful checklist available at www.cem.va.gov/pdf/NCA_NCSO_BeforeYouCallChecklist.pdf to help you organize your documents.

If you cannot find these documents, please ask them for help when you call. It may take several days to check eligibility if you do not have discharge documents.

Note: Discharge documents are not usually needed for scheduling when a veteran or eligible dependent is already interred in a national cemetery.

You will also need the following information about the deceased:

- name
- gender
- Social Security number (SSN) or military service number (veteran ID)
- date of birth
- relationship to the service member or veteran whose military service will be used to decide eligibility
- marital status
- date of death (and zip code and county at the time of death)

You will need the following information about the next of kin (the closest living relative of the deceased):

- name
- relationship to the deceased

- SSN
- phone number
- address

You may also need more information in certain cases:
- If the person was married, you will also need the surviving spouse's status as a veteran, service member, or family member.
- If the person has any children with disabilities, you will need the status and detailed information for any disabled children who may be buried in the future in a national cemetery.
- If the person's spouse passed away previously and was buried in a VA national cemetery, you will need the full name of the spouse as well as the cemetery section and site number where they are buried.

STEP 2: DECIDE ON THE BURIAL DETAILS AND GATHER ALL RELATED INFORMATION

You will need to tell the following information:
- the cemetery where you would prefer the veteran, spouse, or dependent family member to be buried:
  - Find a VA national cemetery (www.cem.va.gov/find-cemetery/all-national.asp).
  - Find a state veteran's cemetery (www.cem.va.gov/find-cemetery).
- the type of burial you would like for the person (casket or cremation) and the size of the casket or cremation urn
- the type of gravesite memorial you would like, such as a headstone, grave marker, niche cover, or medallion
- any religious emblem or optional inscription that you would like on the headstone or marker

If the person is a veteran or reservist, you will also need to tell if you would like burial honors or memorial items, including the following:
- a burial flag
- a Presidential Memorial Certificate (PMC)

413

- other possible military honors beyond the playing of "Taps" and flag folding and presentation

STEP 3: CONTACT THE NATIONAL CEMETERY SCHEDULING OFFICE

The funeral director you have chosen can help you with the following steps:

- For burial in a national cemetery, fax any discharge papers to the NCSO at 866-900-6417. Or scan and email the papers to NCA.Scheduling@va.gov with the person's name you are requesting burial benefits for in the subject line.
- Then call 800-535-1117 (TTY: 711) to confirm the burial application. They are there Monday through Friday, from 8:00 a.m. to 7:30 p.m. ET, and Saturday, from 9:00 a.m. to 5:30 p.m. ET. Be sure to have all the information ready that is listed in steps 1 and 2.

WHEN CAN YOU SCHEDULE A BURIAL?

National cemeteries are open for burials Monday through Friday. When a federal holiday is on a Monday or Friday, national cemeteries will open for burials one day during that holiday weekend.

Note: The National Cemetery Scheduling Office (NCSO) is closed on July 4, Memorial Day, Labor Day, Thanksgiving Day, Christmas Day, and New Year's Day.

WOULD YOU EVER NEED TO CONTACT A NATIONAL CEMETERY DIRECTLY?

Yes, you should contact a national cemetery directly:

- to schedule a burial for an active-duty service member
- to cancel or reschedule a burial
- to change any information you already provided to the scheduling office
- to request a disinterment and/or relocation to another national cemetery

- to get information that is specific to a cemetery, such as what can be inscribed on a headstone, the policy for flowers, and the hours of operation

CAN YOU GET INFORMATION ABOUT THE BURIAL AT SEA PROGRAM?

If you have questions about the Burial at Sea program, please contact the United States Navy Mortuary Affairs office at 866-787-0081 (toll-free).

CAN YOU GET HELP TO PAY FOR BURIAL COSTS?

If you are the spouse of record (the legally recognized spouse) or a designated (legally chosen) family member of a veteran, you may be able to get financial help for burial and funeral costs.[1]

---

[1] "Schedule a Burial for a Veteran or Family Member," U.S. Department of Veterans Affairs (VA), November 7, 2022. Available online. URL: www.va.gov/burials-memorials/schedule-a-burial. Accessed July 31, 2023.

Chapter 46 | **Cremation Services**

Cremation is the second most common method of disposition in the United States and gains popularity every year. It is the most common option in Japan, India, England, and other countries. For most individuals, the selection of cremation is motivated by religious practice and cultural preference.

Additional reasons for choosing cremation over traditional burial are lower cost, ease, more options for memorialization, and environmental considerations.

Cremation is generally less expensive than traditional burial. The price does not include cemetery charges, such as grave space, burial fees, monuments, or markers, which generally add more to the final cost. Although cremation is typically perceived to be a wholly different form of service, most firms provide elements from the traditional burial service. For example, memorial services, where the body is viewed in a rented casket, are becoming more common. Also, many people who preplan and prepay for their funeral services select cremation.

Some consumers perceive cremation to be simpler than traditional burial, and this simplicity appeals to a growing share of the market. There are fewer transactions in the cremation process, and a consumer may only have to interact with a funeral director rather than with cemeteries and other agencies. Funeral directors provide most legal services as part of the cremation fee, reducing the burden on families.

Cremation also provides more options for memorialization. Remains can be stored in an urn at someone's home, a cemetery, or a mausoleum. The remains can also be scattered at sea, in a park, or at other locations (where permitted by law) as per the deceased's request. Finally, cremated remains do not require the relatively large burial plots needed for traditional burial, thereby reducing the cemeteries' pressure on the environment. When cremains are buried, the individual plot is significantly smaller than the plot used in traditional burial.

CREMATION PROCESS

There are different classes of crematories; however, the technology employed by each unit type is essentially the same. The technology has changed little in the latter half of the 20th century. Crematories vary according to size and capacity. They are typically large, front-loaded units that weigh between 20,000 and 30,000 pounds.

Combustion takes place in two chambers at an average rate of 100–150 pounds per hour. Crematories use natural gas, electricity, and propane to power the unit and facilitate the combustion process.

The primary chamber is preheated to about 1,292 °F (700 °C). The body is enclosed in a combustible container, such as a wooden coffin, cardboard box, or plastic bag. The operator increases the temperature to between 1,652 °F (900 °C) and 2,012 °F (1,100 °C). The body stays in the primary chamber for between one and two hours, depending on the body size. After the remains have cooled, the bones are crushed to the consistency of coarse sand. Finally, all the remains are placed in either an urn or a plastic bag for transport.[1]

IMPORTING HUMAN REMAINS FOR BURIAL, ENTOMBMENT, OR CREMATION

The Centers for Disease Control and Prevention (CDC) regulates the importation of human remains and provides guidance for their importation. The requirements are more stringent if the person died from a disease classified as quarantinable in the United States.

Except for cremated remains, human remains intended for burial, entombment, or cremation after entry into the United States

---

[1] "Economic Impact Analysis of Proposed Other Solid Waste Incinerator Regulation," U.S. Environmental Protection Agency (EPA), September 1999. Available online. URL: www3.epa.gov/ttn/ecas/docs/eia_ip/other-solid-waste-incinerator_ip_09-1999.pdf. Accessed August 7, 2023.

must be accompanied by a death certificate stating the cause of death. A death certificate is an official government document that certifies that a death has occurred and provides identifying information about the deceased, including (at a minimum) name, age, and sex. The document must also certify the time, place, and cause of death, if known. If the official government document is not written in English, it must be accompanied by an English language translation of the official government document, the authenticity of which must be attested to by a person licensed to perform acts in legal affairs in the country where the death occurred.

In lieu of a death certificate, a copy of the consular mortuary certificate, the affidavit of the foreign funeral director, and the transit permit together constitute acceptable identification of human remains. If a death certificate is not available on time for returning the remains, the U.S. embassy or consulate should provide a consular mortuary certificate stating whether the person died from a disease classified as quarantinable in the United States. A person transporting human remains must also meet the requirements of the country of origin, air carrier, the Transportation Security Administration (TSA), and Customs and Border Protection (CBP).

EXPORTING HUMAN REMAINS

The CDC does not regulate the exportation of human remains outside the United States although other state and local regulations might apply. The United States Postal Service (USPS) is the only courier legally allowed to ship cremated remains. Exporters of human remains and travelers taking human remains out of the United States should be aware that they must meet the importation requirements of the destination country. Information regarding these requirements can be obtained from the foreign embassy or consulate. Air carriers might also have their own requirements, which the individuals transporting remains outside the United States should be aware of.[2]

---

[2] "Death during Travel," Centers for Disease Control and Prevention (CDC), May 1, 2023. Available online. URL: wwwnc.cdc.gov/travel/yellowbook/2024/environmental-hazards-risks/death-during-travel. Accessed August 7, 2023.

Chapter 47 | The Importance of Death Certification

A death certificate is a permanent record of an individual's death. One purpose of the death certificate is to obtain a simple description of the sequence or process leading to death rather than a record describing all medical conditions present at death.

The causes of death on the death certificate represent a medical opinion that might vary among individual physicians. In signing the death certificate, the physician, medical examiner, or coroner certifies that in his or her medical opinion, the individual died from the reported causes of death. The certifier's opinion and confidence in that opinion are based upon his or her training, knowledge of medicine, available medical history, symptoms, diagnostic tests, and available autopsy results for the decedent. Even if extensive information is available to the certifier, causes of death may be difficult to determine, so the certifier may indicate uncertainty by qualifying the causes on the death certificate.

Cause-of-death data are important for surveillance, research, design of public health and medical interventions, and funding decisions for research and development. While the death certificate is a legal document used for legal, family, and insurance purposes, it may not be the only record used because, in some cases, the death certificate may only be admissible as a proof of death.

DIFFICULTIES IN DEATH CERTIFICATION
Uncertainty

Often, several acceptable ways of writing a cause-of-death statement exist. Optimally, a certifier will be able to provide a simple description of the process leading to death that is etiologically clear and be confident that this is the correct sequence of causes. However, realistically, a description of the process is sometimes difficult because the certifier is not certain.

In this case, the certifier should think through the causes about which he/she is confident and what possible etiologies could have resulted in these conditions. The certifier should select the causes that are suspected to have been involved and use words, such as "probable" or "presumed," to indicate that the description provided is not completely certain. If the initiating condition reported on the death certificate could have arisen from a preexisting condition, but the certifier cannot determine the etiology, then he/she should state that the etiology is unknown, undetermined, or unspecified so that it is clear that the certifier did not have enough information to provide even a qualified etiology.

The Elderly

When preparing a cause-of-death statement for an elderly decedent, the causes should present a clear and distinct etiological sequence, if possible. Causes of death on the death certificate should not include terms such as senescence, old age, infirmity, and advanced age because they have little value for public health or medical research. Age is recorded elsewhere on the death certificate. When malnutrition is involved, the certifier should consider if other medical conditions could have led to malnutrition.

When a number of conditions or multiple organ/system failures result in death, the physician, medical examiner, or coroner should choose a single sequence to describe the process leading to death and list the other conditions in Part II of the certification section. "Multiple system failure" could be included as an "other significant condition," but the systems involved should also be specified. In other instances, conditions listed in Part II of the death certificate may include causes that resulted from the underlying cause but did not fit into the sequence resulting in death.

If the certifier cannot determine a descriptive sequence of causes of death despite carefully considering all the information available and the circumstances of death did not warrant investigation by the medical examiner or coroner, then the death may be reported as "unspecified natural causes." If any potentially lethal medical conditions are known but cannot be cited as a part of the sequence leading to death, then they should be listed as other significant conditions.

Infant Deaths

Maternal conditions may have initiated or affected the sequence that resulted in infant death. These maternal conditions should be reported in the cause-of-death statement in addition to the infant causes.

When sudden infant death syndrome (SIDS) is suspected, a complete investigation should be conducted, typically by a medical examiner. If the infant is under one year of age and no cause of death is determined even after scene investigation, reviewing of clinical history, and a complete autopsy, then the death can be reported as SIDS. If the investigation is not complete, then the death may be reported as presumed to be SIDS.

Avoid Ambiguity

Most certifiers will find themselves, at some point, in a circumstance in which they are unable to provide a simple description of the process of death. In this situation, the certifier should try to provide a clear sequence, qualify the causes about which he/she is uncertain, and be able to explain the certification chosen.

When processes provided in Table 47.1 are reported, additional information about the etiology should be reported if possible.

If the certifier is unable to determine the etiology of a process such as those listed in Table 47.1, then the process must be qualified as being of an unknown, undetermined, probable, presumed, or

Table 47.1. Processes of Death

Cardiovascular		
Acute myocardial infarction	Congestive heart failure	Myocardial infarction
Arrhythmia	Cardiomyopathy	Shock
Atrial fibrillation	Dysrhythmia	Ventricular fibrillation
Cardiac arrest	Heart failure	Ventricular tachycardia
Cardiac dysrhythmia	Hypotension	
Central Nervous System		
Altered mental status	Cerebral edema	Open (or closed) head injury
Anoxic encephalopathy	Dementia (when not otherwise specified)	Seizures
Brain injury	Epidural hematoma	Subdural hematoma
Brain stem herniation	Increased intracranial pressure	Subarachnoid hemorrhage
Cerebrovascular accident	Intracranial hemorrhage	Uncal herniation
Cerebellar tonsillar herniation	Metabolic encephalopathy	
Respiratory		
Aspiration	Pneumonia	Pulmonary insufficiency
Pleural effusions	Pulmonary embolism	Pulmonary edema
Gastrointestinal		
Biliary obstruction	Diarrhea	Hepatic failure
Bowel obstruction	End-stage liver disease	Hepatorenal syndrome
Cirrhosis	Gastrointestinal hemorrhage	Perforated gallbladder
Blood, Renal, and Immune		
Coagulopathy	Hepatorenal syndrome	Renal failure
Disseminated intravascular coagulopathy	Immunosuppression	Thrombocytopenia
End-stage renal disease	Pancytopenia	Urinary tract infection (UTI)

Table 47.1. Continued

Not System-Oriented		
Abdominal hemorrhage	Decubiti	Hyponatremia
Ascites	Dehydration	Multi-organ failure
Anoxia	Exsanguination	Necrotizing soft tissue infection
Bacteremia	Failure to thrive	Peritonitis
Bedridden	Gangrene	Sepsis
Carcinogenesis	Hemothorax	Septic shock
Carcinomatosis	Hyperglycemia	Shock
Chronic bedridden state	Hyperkalemia	Volume depletion

unspecified etiology so that it is clear that a distinct etiology was not inadvertently or carelessly omitted.

The following conditions and types of death might seem to be specific, but when the medical history is examined, further complications of an injury or poisoning may be found (possibly occurring long ago):

- subdural hematoma
- epidural hematoma
- subarachnoid hemorrhage
- fracture
- pulmonary embolism
- thermal burns/chemical burns
- sepsis
- hyperthermia
- hypothermia
- hip fracture
- seizure disorder
- drug or alcohol overdose/drug or alcohol abuse

Is it possible that the underlying cause of death was the result of an injury or poisoning? If it might be, check with the medical examiner/coroner to find out if the death should be reported to him or her.

425

When indicating neoplasms as a cause of death, indicate the following:

- primary site or that the primary site is unknown
- benign or malignant
- cell type or that the cell type is unknown
- grade of a neoplasm
- part or lobe of an organ affected (e.g., a well-differentiated squamous cell carcinoma, lung, left upper lobe)

MEDICAL EXAMINER OR CORONER

The medical examiner/coroner investigates the deaths that are unexpected or unexplained or if an injury or poisoning was involved. State laws often provide guidelines for when a medical examiner/coroner must be notified. In the case of deaths known or suspected to have resulted from injury or poisoning, report the death to the medical examiner/coroner as required by state law. The medical examiner/coroner will either complete the cause-of-death section of the death certificate or waive that responsibility. If the medical examiner/coroner does not accept the case, then the certifier will need to complete the cause-of-death section.[1]

---

[1] "Possible Solutions to Common Problems in Death Certification," Centers for Disease Control and Prevention (CDC), November 6, 2015. Available online. URL: www.cdc.gov/nchs/nvss/writing-cod-statements/death_certification_problems.htm. Accessed August 28, 2023.

Chapter 48 | Grief, Bereavement, and Coping with Loss

GRIEF

Grief is the emotional response to the loss of a loved one. Common grief reactions include the following:
- feeling emotionally numb
- being unable to believe the loss occurred
- having anxiety from the distress of being separated from the loved one
- mourning along with feeling depressed
- a feeling of acceptance

MOURNING

Mourning is the way we show grief in public. The way people mourn is affected by beliefs, religious practices, and culture. Grief and mourning are closely related.

BEREAVEMENT

Bereavement is the period of sadness after the death of a loved one. Grief and mourning occur during the period of bereavement. People who are grieving are described as bereaved.

TYPES OF GRIEF

The three types of grief are as follows.

Anticipatory Grief

Anticipatory grief occurs before death. It is grief that occurs leading up to death. It may be felt by the person dying or the person's family. When a patient experiences distress, pain, and medical complications, it can add to anticipatory grief. Anticipatory grief is different from the grief that occurs after death.

Anticipatory grief does not affect everyone. Research has shown that about one in four patients with incurable cancer feels anticipatory grief. Anticipatory grief is less likely to occur when the patient and family accept death. Talking with someone who is trained in grief and bereavement may help patients and their families come to terms with impending death.

Normal or Common Grief

Normal or common grief begins soon after a loss, and the symptoms go away over time.

Normal grief occurs in most people who have experienced a loss. During normal grief, the bereaved person accepts the loss and continues with daily activities even though it is hard to do. Common emotional reactions include the following:

- emotional numbness, shock, disbelief, or denial, which often occur right after the death, especially if the death was not expected
- anxiety over being separated from a loved one, where the bereaved may wish to bring the person back and become lost in the thoughts of the deceased (Images of death may often occur in the person's thoughts.)
- distress that leads to crying, sighing, having dreams, illusions, and hallucinations of the deceased, as well as looking for places or things that were shared with the deceased
- anger
- periods of sadness, loss of sleep, loss of appetite, fatigue, guilt, and loss of interest in life

Grief bursts or pangs are short periods (20–30 minutes) of very intense distress. These bursts are caused by reminders of the deceased person, such as during holidays, the anniversary of the loved one's death, or when giving away items that belonged to the person. At other times, they seem to happen for no reason.

In normal grief, symptoms will occur less often and will feel less severe as time passes. Recovery time will vary with each person. For most bereaved people, symptoms lessen between six months and two years after the loss. Although many bereaved people have similar responses as they cope with their losses, there is no typical grief response.

Normal grief is different from major depression. When a person grieves, they can have symptoms that overlap with major depression, such as sleep problems, feelings of guilt, repeated thoughts, and lack of interest. Normal grief is different from major depression in the following ways:

- Painful feelings come and go instead of being constant.
- There are feelings of emptiness rather than sadness or not feeling pleasure.
- People have good self-esteem and do not feel worthless or bad about themselves.
- If there are thoughts of suicide, they are focused on the deceased person, such as a wish to join them in death instead of thoughts about oneself.

A bereaved person can be diagnosed with major depression if they have symptoms that occur outside the normal grief process.

Complicated Grief

Complicated grief lasts longer than normal grief. Complicated grief is when symptoms do not improve and last for a long period of time, cause extreme distress, affect multiple areas of their lives, and decrease their ability to take part in daily activities.

FACTORS THAT AFFECT GRIEF

There are factors that affect the response to grief. A person's grief is affected by the following.

Personality, Age, and Gender

The personality, age, and gender of the bereaved may affect whether they are more likely to experience depression with their grief. Studies have found that people with certain personality traits are more likely to have long-lasting depression after a loss. These include people who are dependent on a loved one (such as a spouse) and people who deal with distress by thinking about it all the time.

In general, younger bereaved people have more problems after a loss than older bereaved people do. They have more severe health problems, grief symptoms, and other mental and physical symptoms. Younger bereaved people, however, may recover more quickly than older bereaved people do because they tend to have more resources and social support.

Men have more problems than women do after a spouse's death. Men tend to have worse depression and more health problems than women do after the loss. Some researchers think this may be because men tend to have less social support after a loss.

Culture and Religion

Grief occurs in all cultures. However, some cultures have different beliefs about death that affect the attitudes and practices of the bereaved. They use what will best meet their needs to deal with death.

Some studies show that religion helps people cope better with grief, while other studies show that it does not help or causes more distress. Regular church attendance and social support from a religious setting are linked to positive grief outcomes, such as coping and understanding the loss.

Coping Skills and Mental Health

It may seem that any sudden, unexpected loss might lead to more difficult grief. However, studies have found that bereaved people with high self-esteem and/or a feeling that they have control over life are likely to have a normal grief reaction even after an unexpected loss. Bereaved people with low self-esteem and/or a sense that life cannot be controlled are more likely to have complicated grief after an unexpected loss. This includes more depression and physical problems.

Social Support

A lack of social support increases the chance of having problems coping with a loss. Social support includes the person's family, friends, neighbors, and community members who can give psychological, physical, and financial help. After the death of a close family member, many people have related losses. The death of a spouse, for example, may cause a loss of income and changes in lifestyle and day-to-day living. These are all related to social support.

TREATMENT OF GRIEF
Normal Grief May Not Need to be Treated

Most bereaved people work through grief and recover within the first six months to two years. Researchers are studying whether bereaved people who have normal grief could be helped by treatment. They are also studying whether treatment might prevent complicated grief in people who are likely to have it.

For people who have serious grief reactions or symptoms of distress, treatment may be helpful.

Cognitive Behavioral Therapy May Help People with Complicated Grief

Cognitive behavioral therapy (CBT) helps a person learn skills that change negative thoughts and behaviors about grief.

A clinical trial compared CBT to counseling for complicated grief. Results showed that patients treated with CBT had more improvement in symptoms and general mental distress than those in the counseling group.

Depression Related to Grief Might be Treated with Drugs

There is no standard drug therapy for depression that occurs with grief. The decision to treat grief-related depression with drugs is up to the patient and the health-care professional.

431

Clinical trials of antidepressants for depression related to grief have found that the drugs can help relieve depression. However, they give less relief and take longer to work than they do when used for depression that is not related to grief. Some clinical trials have found that psychotherapy while on antidepressants can improve depression and reduce the intensity of grief.[1]

[1] "Grief, Bereavement, and Loss (PDQ®)—Patient Version," National Cancer Institute (NCI), November 11, 2021. Available online. URL: www.cancer.gov/about-cancer/advanced-cancer/caregivers/planning/bereavement-pdq. Accessed August 7, 2023.

Chapter 49 | **Mourning the Death of a Spouse**

When your spouse dies, your world changes. You are in mourning—feeling grief and sorrow at the loss. You may feel numb, shocked, and fearful. You may feel guilty for being the one who is still alive. At some point, you may even feel angry at your spouse for leaving you. All of these feelings are normal. There are no rules about how you should feel. There is no right or wrong way to mourn.

When you grieve, you can feel both physical and emotional pain. People who are grieving often cry easily and can have:
- trouble sleeping
- little interest in food
- problems with concentration
- a hard time making decisions

In addition to dealing with feelings of loss, you may also need to put your own life back together. This can be hard work. Some people feel better sooner than they expect. Others may take longer.

As time passes, you may still miss your spouse. But, for most people, the intense pain will lessen. There will be good and bad days. You will know you are feeling better when there are more good days than bad. You may feel guilty for laughing at a joke or enjoying a visit with a friend. It is important to understand that it can be a common feeling.

FINDING A SUPPORT SYSTEM

There are many ways to grieve and learn in order to accept loss. Try not to ignore your grief. Support may be available until you can manage your grief on your own. It is especially important to get help with your loss if you feel overwhelmed or very depressed by it.

Family and compassionate friends can be a great support. They are grieving, too, and some people find that sharing memories is one way to help each other. Feel free to share stories about the one who is gone. Sometimes, people hesitate to bring up the loss or mention the dead person's name because they worry that it can be hurtful. But people may find it helpful to talk directly about their loss. You are all coping with the death of someone you cared for.

For some people, mourning can go on so long that it becomes unhealthy. This can be a sign of serious depression and anxiety. Talk with your doctor if sadness keeps you from carrying on with your day-to-day life.

HOW GRIEF COUNSELING CAN HELP

Sometimes, people find grief counseling makes it easier to work through their sorrow. Regular talk therapy with a grief counselor or therapist can help people learn to accept a death and, in time, start a new life.

There are also support groups where grieving people help each other. These groups can be specialized—parents who have lost children or people who have lost spouses, for example—or they can be for anyone learning to manage grief. Check with religious groups, local hospitals, nursing homes, funeral homes, or your doctor to find support groups in your area.

An essential part of hospice is providing grief counseling, called "bereavement support," to the family of someone who was under their care. You can also ask hospice workers for bereavement support, even if hospice was not used before the death.

Remember to take good care of yourself. You might know that grief affects how you feel emotionally, but you may not realize that it can also have physical effects. The stress of the death and your grief could even make you sick. Eat well, exercise, get enough sleep, and get back to doing things you used to enjoy, such as going to the movies, walking, or reading. Accept offers of help or companionship from friends and family. It is good for you and for them.

If you have children, remember that they are grieving, too. It will take time for the whole family to adjust to life without your spouse. You may find that your relationship with your children and their relationships with each other have changed. Open, honest communication is important.

Mourning takes time. It is common to have roller-coaster emotions for a while.

TAKING CARE OF YOURSELF WHILE GRIEVING

In the beginning, you may find that taking care of details and keeping busy help. For a while, family and friends may be around to assist you. But there comes a time when you will have to face the change in your life.

Here are some ideas to keep in mind:

- **Take care of yourself**. Grief can be hard on your health. Exercise regularly, eat healthy food, and get enough sleep. Bad habits, such as drinking too much alcohol or smoking, can put your health at risk.
- **Try to eat right**. Some widowed people lose interest in cooking and eating. It may help to have lunch with friends. Sometimes, eating at home alone feels too quiet. Turning on the radio or TV during meals can help. For information on nutrition and cooking for one, look for helpful books at your local library or bookstore or online.
- **Talk with caring friends**. Let family and friends know when you want to talk about your spouse. They may be grieving, too, and may welcome the chance to share memories. When possible, accept their offers of help and company.
- **Visit with members of your religious community**. Many people who are grieving find comfort in their faith. Praying, talking with others of your faith, reading religious or spiritual texts, or listening to uplifting music may also bring comfort.
- **See your doctor**. Keep up with visits to your health-care provider. If it has been a while, schedule a

physical visit and keep your doctor up-to-date on any preexisting medical conditions and any new health issues that may be of concern. Let your health-care provider know if you are having trouble taking care of your everyday activities, such as getting dressed or fixing meals.

WHAT ARE THE SIGNS OF COMPLICATED GRIEF?

Complicated grief is a condition that occurs in about 7 percent of people who have recently lost a close loved one. People with this condition may be unable to comprehend the loss; experience intense, prolonged grief; and have trouble resuming their own life. Signs of complicated grief may include overly negative emotions, dramatically restricting your life to try to avoid places you went with the deceased, and being unable to find meaning or a purpose in life.

Complicated grief can be a serious condition, and those who have it may need additional help to overcome the loss. Support groups, professionals, and close loved ones can help comfort and support someone with this condition.

DOES EVERYONE FEEL THE SAME WAY AFTER DEATH?

Men and women share many of the same feelings when a spouse dies. Both may deal with the pain of loss, and both may worry about the future. But there can also be differences.

Many married couples divide their household tasks. One person may pay bills and handle car repairs, while the other person may cook meals and mow the lawn. Splitting up jobs often works well until there is only one person who has to do it all. Learning to manage new tasks—from chores to household repairs to finances—takes time, but it can be done.

Being alone can increase concerns about safety. It is a good idea to make sure there are working locks on the doors and windows. If you need help, ask your family or friends.

Facing the future without a husband or wife can be scary. Many people have never lived alone. Those who are both widowed and retired may feel very lonely and become depressed. Talk with your doctor about how you are feeling.

MAKE PLANS AND BE ACTIVE

After years of being part of a couple, it can be upsetting to be alone. Many people find that it helps to have things to do every day. Whether you are still working or are retired, write down your weekly plans. You might include the following:

- Take a walk with a friend.
- Visit the library.
- Try to be a volunteer.
- Try an exercise class.
- Join a singing group.
- Join a bowling league.
- Offer to watch your grandchildren.
- Consider adopting a pet.
- Take a class at a nearby senior center, college, or recreation center.
- Stay in touch with family and friends, either in person or online.

GETTING YOUR LEGAL AND FINANCIAL PAPERWORK IN ORDER

When you feel stronger, you should think about getting your legal and financial affairs in order. For example, you might need to do the following:

- Write a new will and update your advance care planning.
- Look into a durable power of attorney for legal matters and health care in case you are unable to make your own medical decisions in the future.
- Put joint property (such as a house or car) in your name.
- Check on changes you might need to make to your health insurance as well as to your life, car, and homeowner's insurance.
- Sign up for Medicare by your 65th birthday.

- Make a list of bills you will need to pay in the next few months, for instance, state and federal taxes and your rent or mortgage.

When you are ready, go through your husband or wife's clothes and other personal items. It may be hard to give away those belongings. Instead of parting with everything at once, you might make three piles: one to keep, one to give away, and one "not sure." Ask your children or others to help. Think about setting aside items, such as a special piece of clothing, watch, favorite book, or picture, to give to your children or grandchildren as personal reminders of your spouse.

GOING OUT AFTER THE DEATH OF A SPOUSE

Having a social life on your own can be tough. It may be hard to think about going to parties or other social events by yourself. It can be hard to think about coming home alone.

You may be anxious about dating. Many people miss the feeling of closeness that marriage brings. After some time, some are ready to have a social life again.

Here are some things to remember:
- Go at a comfortable pace, as there is no rush.
- Make the first move when it comes to planning things to do.
- Try group activities, such as inviting friends for a potluck dinner or going to a senior center.
- Think about informal outings with married friends, such as walks, picnics, or movies, rather than couple's events that remind you of the past.
- Find an activity you like in which you may have fun and meet people who like to do the same thing.
- Develop meaningful relationships with friends and family members of all ages.
- Find comforting companionship, such as pets, as many people do.[1]

---

[1] National Institute on Aging (NIA), "Mourning the Death of a Spouse," National Institutes of Health (NIH), August 20, 2020. Available online. URL: www.nia.nih.gov/health/mourning-death-spouse. Accessed August 31, 2023.

Part 9 | **Mortality Statistics**

Chapter 50 | **Leading Causes of Death and Mortality Trends in the United States**

DEATHS AND MORTALITY

The following death and mortality data for the United States are from the National Vital Statistics System, Mortality (NVSS-M):

- number of deaths: 3,464,231
- death rate: 1,043.8 deaths per 100,000 population
- life expectancy: 76.4 years
- infant mortality rate (IMR): 5.44 deaths per 1,000 live births[1]

HOW LONG CAN WE EXPECT TO LIVE?

In 2021, life expectancy at birth was 76.4 years for the total U.S. population—a decrease of 0.6 years from 77.0 years in 2020 (see Figure 50.1). For males, life expectancy decreased by 0.7 years from 74.2 in 2020 to 73.5 in 2021. For females, life expectancy decreased by 0.6 years from 79.9 in 2020 to 79.3 in 2021.

In 2021, the difference in life expectancy between females and males was 5.8 years, an increase of 0.1 years from 2020.

In 2021, life expectancy at age 65 for the total population was 18.4 years, a decrease of 0.1 years from 2020. For females, life

---

[1] "Deaths and Mortality," Centers for Disease Control and Prevention (CDC), January 17, 2023. Available online. URL: www.cdc.gov/nchs/fastats/deaths.htm. Accessed September 1, 2023.

expectancy at age 65 decreased by 0.1 years from 19.8 in 2020 to 19.7 years in 2021. For males, life expectancy at age 65 was 17.0 years in 2021, unchanged from 2020. The difference in life expectancy at age 65 between females and males decreased by 0.1 years from 2.8 years in 2020 to 2.7 years in 2021.

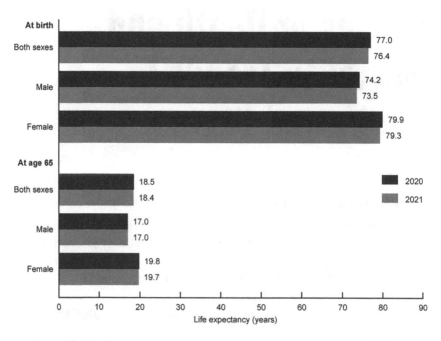

Figure 50.1. Life Expectancy at Birth and Age 65, by Sex in the United States, 2020 and 2021

National Center for Health Statistics (NCHS), National Vital Statistics System, Mortality (NVSS-M)

WHAT ARE THE AGE-ADJUSTED DEATH RATES FOR RACE-ETHNICITY-SEX GROUPS?

The age-adjusted death rate for the total population increased by 5.3 percent from 835.4 deaths per 100,000 U.S. standard population in 2020 to 879.7 in 2021 (see Figure 50.2).

From 2020 to 2021, age-adjusted death rates, corrected for race and ethnicity misclassification, increased by 2.3 percent for Hispanic females (586.6 to 599.8), 6.1 percent for non-Hispanic American-Indian or Alaska Native (AIAN) males (1,618.9 to 1,717.5), 7.3 percent for non-Hispanic AIAN females (1,152.9 to

1,236.6), 1.3 percent for non-Hispanic Black females (910.0 to 921.9), 7.2 percent for non-Hispanic White males (984.6 to 1,055.3), and 6.9 percent for non-Hispanic White females (702.3 to 750.6).

Age-adjusted death rates decreased by 2.1 percent (from 934.8 in 2020 to 915.6 in 2021) for Hispanic males and 1.8 percent (1,405.6 to 1,380.2) for non-Hispanic Black males.

The age-adjusted rates for non-Hispanic-Asian males and non-Hispanic Asian females in 2021 were not significantly different from the rates in 2020.

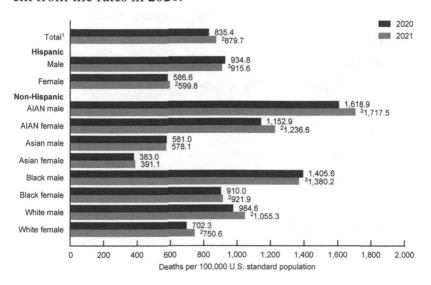

Figure 50.2. Age-Adjusted Death Rate by Race and Hispanic Origin and Sex in the United States, 2020 and 2021

National Center for Health Statistics (NCHS), National Vital Statistics System, Mortality (NVSS-M)
[1]Includes races and origins not shown separately.
[2]Statistically significant increase from 2020 to 2021 (p < 0.05).
[3]Statistically significant decrease from 2020 to 2021 (p < 0.05).
Notes: *AIAN is American Indian or Alaska Native. Race groups are single race. Data by race and Hispanic origin are adjusted for race and Hispanic origin misclassification on death certificates. Adjusted data may differ from data shown in other reports that have not been adjusted for misclassification.*

DID AGE-SPECIFIC DEATH RATES IN 2021 CHANGE FROM 2020 FOR THOSE AGED ONE YEAR AND OVER?

From 2020 to 2021, death rates increased for each age group one year and over (see Figure 50.3).

Age-specific rates increased by 10.1 percent for age group 1–4 (from 22.7 deaths per 100,000 population in 2020 to 25.0 in 2021), 4.4 percent for 5–14 (13.7 to 14.3), 5.6 percent for 15–24 (84.2 to 88.9), 13.4 percent for 25–34 (159.5 to 180.8), and 16.1 percent for 35–44 (248.0 to 287.9).

Rates increased by 12.1 percent for 45–54 (473.5 to 531.0), 7.5 percent for 55–64 (1,038.9 to 1,117.1), 3.8 percent for 65–74 (2,072.3 to 2,151.3), 2.4 percent for 75–84 (4,997.0 to 5,119.4), and 3.5 percent for 85 and over (15,210.9 to 15,743.3).

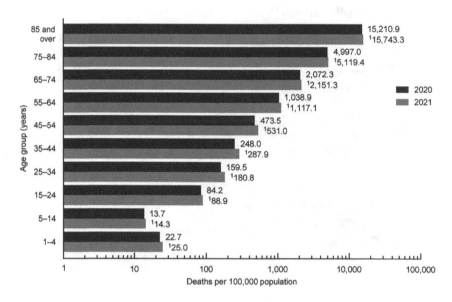

Figure 50.3. Death Rate for Ages One Year and Over in the United States, 2020 and 2021

National Center for Health Statistics (NCHS), National Vital Statistics System, Mortality (NVSS-M)
[1]Statistically significant increase from 2020 to 2021 (p < 0.05).
***Notes**: Rates are plotted on a logarithmic scale.*

WHAT ARE THE DEATH RATES FOR THE LEADING CAUSES OF DEATH?

In 2021, 9 of the 10 leading causes of death remained the same as in 2020. The top leading cause in 2021 was heart disease, followed by cancer and coronavirus disease 2019 (COVID-19; see Figure 50.4).

Chronic liver disease (CLD) and cirrhosis became the ninth leading cause of death in 2021, while influenza and pneumonia

Leading Causes of Death and Mortality Trends in the United States

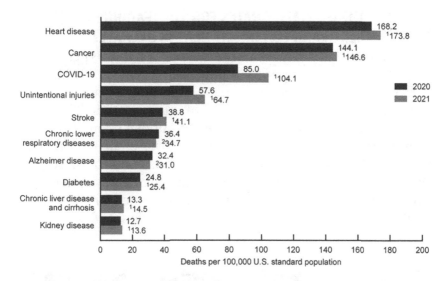

Figure 50.4. Age-Adjusted Death Rate for the 10 Leading Causes of Death in 2021 in the United States, 2020 and 2021

National Center for Health Statistics (NCHS), National Vital Statistics System, Mortality (NVSS-M)
[1]Statistically significant increase from 2020 to 2021 (p < 0.05).
[2]Statistically significant decrease from 2020 to 2021 (p < 0.05).
Notes: *A total of 3,464,231 resident deaths were registered in the United States in 2021. The 10 leading causes of death accounted for 74.5 percent of all U.S. deaths in 2021. Causes of death are ranked according to the number of deaths. Rankings for 2020 data are not shown.*

dropped from the list of 10 leading causes. The remaining leading causes in 2021 (unintentional injuries, stroke, chronic lower respiratory diseases (CLRD), Alzheimer disease (AD), diabetes, and kidney disease) remained at the same ranks as in 2020.

From 2020 to 2021, age-adjusted death rates increased for 8 of the 10 leading causes of death and decreased for 2. The rate increased by 3.3 percent for heart disease (from 168.2 in 2020 to 173.8 in 2021), 1.7 percent for cancer (144.1 to 146.6), 22.5 percent for COVID-19 (85.0 to 104.1), 12.3 percent for unintentional injuries (57.6 to 64.7), 5.9 percent for stroke (38.8 to 41.1), 2.4 percent for diabetes (24.8 to 25.4), 9.0 percent for chronic liver disease (CLD) and cirrhosis (13.3 to 14.5), and 7.1 percent for kidney disease (12.7 to 13.6).

Rates decreased by 4.7 percent for CLRD (36.4 to 34.7) and 4.3 percent for AD (32.4 to 31.0).

WHAT ARE THE MORTALITY RATES FOR THE LEADING CAUSES OF INFANT DEATH AND FOR INFANT DEATHS OVERALL?

The infant mortality rate in 2021 of 543.6 infant deaths per 100,000 live births did not change significantly from the rate in 2020 (541.9).

Causes of infant death are ranked according to the number of infant deaths. The 10 leading causes of infant death in 2021 (congenital malformations, low birth weight, sudden infant death syndrome (SIDS), unintentional injuries, maternal complications, cord and placental complications, bacterial sepsis of newborn, respiratory distress of newborn, diseases of the circulatory system, and intrauterine hypoxia and birth asphyxia) accounted for 66.2 percent of all infant deaths in the United States (see Figure 50.5).

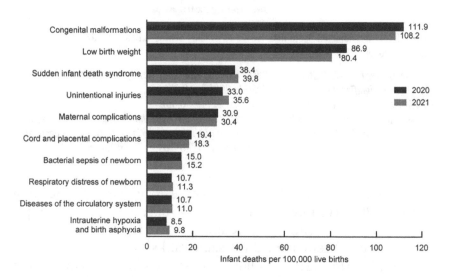

Figure 50.5. Infant Mortality Rate for the 10 Leading Causes of Infant Death in 2021 in the United States, 2020 and 2021

National Center for Health Statistics (NCHS), National Vital Statistics System, Mortality (NVSS-M)
[1]Statistically significant decrease from 2020 to 2021 (p < 0.05)
Notes: *A total of 19,920 deaths occurred in children under the age of one year in the United States in 2021, with an infant mortality rate (IMR) of 543.6 infant deaths per 100,000 live births. The 10 leading causes of infant death in 2021 accounted for 66.2 percent of all U.S. infant deaths. A total of 19,582 infant deaths occurred in 2020, with an IMR of 541.9 infant deaths per 100,000 live births. Rankings for 2020 data are not shown. Causes of death are ranked according to the number of deaths.*

Leading Causes of Death and Mortality Trends in the United States

In 2021, intrauterine hypoxia and birth asphyxia became the 10th leading cause of infant death, replacing neonatal hemorrhage, which dropped from the list. The IMR for low birth weight decreased by 7.5 percent from 86.9 in 2020 to 80.4 in 2021. Mortality rates for the other leading causes of infant death did not change significantly.[2]

[2] "Mortality in the United States, 2021," Centers for Disease Control and Prevention (CDC), December 8, 2022. Available online. URL: www.cdc.gov/nchs/products/databriefs/db456.htm. Accessed September 1, 2023.

Chapter 51 | **Exploring Life Expectancy**

LIVING LONGER: HISTORICAL AND PROJECTED LIFE EXPECTANCY IN THE UNITED STATES, 1960–2060

Over the past four decades, life expectancy in the United States has largely risen although certain groups have experienced slight decreases in their life expectancy, gaining the attention of mortality experts and the media. The headlines draw attention to the role of the opioid epidemic in this unusual downturn in life expectancy among non-Hispanic White adults. In considering what the future of the U.S. population may look like, we must address historical and recent shifts in life expectancy and understand that these shifts are the result of complex social, cultural, biological, and economic forces. Looking forward, we seek to uncover how life expectancy might change in the coming decades and assess how these changes might look across the various race, ethnic, and nativity groups that make up the U.S. population.

The U.S. Census Bureau's 2017 National Population Projections is used to examine potential mortality and life expectancy changes in the coming decades. To provide historical context, the life expectancy data from the National Center for Health Statistics (NCHS) is used. Here, projections of life expectancy from 2017 to 2060 are included, and projected differences in mortality for men and women and for different race and Hispanic origin groups in the United States are explored. And projected life expectancy differences between the native- and foreign-born populations are also focused. The mortality projections covered here are based on the first nativity-specific life tables and life expectancy to be published by the Census Bureau.

449

Projections of life expectancy can provide essential information on population aging, guide the future of U.S. public health, and gauge potential impacts on health-care systems. As a result, they can help improve our understanding of social welfare and better inform policy planning. In addition to presenting mortality patterns for the total population, depicting life expectancy patterns by characteristics, such as sex, race, Hispanic origin, and nativity, provides a more accurate story of current and future population health within the United States.

- Americans are projected to have longer life expectancy in the coming decades. By 2060, life expectancy for the total population is projected to increase by about six years, from 79.7 in 2017 to 85.6 in 2060.
- Increases in life expectancy are projected to be larger for men than women although women are still projected to live longer than men do, on average, in 2060.
- All racial and ethnic groups are projected to have longer life expectancy in the coming decades, but the greatest gains will be to native-born men who are non-Hispanic Black alone and non-Hispanic American Indian or Alaska Native alone.
- Among the native-born population, Hispanic women had the longest life expectancy, 83.3 years, of any race or Hispanic origin group in the United States in 2017. They are projected to continue to have the longest life expectancy, 87.8 years, in 2060.
- In 2060, foreign-born men and women are projected to continue having longer life expectancy than their native-born peers, regardless of race or Hispanic origin.

PROJECTING MORTALITY BY NATIVITY, RACE, AND HISPANIC ORIGIN

Nativity is a demographic characteristic that identifies if an individual is native- or foreign-born. The U.S. Census Bureau uses the following definitions for nativity status:

- **Native-born or native-born population**. Anyone who is a U.S. citizen at birth, including people born in the United States, Puerto Rico, or a U.S. Island Area (Guam, the Commonwealth of the Northern Mariana Islands, and the U.S. Virgin Islands) or born abroad to a U.S. citizen parent or parents.

- **Foreign-born or foreign-born population.** Anyone who is not a U.S. citizen at birth, which includes non-citizen U.S. nationals, naturalized U.S. citizens, lawful permanent residents (immigrants), temporary migrants (such as foreign students), humanitarian migrants (such as refugees and asylees), and unauthorized migrants.

For the purposes of the 2017 National Population Projections, those born in the United States or in U.S. territories are considered native-born while those born elsewhere are considered foreign-born.

One of the innovations in the 2017 National Population Projections series was the inclusion of nativity as a characteristic in the mortality measures. Similar to projecting mortality by sex, race, and Hispanic origin, projecting mortality rates by nativity requires additional information from administrative records, specifically about the place of birth of the deceased. This addition improves the population projections by accounting for the different mortality patterns of the native- and foreign-born.

The 2017 National Population Projections use historical vital statistics data to inform projected mortality rates by sex, nativity, race, and Hispanic origin. The denominators of the mortality rates contain bridged population estimates to maintain continuity with race and Hispanic origin classifications of vital records over time. Because current population estimates adhere to revised 1997 Office of Management and Budget (OMB) standards for race and ethnicity, which allow for the reporting of more than one race, estimates for multiple-race people must be bridged back to single-race categories in accordance with 1977 OMB standards to ensure historical continuity. Furthermore, due to concerns about the quality of race reporting in death data over the time series, non-Hispanic race groups with similar mortality patterns were collapsed into two categories. As a result, mortality rates were produced for three races and Hispanic origin groups for the projected data:

- **Group 1**. Non-Hispanic White alone, non-Hispanic Asian alone, and non-Hispanic Native Hawaiian or other Pacific Islander alone.
- **Group 2**. Non-Hispanic Black or African American alone and non-Hispanic American Indian or Alaska Native alone.
- **Group 3**. Hispanic or Latino (of any race).

Here, projected mortality trends by race and ethnicity will be based on these groupings. When observed or historical NCHS data and other citations are used, these groupings do not apply.[1]

---

[1] "Living Longer: Historical and Projected Life Expectancy in the United States, 1960 to 2060," United States Census Bureau, February 1, 2020. Available online. URL: www.census.gov/content/dam/Census/library/publications/2020/demo/p25-1145.pdf. Accessed September 7, 2023.

Chapter 52 | **Maternal Mortality Trends**

The maternal mortality rates for 2021 are based on data from the National Vital Statistics System (NVSS). Maternal death is defined by the World Health Organization (WHO) as "the death of a woman while pregnant or within 42 days of termination of pregnancy, irrespective of the duration and the site of the pregnancy, from any cause related to or aggravated by the pregnancy or its management, but not from accidental or incidental causes." Maternal mortality rates, which are the number of maternal deaths per 100,000 live births, are shown in the figures by age group, race, and Hispanic origin.

In 2021, 1,205 women died of maternal causes in the United States, compared with 861 in 2020 and 754 in 2019. The maternal mortality rate for 2021 was 32.9 deaths per 100,000 live births, compared with a rate of 23.8 in 2020 and 20.1 in 2019.

In 2021, the maternal mortality rate for non-Hispanic Black (subsequently, Black) women was 69.9 deaths per 100,000 live births, 2.6 times the rate for non-Hispanic White (subsequently, White) women (26.6; see Figure 52.1). Rates for Black women were significantly higher than rates for White and Hispanic women. The increases from 2020 to 2021 for all races and Hispanic origin groups were significant.

Rates increased with maternal age. Rates in 2021 were 20.4 deaths per 100,000 live births for women under age 25, 31.3 for those aged 25–39, and 138.5 for those aged 40 and over (see Figure 52.2). The rate for women aged 40 and over was 6.8 times higher than the rate for women under age 25. Differences in the rates between age groups were statistically significant. The increases in the rates

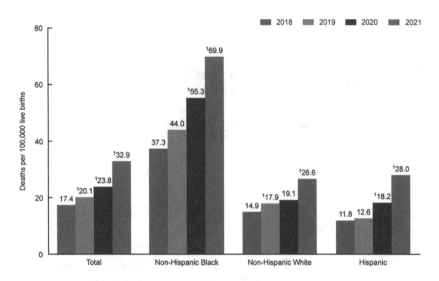

Figure 52.1. Maternal Mortality Rates, by Race and Hispanic Origin: United States, 2018–2021

Center for Health Statistics (NCHS), National Vital Statistics System, Mortality (NVSS-M)
[1]Statistically significant increase from the previous year (p < 0.05)
***Notes**: Race groups are single race.*

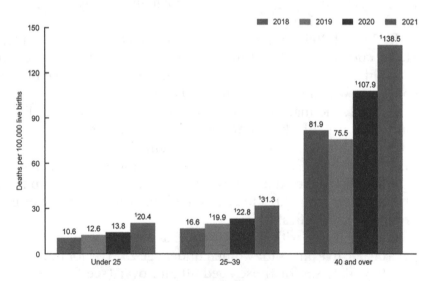

Figure 52.2. Maternal Mortality Rates, by Age Group: United States, 2018–2021

Center for Health Statistics (NCHS), National Vital Statistics System, Mortality (NVSS-M)
[1]Statistically significant increase from the previous year (p < 0.05)

between 2020 and 2021 for each of these age groups were statistically significant.

DATA SOURCE AND METHODS

Data are from the NVSS mortality file. Consistent with previous reports, the number of maternal deaths does not include all deaths occurring to pregnant or recently pregnant women but only deaths with the underlying cause of death assigned to International Statistical Classification of Diseases, 10th Revision code numbers A34, O00–O95, and O98–O99. Maternal mortality rates are per 100,000 live births, based on data from the NVSS natality file. Maternal mortality rates fluctuate from year to year because of the relatively small number of these events and possibly due to issues with the reporting of maternal deaths on death certificates. Efforts to improve data quality are ongoing, and these data will continue to be evaluated for possible errors. Data are shown for only the three largest race and Hispanic origin groups for which statistically reliable rates can be calculated.[1]

---

[1] "Maternal Mortality Rates in the United States, 2021," Centers for Disease Control and Prevention (CDC), March 16, 2023. Available online. URL: www.cdc.gov/nchs/data/hestat/maternal-mortality/2021/maternal-mortality-rates-2021.htm. Accessed September 7, 2023.

Chapter 53 | Work-Related Deaths and Occupational Health

There were 5,190 fatal work injuries recorded in the United States in 2021, an 8.9 percent increase from 4,764 in 2020, the U.S. Bureau of Labor Statistics (BLS) reported (see Figure 53.1). The fatal work injury rate was 3.6 fatalities per 100,000 full-time equivalent (FTE) workers, up from 3.4 per 100,000 FTE in 2020 and up from the 2019 prepandemic rate of 3.5 (see Figure 53.2). These data are from the Census of Fatal Occupational Injuries (CFOI).

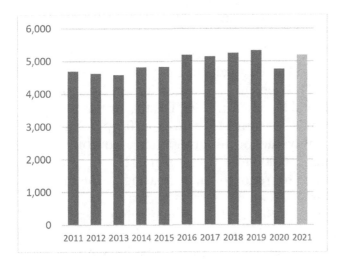

Figure 53.1. Number of Fatal Work Injuries, 2011–2021

U.S. Bureau of Labor Statistics (BLS), U.S. Department of Labor (DOL)

457

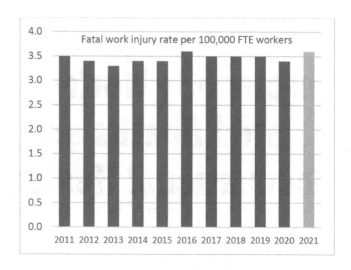

Figure 53.2. Fatal Work Injury Rate, 2011–2021

U.S. Bureau of Labor Statistics (BLS), U.S. Department of Labor (DOL)

CENSUS OF FATAL OCCUPATIONAL INJURIES IN 2021

- The 3.6 fatal occupational injury rate in 2021 represents the highest annual rate since 2016.
- A worker died every 101 minutes from a work-related injury in 2021.
- The share of Black or African-American workers fatally injured on the job reached an all-time high in 2021, increasing from 11.4 percent of total fatalities in 2020 to 12.6 percent of total fatalities in 2021. Deaths for this group climbed to 653 in 2021 from 541 in 2020, a 20.7 percent increase. The fatality rate for this group increased from 3.5 in 2020 to 4.0 per 100,000 FTE workers in 2021.
- Suicides continued to trend down, decreasing to 236 in 2021 from 259 in 2020, an 8.9 percent decrease.
- Workers in transportation and material moving occupations experienced a series high of 1,523 fatal work injuries in 2021 and represented the occupational group with the highest number of fatalities. This is an increase of 18.8 percent from 2020.

- Transportation incidents remained the most frequent type of fatal event in 2021, with 1,982 fatal injuries, an increase of 11.5 percent from 2020. This major category accounted for 38.2 percent of all work-related fatalities in 2021.

WORKER CHARACTERISTICS

- Black or African-American workers as well as Hispanic or Latinx workers had fatality rates (4.0 and 4.5 per 100,000 FTE workers, respectively) in 2021 that were higher than the all-worker rate of 3.6. Transportation incidents were the highest cause of fatalities within both of these groups (267 for Black or African-American workers and 383 for Hispanic or Latinx workers).
- The second highest cause of fatalities to Black or African-American workers was injuries due to violence and other injuries by persons or animals (155), whereas for Hispanic or Latinx workers, it was falls, slips, or trips (272). Almost a quarter of Black or African-American workplace fatalities (23.7%) are a result of violence and other injuries by persons or animals as opposed to 14.7 percent for all workers.
- Women made up 8.6 percent of all workplace fatalities but represented 14.5 percent of intentional injuries by a person in 2021.
- In 2021, workers between the ages of 45 and 54 suffered 1,087 workplace fatalities, a 13.9 percent increase from 2020. This age group accounted for just over one-fifth of the total fatalities for the year (20.9%).

FATAL EVENT OR EXPOSURE

- Despite experiencing an increase from 2020 to 2021, transportation incidents are still down 6.6 percent from 2019 when there were 2,122 fatalities (see Figure 53.3).
- Fatalities due to violence and other injuries by persons or animals increased to 761 fatalities in 2021 from 705 fatalities in 2020 (7.9%). The largest subcategory, intentional injuries by person, increased 10.3 percent to 718 in 2021.

- Exposure to harmful substances or environments led to 798 worker fatalities in 2021, the highest figure since the series began in 2011. This major event category experienced the largest increase in fatalities in 2021, increasing 18.8 percent from 2020. Unintentional overdose from nonmedical use of drugs or alcohol accounted for 58.1 percent of these fatalities (464 deaths), up from 57.7 percent of this category's total in 2020.
- Work-related fatalities due to falls, slips, and trips increased by 5.6 percent in 2021, from 805 fatalities in 2020 to 850 in 2021. Falls, slips, and trips in construction and extraction occupations accounted for 370 of these fatalities in 2021, an increase of 7.2 percent from 2020 when there were 345 fatalities. Despite the increase, this is still down 9.3 percent from 2019 when construction and extraction occupations experienced 408 fatalities due to this event.

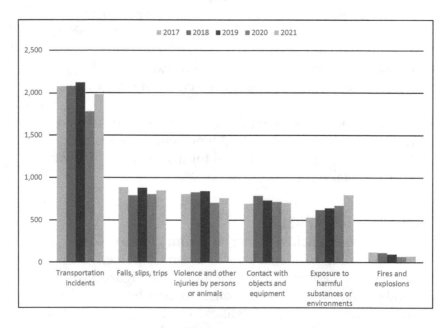

Figure 53.3. Fatal Work Injuries by Major Event or Exposure, 2017–2021

U.S. Bureau of Labor Statistics (BLS), U.S. Department of Labor (DOL)

OCCUPATION

- There was a 16.3 percent increase in deaths for driver/sales workers and truck drivers that went up to 1,032 deaths in 2021 from 887 deaths in 2020. This was the primary factor behind the increase in fatalities of workers in transportation and material moving occupations, which reached a series high in 2021 (see Figure 53.4).

- Construction and extraction occupations had the second most occupational deaths (951) in 2021 despite experiencing a 2.6 percent decrease in fatalities from 2020. The fatality rate for this occupation also decreased from 13.5 deaths per 100,000 FTE workers in 2020 to 12.3 in 2021.

- Protective service occupations (such as firefighters, law enforcement workers, police and sheriff's patrol officers, and transit and railroad police) had a 31.9 percent increase in fatalities in 2021, increasing to 302 from 229 in 2020. Almost half (45.4%) of these fatalities are due to homicides (116) and suicides (21). About one-third

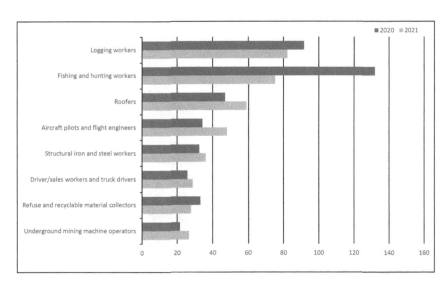

Figure 53.4. Fatal Work Injury Rates per 100,000 Full-Time Equivalent Workers by Selected Occupations, 2020–2021

U.S. Bureau of Labor Statistics (BLS), U.S. Department of Labor (DOL)

(33.4%) are due to transportation incidents, representing the highest count since 2016.

- Installation, maintenance, and repair occupations had 475 fatalities in 2021, an increase of 20.9 percent. Almost one-third of these deaths (152) were to vehicle and mobile equipment mechanics, installers, and repairers.
- The fatal injury rate for fishing and hunting workers decreased from 132.1 per 100,000 FTEs in 2020 to 75.2 in 2021.[1]

---

[1] U.S. Bureau of Labor Statistics (BLS), "National Census of Fatal Occupational Injuries in 2021," U.S. Department of Labor (DOL), December 16, 2022. Available online. URL: www.bls.gov/news.release/pdf/cfoi.pdf. Accessed August 10, 2023.

Chapter 54 | Suicide Facts and Statistics

SUICIDE DATA AND STATISTICS

Suicide rates increased by 37 percent between 2000 and 2018 and decreased by 5 percent between 2018 and 2020. However, rates nearly returned to their peak in 2021.

Suicide Rates by Demographic Characteristics

Overall, the number of deaths by suicide increased by 2.6 percent from 2021 to 2022 provisional data but decreased among American-Indian/Alaska Native people and youth. Figure 54.1 describes the overall suicide deaths from 2021 to 2022 in the United States by demographic characteristics.

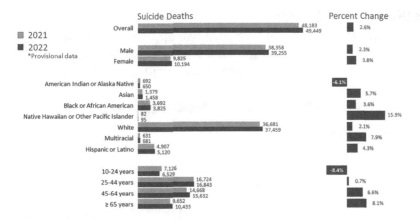

Figure 54.1. Suicide Deaths in the United States Overall and by Select Demographic Characteristics, 2021–2022

Centers for Disease Control and Prevention (CDC)

Racial/Ethnic Disparities in Suicide

Some groups have disproportionately high rates of suicide. The racial/ethnic groups with the highest rates in 2021 were non-Hispanic American-Indian and Alaska Native people and non-Hispanic White people (see Figure 54.2).

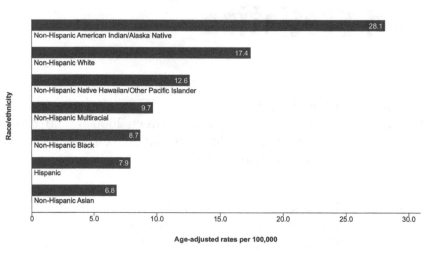

Figure 54.2. Racial and Ethnic Disparities in Suicide

Centers for Disease Control and Prevention (CDC)

Sex Disparities in Suicide

The suicide rate among males in 2021 was approximately four times higher than the rate among females. Males make up 50 percent of the population but nearly 80 percent of suicides (see Figure 54.3).

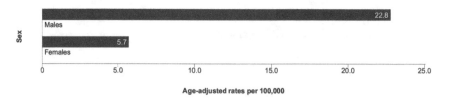

Figure 54.3. Sex Disparities in Suicide

Centers for Disease Control and Prevention (CDC)

Age Disparities in Suicide

People aged 85 and older have the highest rates of suicide (see Figure 54.4).

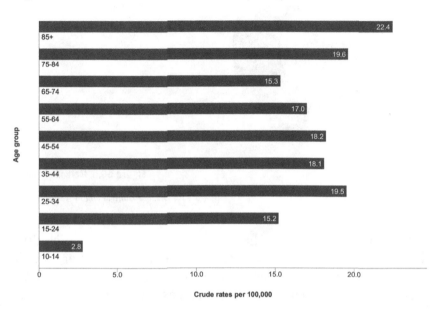

Figure 54.4. Age Disparities in Suicide

Centers for Disease Control and Prevention (CDC)

Method of Suicide

Using firearms is the most common method of suicide. Firearms are used in more than 50 percent of suicides (see Figure 54.5).[1]

SUICIDE IS A LEADING CAUSE OF DEATH

Suicide is death caused by injuring oneself with the intent to die. A suicide attempt is when someone harms themselves with any intent to end their lives, but they do not die as a result of their actions.

Many factors can increase the risk for suicide or protect against it. Suicide is connected to other forms of injury and violence.

---

[1] "Suicide Data and Statistics," Centers for Disease Control and Prevention (CDC), August 10, 2023. Available online. URL: www.cdc.gov/suicide/suicide-data-statistics.html. Accessed September 1, 2023.

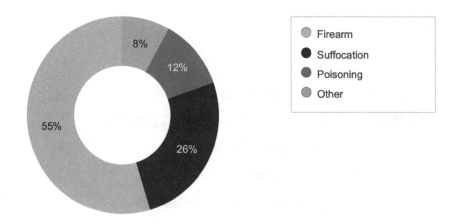

Figure 54.5. Method of Suicide

Centers for Disease Control and Prevention (CDC)

For example, people who have experienced violence, including child abuse, bullying, or sexual violence, have a higher suicide risk. Being connected to family and community support and having easy access to health care can decrease suicidal thoughts and behaviors.

SUICIDE HAS FAR-REACHING IMPACTS

Suicide and suicide attempts cause serious emotional, physical, and economic impacts. People who attempt suicide and survive may experience serious injuries that can have long-term effects on their health. They may also experience depression and other mental health concerns.

Suicide and suicide attempts affect the health and well-being of friends, loved ones, coworkers, and the community. When people die by suicide, their surviving family and friends may experience prolonged grief, shock, anger, guilt, symptoms of depression or anxiety, and even thoughts of suicide themselves.

The financial toll of suicide on society is also costly. In 2020, suicide and nonfatal self-harm cost the nation over $500 billion in medical costs, work loss costs, value of statistical life, and quality-of-life costs.

Suicidal behavior also has a far-reaching impact. There were 46,412 suicides among adults in 2021. But suicides are just the tip of the iceberg. For every suicide death*, there were about:
- 3 hospitalizations for self-harm
- 8 emergency department visits related to suicide
- 38 self-reported suicide attempts in 2020
- 265 people who seriously considered suicide in 2020

*This is based on the latest year of available data for adults aged 18 and older.

SUICIDE PREVENTION RESOURCE FOR ACTION

Suicide is preventable, and everyone has a role to play to save lives and create healthy and strong individuals, families, and communities. Suicide prevention requires a comprehensive public health approach. The Centers for Disease Control and Prevention (CDC) developed the Suicide Prevention Resource for Action (Prevention Resource), which provides information on the best available evidence for suicide prevention. States and communities can use the Prevention Resource to help make decisions about suicide prevention activities. Strategies range from those designed to support people at increased risk to a focus on the whole population, regardless of risk:
- Strengthen economic supports:
  - Improve household financial security.
  - Stabilize housing.
- Create protective environments:
  - Reduce access to lethal means among persons at risk of suicide.
  - Create healthy organizational policies and culture.
  - Reduce substance use through community-based policies and practices.
- Improve access and delivery of suicide care:
  - Cover mental health conditions in health insurance policies.
  - Increase provider availability in underserved areas.
  - Provide rapid and remote access to help.
  - Create safer suicide care through systems change.

- Promote healthy connections:
  - Promote healthy peer norms.
  - Engage community members in shared activities.
- Teach coping and problem-solving skills:
  - Support social-emotional learning programs.
  - Teach parenting skills to improve family relationships.
  - Support resilience through education programs.
- Identify and support people at risk:
  - Train gatekeepers.
  - Respond to crises.
  - Plan for safety and follow-up after an attempt.
  - Provide therapeutic approaches.
- Lessen harm and prevent future risk:
  - Intervene after a suicide (postvention).
  - Report and message about suicide safely.[2]

---

[2] "Facts about Suicide," Centers for Disease Control and Prevention (CDC), May 8, 2023. Available online. URL: www.cdc.gov/suicide/facts/index.html. Accessed September 1, 2023.

Chapter 55 | **Alcohol-Attributable Deaths and Public Health Impact**

ALCOHOL-RELATED EMERGENCIES AND DEATHS IN THE UNITED STATES

- The rate of all alcohol-related emergency department visits increased by 47.0 percent between 2006 and 2014, which translates to an average annual increase of 210,000 alcohol-related emergency department visits.
- Alcohol contributes to approximately 18.5 percent of emergency department visits and 22.1 percent of overdose deaths related to prescription opioids.
- It is estimated that more than 140,000 people (approximately 97,000 men and 43,000 women) die from alcohol-related causes annually, making alcohol the fourth-leading preventable cause of death in the United States behind tobacco, poor diet and physical inactivity, and illegal drugs.
- An analysis of death certificates from 2019 and 2020 showed that deaths involving alcohol rose from approximately 79,000 to more than 99,000, a 25.5 percent increase.
- Between 2015 and 2019, the leading causes of alcohol-attributable deaths due to chronic conditions in the United States were liver diseases (e.g., alcohol-associated liver diseases and unspecified liver cirrhosis), cardiovascular diseases (CVD), cancers of various types

(e.g., organs of the upper respiratory and digestive tracts, liver, colon, and breast), and alcohol use disorder (AUD).

- In 2021, alcohol-impaired driving fatalities accounted for 13,384 deaths (or 31% of overall driving fatalities).
- According to the most recent estimate from the Centers for Disease Control and Prevention (CDC), 21.0 percent of suicide decedents have blood alcohol concentrations of 0.1 percent or more.
- Among people who die by suicide, AUD is the second most common mental disorder and is involved in roughly one in four deaths by suicide.

Death Involving Alcohol

- Death certificates listing alcohol increased by 25.5 percent from 78,927 in 2019 to 99,017 in 2020, the first year of the pandemic, and 10 percent more to 108,891 in 2021.
- Alcohol was listed in one in six (16%) of drug overdose deaths in 2020 and 2021.
- Alcohol-related traffic fatalities increased by 14 percent to 11,654 in 2020—the highest since 2008.

Impact of Alcohol and Opioids in the United States
ALCOHOL

- past-year use percentage of the population:
  - 174,339,000 (62.3%)
- Diagnostic and Statistical Manual of Mental Disorders and Alcohol Use Disorder (DSM-AUD) percentage of the population:
  - 29,544,000 (10.6%)
- emergency department visits:
  - 1,714,757: primary reason
  - 4,936,690: all alcohol-related
- 140,557 annual deaths:
  - 58,277: acute (e.g., injury)
  - 82,279: chronic (e.g., liver disease)

OPIOIDS

- past-year misuse percentage of the population:
  - 9,117,000 (3.3%)
- opioid use disorder (OUD) percentage of the population:
  - 5,559,000 (0.9%)
- emergency department visits:
  - 408,079: primary reason
  - 1,461,770: all opioid-related
- 80,411 annual deaths:
  - 58,277: acute (e.g., injury)
  - 82,279: chronic (e.g., liver disease)[1]

EVERYONE CAN HELP PREVENT EXCESSIVE ALCOHOL USE

You can do the following:

- Choose not to drink or to drink in moderation by limiting intake to two drinks or less in a day (if you are a man) and one drink or less in a day (if you are a woman) on days when alcohol is consumed. Some people should not drink any alcohol, including the following:
  - pregnant or probably pregnant
  - younger than 21 years
  - having certain medical conditions or taking certain medicines that can interact with alcohol
  - recovering from AUD or unable to control the amount they drink.
- Check your drinking and learn more about the benefits of drinking less alcohol.
- Support effective community strategies to prevent excessive alcohol use, such as those recommended by the Community Preventive Services Task Force (CPSTF).

---

[1] "Alcohol-Related Emergencies and Deaths in the United States," National Institute on Alcohol Abuse and Alcoholism (NIAAA), 2023. Available online. URL: www.niaaa.nih.gov/alcohols-effects-health/alcohol-topics/alcohol-facts-and-statistics/alcohol-related-emergencies-and-deaths-united-states. Accessed August 11, 2023.

- Do not serve or provide alcohol to anyone who should not be drinking, including people younger than 21 or those who have already consumed too much.
- Talk with your health-care provider about your drinking behavior and request counseling if you drink too much.

States and communities can include the following:
- Implement effective strategies for preventing excessive alcohol use to reduce the availability and accessibility of alcohol and increase its price, including regulating the number and concentration of alcohol outlets, limiting days and hours of alcohol sales, and avoiding further privatization of alcohol sales. Check out the CDC's alcohol outlet density measurement resources.
- Enforce existing laws and regulations about alcohol sales and service.
- Partner with law enforcement, community groups, health departments, doctors, nurses, and other health-care providers to reduce excessive drinking and related harms.
- Track the role of alcohol in injuries and deaths with more routine alcohol toxicology testing among patients and people who have died.
- Routinely monitor and report on measures of excessive alcohol use and the status of effective alcohol policies.[2]

[2] "Deaths from Excessive Alcohol Use in the United States," Centers for Disease Control and Prevention (CDC), July 6, 2022. Available online. URL: www.cdc.gov/alcohol/features/excessive-alcohol-deaths.html. Accessed August 11, 2023.

Part 10 | **Additional Help and Information**

Chapter 56 | **Glossary of End-of-Life Terms**

accelerated death benefit (ADB): A life insurance policy feature that lets you use some of the policy's death benefit prior to death.

activities of daily living (ADLs): Basic actions that independently functioning individuals perform on a daily basis.

acute care: A health care approach that focuses on achieving rapid recovery. This type of care is often provided in hospitals, emergency rooms, specialized clinics, and specific doctor's offices. It offers intensive, short-term medical attention to individuals facing severe health issues.

adult day services (ADS): Services provided during the day at a community-based center. Programs address the individual needs of functionally or cognitively impaired adults. These structured, comprehensive programs provide social and support services in a protective setting during any part of the day, but not 24-hour care. Many adult day service programs include health-related services.

advanced directive: Legal document that specifies whether you would like to be kept on artificial life support if you become permanently unconscious or are otherwise dying and unable to speak for yourself. It also specifies other aspects of health care you would like under those circumstances.

Alzheimer disease (AD): Progressive, degenerative form of dementia that causes severe intellectual deterioration. The first symptoms are impaired memory, followed by impaired thought and speech, and finally complete helplessness.

amino acid: One of several molecules that join together to form proteins. There are 20 common amino acids found in proteins.

anemia: A condition in which the number of red blood cells is below normal.

This glossary contains terms excerpted from documents produced by several sources deemed reliable.

anesthetic: A drug that causes insensitivity to pain and is used for surgeries and other medical procedures.

annuity: A financial contract wherein an individual provides funds to an insurance company. In return, they receive regular payments. These payments can be guaranteed for a specific period or for the lifetime of the person. Various types of annuities are available, including fixed and variable options.

anxiety: Feelings of fear, dread, and uneasiness that may occur as a reaction to stress. A person with anxiety may sweat, feel restless and tense, and have a rapid heartbeat.

aspiration: The removal of fluid or tissue through a needle. Also, the accidental breathing in of food or fluid into the lungs.

assisted living facility: Residential living arrangement that provides individualized personal care, assistance with activities of daily living, help with medications, and services, such as laundry and housekeeping. Facilities may also provide health and medical care, but care is not as intensive as care offered at a nursing home.

assistive device: Tools that enable individuals with disabilities to perform essential job functions (e.g., telephone headsets, adapted computer keyboards, and enhanced computer monitors).

assistive technology: Products, devices, or equipment that help maintain, increase, or improve the functional capabilities of people with disabilities.

bacteria: A large group of single-cell microorganisms. Some cause infections and diseases in animals and humans.

biomarker: A specific physical trait or a measurable biologically produced change in the body connected with a disease or health condition.

board and care home: Residential private homes designed to provide housing, meals, housekeeping, personal care services, and support to frail or disabled residents. At least one caregiver is on the premises at all times. In many states, board and care homes are licensed or certified and must meet criteria for facility safety, types of services provided, and the number and type of residents they can care for.

brain tumor: The growth of abnormal cells in the tissues of the brain. Brain tumors can be benign (not cancer) or malignant (cancer).

calorie: A unit of energy in food. Carbohydrates, fats, protein, and alcohol in the foods and drinks we eat provide food energy or "calories."

cardiopulmonary resuscitation (CPR): Combination of rescue breathing (mouth-to-mouth resuscitation) and chest compressions used if someone is not breathing or circulating blood adequately. CPR can restore the circulation of oxygen-rich blood to the brain.

caregiver: A caregiver is anyone who helps care for an elderly individual or person with a disability who lives at home. Caregivers usually provide assistance with activities of daily living and other essential activities such as shopping, meal preparation, and housework.

central nervous system (CNS): Comprises the nerves in the brain and spinal cord. These nerves are used to send electrical impulses throughout the body, resulting in voluntary and reflexive movement. Information about the environment is received by the senses and sent to the CNS, which causes the body to respond appropriately.

charitable remainder trust (CRT): Special tax-exempt irrevocable trust written to comply with federal tax laws and regulations. You transfer cash or assets into the trust and may receive some income from it for life or a specified number of years (not to exceed 20).

chemotherapy: Treatment with anticancer drugs.

cholesterol: A fatty substance present in all parts of the body. It is a component of cell membranes and is used to make vitamin D and some hormones. Some cholesterol in the body is produced by the liver, and some is derived from food, particularly animal products.

chronic disease: A disease that has one or more of the following characteristics: is permanent, leaves residual disability, is caused by nonreversible pathological alteration, requires special training of the patient for rehabilitation, or may be expected to require a long period of supervision, observation, or care.

chronically ill: Having a long-lasting or recurrent illness or condition that causes you to need help with activities of daily living and often other health and support services. The condition is expected to last for at least 90 consecutive days.

cognitive impairment: Deficiency in short- or long-term memory; orientation to person, place, and time; deductive or abstract reasoning; or judgment as it relates to safety awareness. Alzheimer disease is an example of a cognitive impairment.

community-based services: Services and service settings in the community, such as adult day services, home-delivered meals, or transportation services. Often referred to as home- and community-based services, they are designed to help older people and people with disabilities stay in their homes as independently as possible.

computed tomography (CT): A procedure for taking x-ray images from many different angles and then assembling them into a cross-section of the body. This technique is generally used to visualize bone.

constipation: A decrease in the frequency of stools or bowel movements with hardening of the stool. Some forms of osteogenesis imperfecta are associated with increased risk for constipation caused by increased perspiration, growth impairment, pelvic malformation, and diminished physical activity.

continuing care retirement communities (CCRCs): Communities that often require an entrance fee along with monthly fees. They offer a variety of housing options, ranging from independent living units to nursing homes. These communities are designed to accommodate individuals as their care needs change.

dehydration: Excessive loss of body water that the body needs to carry on normal functions at an optimal level.

depression: A mental condition marked by ongoing feelings of sadness, despair, loss of energy, and difficulty dealing with normal daily life. Other symptoms of depression include feelings of worthlessness and hopelessness, loss of pleasure in activities, changes in eating or sleeping habits, and thoughts of death or suicide.

diabetes: A disease in which blood glucose (blood sugar) levels are above normal. There are two main types of diabetes. Type 1 diabetes is caused by a problem with the body's defense system, called the "immune system." This form of diabetes usually starts in childhood or adolescence. Type 2 diabetes is the most common form of diabetes. It starts most often in adulthood.

diet: What a person eats and drinks. Any type of eating plan.

disorder: In medicine, a disturbance of normal functioning of the mind or body. Disorders may be caused by genetic factors, disease, or trauma.

durable power of attorney: Legal document that gives someone else the authority to act on your behalf on matters that you specify. The power can be specific to a certain task or broad to cover many financial duties. You can specify if you want the power to start immediately or upon mental incapacity. For the document to be valid, you must sign it before you become disabled.

fracture: Broken bone. People with osteoporosis, osteogenesis imperfecta, and Paget disease are at greater risk for bone fracture.

glucose: A major source of energy for our bodies and a building block for many carbohydrates. The food digestion process breaks down carbohydrates in foods and drinks into glucose. After digestion, glucose is carried in the blood and goes to body cells where it is used for energy or stored.

group home: Residential private homes designed to provide housing, meals, housekeeping, personal care services, and support to frail or disabled residents. At least one caregiver is onsite at all times. In many states, group homes are licensed or certified and must meet criteria for facility safety, types of services provided, and the number and type of residents they can care for.

hearing aid: An electronic device designed to amplify sound for individual with hearing impairment; it usually consists of a microphone, amplifier, and receiver.

heart disease: A number of abnormal conditions affecting the heart and the blood vessels in the heart. The most common type of heart disease is coronary artery disease, which is the gradual buildup of plaques in the coronary arteries, the blood vessels that bring blood to the heart. This disease develops slowly and silently, over decades. It can go virtually unnoticed until it produces a heart attack.

high blood pressure: Your blood pressure rises and falls throughout the day. Optimal blood pressure is less than 120/80 mmHg. When blood pressure stays high—greater than or equal to 140/90 mmHg—you have high blood pressure, also called "hypertension." With high blood pressure, the heart works harder; your arteries take a beating; and your chances of a stroke, heart attack, and kidney problems are greater.

hospice care: Short-term, supportive care for individuals who are terminally ill (have a life expectancy of six months or less). Hospice care focuses on pain management and emotional, physical, and spiritual support for the patient and family. It can be provided at home or in a hospital, nursing home, or hospice facility. Medicare typically pays for hospice care. Hospice care is not usually considered long-term care.

human immunodeficiency virus (HIV): A virus that infects and destroys the body's immune cells and causes a disease called "acquired immunodeficiency syndrome" (AIDS).

hydration: The amount of fluid in your body. It is important to replace any fluid your body loses during physical activity.

immune system: A complex system of cellular and molecular components having the primary function of distinguishing self from not self and defense against foreign organisms or substances.

informal caregiver: Any person who provides long-term-care services without pay.

living will: Legal document that specifies whether you would like to be kept on artificial life support if you become permanently unconscious or are otherwise dying and unable to speak for yourself. It also specifies other aspects of health care you would like under those circumstances.

long-term care: Services and supports necessary to meet health or personal care needs over an extended period of time.

long-term-care insurance: Insurance policy designed to offer financial support to pay for long-term-care services.

magnetic resonance imaging (MRI): A noninvasive procedure that uses magnetic fields and radio waves to produce three-dimensional computerized images of areas inside the body.

Medicaid: Joint federal and state public assistance program for financing health care for low-income people. It pays for health-care services for those with low incomes or very high medical bills relative to income and assets. It is the largest public payer of long-term-care services.

Medicare: Federal program that provides hospital and medical expense benefits for people over the age of 65 or those meeting specific disability standards. Benefits for nursing home and home health services are limited.

nursing home: Licensed facility that provides general nursing care to those who are chronically ill or unable to take care of daily living needs.

nutrition: The taking in and use of food and other nourishing material by the body. Nutrition is a three-part process. First, food or drink is consumed. Second, the body breaks down the food or drink into nutrients.

organ: A part of the body that performs a specific function. For example, the heart is an organ.

over-the-counter (OTC): Diseases, including ulcerative colitis (UC) and Crohn's disease, that cause swelling in the intestine and/or digestive tract, which may result in diarrhea, abdominal pain, fever, and weight loss. People with inflammatory bowel disease (IBD) are at an increased risk for osteoporosis.

personal care: Nonskilled service or care, such as help with bathing, dressing, eating, getting in and out of bed or chair, moving around, and using the bathroom.

physical activity: Any bodily movement that is produced by the contraction of skeletal muscle and that substantially increases energy expenditure.

prognosis: The likely outcome or course of a disease; the chance of recovery or recurrence.

radiation: Energy moving in the form of particles or waves. Familiar radiations are heat, light, radio, and microwaves. Ionizing radiation is used in medical imaging and cancer treatment and can alter atomic structures.

respite care: Temporary care that is intended to provide time off for those who care for someone on a regular basis. Respite care is typically 14–21 days of care per year and can be provided in a nursing home, in an adult day service center, or at home by a private party.

side effect: A problem that occurs when treatment affects healthy tissues or organs. Some common side effects of cancer treatment are fatigue, pain, nausea, vomiting, decreased blood cell counts, hair loss, and mouth sores.

steroid: Any of a group of lipids (fats) that have a certain chemical structure. Steroids occur naturally in plants and animals, or they may be made in the laboratory.

stroke: Caused by a lack of blood to the brain, resulting in the sudden loss of speech, language, or the ability to move a body part and, if severe enough, death.

Supplemental Security Income (SSI): A program administered by the Social Security Administration (SSA) that provides financial assistance to needy persons who are disabled or aged 65 or older. Many states provide Medicaid without further application to persons who are eligible for SSI.

tai chi: A form of traditional Chinese mind/body exercise and meditation that uses slow sets of body movements and controlled breathing. While it is known for improving balance and strength, it also promotes relaxation and stress reduction, contributing to mental well-being in addition to physical health.

tobacco: A plant with leaves that have high levels of the addictive chemical nicotine. After harvesting, tobacco leaves are cured, aged, and processed in various ways. The resulting products may be smoked (in cigarettes, cigars, and pipes), applied to the gums (as dipping and chewing tobacco), or inhaled (as snuff).

transfer of assets: Giving away property for less than it is worth or for the sole purpose of becoming eligible for Medicaid. Transferring assets during the look-back period results in disqualification for Medicaid payment of long-term-care services for a penalty period.

urinary tract infection (UTI): An infection anywhere in the urinary tract or organs that collect and store urine and release it from your body (the kidneys, ureters, bladder, and urethra).

x-ray: A type of high-energy radiation. In low doses, x-rays are used to diagnose diseases by making pictures of the inside of the body.

yoga: A multifaceted system of practices used to balance the mind and body through exercise, meditation (focusing thoughts), and control of breathing and emotions.

Chapter 57 | **Support Groups for End-of-Life Concerns**

American Association of Suicidology (AAS)
448 Walton Ave., Ste. 790
Hummelstown, PA 17036
Toll-Free: 888-9 PREVENT (888-977-3836)
Website: suicidology.org
Email: info@suicidology.org

American Cancer Society (ACS)
3380 Chastain Meadows Pkwy., N.W., Ste. 200
Kennesaw, GA 30144
Toll-Free: 800-227-2345
Website: www.cancer.org

The Compassionate Friends (TCF)
48660 Pontiac Trl., Ste. 930808
Wixom, MI 48393
Toll-Free: 877-969-0010
Website: www.compassionatefriends.org
Email: nationaloffice@compassionatefriends.org

Resources in this chapter were compiled from several sources deemed reliable; all contact information was verified and updated in September 2023.

First Candle
21 Locust Ave., Ste. 2B
New Canaan, CT 06840
Toll-Free: 800-221-7437
Phone: 203-966-1300
Website: www.firstcandle.org
Email: info@firstcandle.org

GriefShare
P.O. Box 1739
Wake Forest, NC 27588-1739
Toll-Free: 800-395-5755
Phone: 919-562-2112
Fax: 919-562-2114
Website: www.griefshare.org
Email: info@griefshare.org

The Leukemia & Lymphoma Society (LLS)
3 International Dr., Ste. 200
Rye Brook, NY 10573
Toll-Free: 888-557-7177
Website: www.lls.org
Email: customersupport@lls.org

National Hospice and Palliative Care Organization (NHPCO)
1731 King St.
Alexandria, VA 22314
Phone: 703-837-1500
Fax: 703-837-1233
Website: www.nhpco.org

Share Pregnancy and Infant Loss Support
1600 Heritage Landing, Ste. 109
St. Peters, MO 63303
Toll-Free: 800-821-6819
Website: nationalshare.org
Email: info@nationalshare.org

Suicide Prevention Resource Center (SPRC)
1000 N.E. 13th St., Ste. 4900
Nicholson Twr.
Oklahoma City, OK 73104
Website: www.sprc.org

Tragedy Assistance Program for Survivors, Inc. (TAPS)
3033 Wilson Blvd., 3rd Fl.
Arlington, VA 22201
Toll-Free: 800-959-TAPS (800-959-8277)
Phone: 202-588-8277
Fax: 571-385-2524
Website: www.taps.org
Email: info@taps.org

Well Spouse® Association (WSA)
63 W. Main St., Ste. H
Freehold, NJ 07728
Phone: 732-577-8899
Website: wellspouse.org
Email: info@wellspouse.org

Yellow Ribbon Suicide Prevention Program®
Westminster Public Schools, Hidden Lake HS
7300 Lowell Blvd., Ste. 35
Westminster, CO 80030
Toll-Free: 800-273-8255
Phone: 303-429-3530
Website: yellowribbon.org
Email: ask4help@yellowribbon.org

Chapter 58 | Resources for Information about Death and Dying

GOVERNMENT AGENCIES

Administration for Community Living (ACL)
330 C St., S.W.
Washington, DC 20201
Toll-Free: 800-677-1116
Phone: 202-401-4634
Website: www.acl.gov
Email: aclinfo@acl.hhs.gov

Agency for Healthcare Research and Quality (AHRQ)
5600 Fishers Ln.
7th Fl. Rockville, MD 20857
Phone: 301-427-1364
Website: www.ahrq.gov

Alzheimer's Disease Education and Referral Center (ADEAR)
National Institute on Aging (NIA)
P.O. Box 8057
Gaithersburg, MD 20898
Toll-Free: 800-438-4380
Website: www.nia.nih.gov/health/about-adear-center
Email: adear@nia.nih.gov

Centers for Disease Control and Prevention (CDC)
1600 Clifton Rd.
Atlanta, GA 30329-4027
Toll-Free: 800-CDC-INFO
(800-232-4636)
Toll-Free TTY: 888-232-6348
Website: www.cdc.gov

Resources in this chapter were compiled from several sources deemed reliable; all contact information was verified and updated in September 2023.

Centers for Medicare & Medicaid Services (CMS)

7500 Security Blvd.
Baltimore, MD 21244
Toll-Free: 877-267-2323
Phone: 410-786-3000
TTY: 410-786-0727
Toll-Free TTY: 866-226-1819
Website: www.cms.gov
Email: omh@cms.hhs.gov

Eunice Kennedy Shriver National Institute of Child Health and Human Development (NICHD)

P.O. Box 3006
Rockville, MD 20847
Toll-Free: 800-370-2943
Website: www.nichd.nih.gov
Email: NICHDInformation
ResourceCenter@mail.nih.gov

Federal Trade Commission (FTC)

600 Pennsylvania Ave., N.W.
Washington, DC 20580
Phone: 202-326-2222
Website: www.ftc.gov

HIVinfo, National Institutes of Health (NIH)

5601 Fishers Ln., BG 5601 Fl.,
Rm. 2F02
MSC 9840
Rockville, MD 20892-9840
Toll-Free: 800-HIV-0440
(800-448-0440)
Phone: 301-315-2816
Toll-Free TTY: 888-480-3739
Website: hivinfo.nih.gov
Email: HIVinfo@NIH.gov

Internal Revenue Service (IRS)

1111 Constitution Ave., N.W.
Washington, DC 20224
Toll-Free: 800-829-1040
Phone: 267-941-1000
Toll-Free TTY/TDD: 800-829-4059
Fax: 681-247-3101
Website: www.irs.gov
Email: nhqjbea@irs.gov

National Cancer Institute (NCI)

9609 Medical Center Dr.
Rockville, MD 20850
Toll-Free: 800-4-CANCER
(800-422-6237)
Website: www.cancer.gov
Email: NCIinfo@nih.gov

National Heart, Lung, and Blood Institute (NHLBI)

31 Center Dr. Bldg. 31
Bethesda, MD 20892
Toll-Free: 877-NHLBI4U
(877-645-2448)
Website: www.nhlbi.nih.gov
Email: nhlbiinfo@nhlbi.nih.gov

National Institute on Aging (NIA)

P.O. Box 8057
Gaithersburg, MD 20898
Toll-Free: 800-222-2225
Toll-Free TTY: 800-222-4225
Website: www.nia.nih.gov
Email: niaic@nia.nih.gov

National Institutes of Health (NIH)
9000 Rockville Pike
Bethesda, MD 20892
Phone: 301-496-4000
TTY: 301-402-9612
Website: www.nih.gov
Email: olib@od.nih.gov

NIH News in Health
9000 Rockville Pike
Bldg. 31, Rm. 5B52
Bethesda, MD 20892-2094
Phone: 301-451-8224
Website: newsinhealth.nih.gov
Email: nihnewsinhealth@od.nih.
gov

Substance Abuse and Mental Health Services Administration (SAMHSA)
5600 Fishers Ln.
Rockville, MD 20857
Toll-Free: 877-SAMHSA-7
(877-726-4727)
Toll-Free TTY: 800-487-4889
Website: www.samhsa.gov
Email: SAMHSAInfo@samhsa.hhs.
gov

U.S. Bureau of Labor Statistics (BLS)
2 Massachusetts Ave., N.E.
Postal Square Bldg.
Washington, DC 20212-0001
Phone: 202-691-5200
Website: www.bls.gov

U.S. Department of Health and Human Services (HHS)
200 Independence Ave., S.W.
Hubert H. Humphrey Bldg.
Washington, DC 20201
Toll-Free: 877-696-6775
Website: www.hhs.gov

U.S. Department of Labor (DOL)
200 Constitution Ave., N.W.
Washington, DC 20210
Toll-Free: 866-4-USA-DOL
(866-487-2365)
Website: www.dol.gov

U.S. Department of Veterans Affairs (VA)
810 Vermont Ave., N.W.
Washington, DC 20420
Toll-Free: 800-698-2411
Website: www.va.gov

U.S. Environmental Protection Agency (EPA)
1200 Pennsylvania Ave., N.W.
Washington, DC 20460
Phone: 202-564-4700
Website: www.epa.gov

U.S. Food and Drug Administration (FDA)
10903 New Hampshire Ave.
Silver Spring, MD 20993-0002
Toll-Free: 888-INFO-FDA
(888-463-6332)
Website: www.fda.gov

U.S. Social Security Administration (SSA)
1100 W. High Rise
6401 Security Blvd.
Baltimore, MD 21235
Toll-Free: 800-772-1213
Toll-Free TTY: 800-325-0778
Website: www.ssa.gov

PRIVATE AGENCIES

ADvancing States
241 18th St., S., Ste. 403
Arlington, VA 22202
Phone: 202-898-2578
Fax: 202-898-2583
Website: www.advancingstates.org
Email: info@advancingstates.org

ALS Association
1300 Wilson Blvd., Ste. 600
Arlington, VA 22209
Toll-Free: 800-782-4747
Website: www.als.org
Email: alsinfo@als.org

Alzheimer's Association®
225 N. Michigan Ave. 17th Fl.
Chicago, IL 60601
Toll-Free: 800-272-3900
Website: www.alz.org

American Academy of Hospice and Palliative Medicine (AAHPM)
8735 W. Higgins Rd., Ste. 300
Chicago, IL 60631
Phone: 847-375-4712
Fax: 847-375-6475
Website: aahpm.org
Email: info@aahpm.org

American Association of Retired People (AARP)
3200 E. Carson St.
Lakewood, CA 90712
Toll-Free: 888-OUR-AARP
(888-687-2277)
Phone: 202-434-3525
Toll-Free TTY: 877-434-7598
Website: www.aarp.org

American Chronic Pain Association (ACPA)
11936 W. 119th St., Ste. 216
Overland Park, KS 66213
Phone: 913-991-4740
Website: www.acpanow.com
Email: acpa@theACPA.org

American Pain Society (APS)
210 E. 10th St.
Kansas City, MO 64106
Website: americanpainsociety.org

Association for Death Education and Counseling (ADEC)
9462 Brownsboro Rd., Ste. 164
Louisville, KY 40241
Phone: 502-931-2332
Website: www.adec.org
Email: adec@adec.org

Bereaved Parents of the USA (BPUSA)
5 Vanek Rd.
Poughkeepsie, NY 12603-5403
Website: bereavedparentsusa.org
Email: bpusachapterdevelopment@gmail.com

Board of Chaplaincy Certification, Inc., Association of Professional Chaplains®
2800 W. Higgins Rd., Ste. 295
Hoffman Estates, IL 60169
Phone: 847-240-1014
Fax: 847-240-1015
Website: www.apchaplains.org/bcci-site
Email: info@apchaplains.org

CancerCare®
275 Seventh Ave., 22nd Fl.
New York, NY 10001
Toll-Free: 800-813-HOPE
(800-813-4673)
Phone: 212-712-8400
Fax: 212-712-8495
Website: www.cancercare.org
Email: info@cancercare.org

Caregiver Action Network (CAN)
1150 Connecticut Ave., N.W. Ste. 501
Washington, DC 20036-3904
Toll-Free: 855-227-3640
Phone: 202-454-3970
Website: caregiveraction.org
Email: info@caregiveraction.org

CARF (Commission on Accreditation of Rehabilitation Facilities) International
6951 E. Southpoint Rd.
Tucson, AZ 85756-9407
Toll-Free: 888-281-6531
Phone: 520-325-1044
Fax: 520-318-1129
Website: www.carf.org

Children's Hospice International (CHI)
1800 Diagonal Rd., Ste. 600
Alexandria, VA 22314
Phone: 703-684-0330
Website: www.chionline.org
Email: Info@CHIonline.org

Compassion & Choices
101 S.W. Madison St., Ste. 8009
Portland, OR 97207
Toll-Free: 800-247-7421
Website: compassionandchoices.
org

Death Penalty Information Center
1701 K St., N.W., Ste. 205
Washington, DC 20006
Phone: 202-289-2275
Website: deathpenaltyinfo.org
Email: dpic@deathpenaltyinfo.org

Death with Dignity
P.O. Box 2009
Portland, OR 97208
Phone: 503-389-3260
Website: deathwithdignity.org
Email: info@deathwithdignity.org

Dougy Center
P.O. Box 86852
Portland, OR 97286
Phone: 503-775-5683
Website: www.dougy.org
Email: help@dougy.org

Family Caregiver Alliance® (FCA)
235 Montgomery St., Ste. 930
San Francisco, CA 94104
Toll-Free: 800-445-8106
Phone: 415-434-3388
Website: www.caregiver.org
Email: info@caregiver.org

Funeral Service Foundation
13625 Bishop's Dr.
Brookfield, WI 53005
Toll-Free: 877-402-5900
Website: www.
funeralservicefoundation.org

The GW Institute for Spirituality and Health (GWish)
2600 Virginia Ave., N.W., Ste. 300
Washington, DC 20037
Phone: 202-994-6220
Website: gwish.smhs.gwu.edu
Email: gwish@gwu.edu

Health In Aging
40 Fulton St., Ste. 809
New York, NY 10038
Phone: 212-308-1414
Website: www.healthinaging.org
Email: info@healthinaging.org

Hospice Foundation of America (HFA)
1707 L St., N.W., Ste. 220
Washington, DC 20036
Toll-Free: 800-854-3402
Phone: 202-457-5811
Website: hospicefoundation.org
Email: info@hospicefoundation.org

International Cemetery, Cremation & Funeral Association (ICCFA)

107 Carpenter Dr., Ste. 100
Sterling, VA 20164
Toll-Free: 800-645-7700
Phone: 703-391-8400
Fax: 703-391-8416
Website: iccfa.com
Email: hq@iccfa.com

Joint Commission Resources (JCR)

1 Renaissance Blvd., Ste. 401
Oakbrook Terrace, IL 60181
Toll-Free: 877-223-6866
Phone: 630-268-7400
Website: www.jcrinc.com
Email: jcrcustomerservice@jcrinc.com

National Association for Home Care & Hospice (NAHC)

228 7th St., S.E.
Washington, DC 20003
Phone: 202-547-7424
Fax: 202-547-3540
Website: www.nahc.org

National Association of Catholic Chaplains (NACC)

4915 S. Howell Ave., Ste. 501
Milwaukee, WI 53207
Phone: 414-483-4898
Fax: 414-483-6712
Website: www.nacc.org
Email: info@nacc.org

National Funeral Directors Association (NFDA)

13625 Bishop's Dr.
Brookfield, WI 53005
Toll-Free: 800-228-6332
Phone: 262-789-1880
Fax: 262-789-6977
Website: www.nfda.org
Email: nfda@nfda.org

Neptune Society

100 N.W. 70th Ave., Ste. 100
Plantation, FL 33317
Toll-Free: 800-NEPTUNE
(800-637-8863)
Phone: 954-556-9400
Fax: 954-828-9901
Website: www.neptunesociety.com

Safe Kids Worldwide

1 Inventa Pl.
6th Fl., W.
Silver Spring, MD 20910
Phone: 202-662-0600
Website: www.safekids.org
Email: info@safekids.org

Society of Critical Care Medicine (SCCM)

500 Midway Dr.
Mount Prospect, IL 60056
Phone: 847-827-6888
Fax: 847-439-7226
Website: www.sccm.org
Email: support@sccm.org

USAging
1100 New Jersey Ave., S.E., Ste. 350
Washington, DC 20003
Phone: 202-872-0888
Fax: 202-872-0057
Website: www.usaging.org
Email: info@usaging.org

Visiting Nurse Associations of America (VNAA)
2519 Connecticut Ave., N.W.
Washington, DC 20008
Phone: 202-508-9498
Website: www.vnaa.org
Email: vnaa@vnaa.org

INDEX

INDEX

Page numbers followed by "n" refer to citation information; by "t" indicate tables; and by "f" indicate figures.

Index

Index

Index

Index

Index

Index

Index

Index

Index

Index